D0887932

OXFORD MEDICAL PUBLICATIONS

# Oxford Handbook of
# **Dental Patient Care**

# Oxford Handbook of
# Dental Patient Care

## Second edition

## Crispian Scully

Eastman Dental Institute,
University College London,
University of London, UK
Visiting Professor, University of Helsinki, Finland

## Athanasios Kalantzis

Maxillofacial Unit,
United Lincolnshire Hospitals, Lincoln, UK

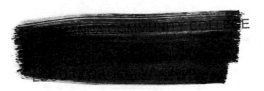

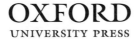

OXFORD
UNIVERSITY PRESS

# OXFORD
UNIVERSITY PRESS

Great Clarendon Street, Oxford OX2 6DP

Oxford University Press is a department of the University of Oxford.
It furthers the University's objective of excellence in research, scholarship,
and education by publishing worldwide in

Oxford New York

Auckland Cape Town Dar es Salaam Hong Kong Karachi
Kuala Lumpur Madrid Melbourne Mexico City Nairobi
New Delhi Shanghai Taipei Toronto

With offices in

Argentina Austria Brazil Chile Czech Republic France Greece
Guatemala Hungary Italy Japan Poland Portugal Singapore
South Korea Switzerland Thailand Turkey Ukraine Vietnam

Oxford is a registered trade mark of Oxford University Press
in the UK and in certain other countries

Published in the United States
by Oxford University Press Inc., New York

© Crispian Scully, 2005

The moral rights of the authors have been asserted
Database right Oxford University Press (maker)

First published 1998
Second edition published 2005

British Library Cataloguing in Publication Data
Data available

Library of Congress Cataloging in Publication Data
Data available

Typeset by Newgen Imaging Systems (P) Ltd, Chennai, India
Printed in Italy
on acid-free paper by
Legoprint S.p.A.

ISBN 0–19–856623–9  978–0–19–856623–6

10 9 8 7 6 5 4 3 2 1

# Preface to the second edition

This edition has been completely updated and re-organized, taking into consideration the fact that most dentists in the UK now must spend a year in hospital as part of their general professional training. Recognizing the difficulties they experience (and shortcomings of the undergraduate training), relevant chapters have been added on *History, examination, and investigations*. The curriculum for the MFDS exam has been taken into account. An extensive chapter on *Relevant medicine* with dental aspects of the most relevant diseases, such as management of diabetic patients, infective endocarditis prophylaxis, corticosteroid cover, etc. has been added, as has a new chapter on *Special care groups*. The chapter on *Being a professional* has been extended with new information on clinical governance, evidence-based dentistry, clinical guidelines, etc.

CS
AK
2005

# Dedication

This work is dedicated to Dimitris and Eleftheria Kalantzis, and Zoe and Frances Scully, and to the memory of Anastasia Boucoumanis.

# Preface to the first edition

From the rather sheltered academic environment of the university, the graduate dental provider is thrown into the world to deal with often difficult and sometimes worrying clinical problems. Faced with making his or her own decisions, often with minimal background experience, and building relationships with patients and professional colleagues, the transition from being a student with few responsibilities, to a qualified person can be traumatic. Enthusiasm is often at a maximum at a time when experience is limited: hopefully, the new graduate will have insight and recognize their strengths and limitations. Although a major change at this time of transition is from discussing the academic aspects of management to putting concepts into practice, documentation of the more practical aspects of patient management is not readily available. The person who is a resident, working in a general hospital, or who is treating medically or physically handicapped patients is often made more acutely aware of these shortcomings. There may even be more senior members of the profession who, like us, find it difficult reliably to recall data from memory, particularly with the introduction of new drugs, new units, and so on.

The object of this book is to help in these situations by presenting some of the more practical aspects of diagnosis and management, mainly in note and tabular form, primarily for staff in hospital positions. It is a relatively brief synopsis, designed as a pocket companion or *aide-mémoire* that should complement the basic undergraduate training. The book covers many of the areas of dentistry that overlap with, or border on, other specialties in the field of medicine and surgery, but does not attempt to duplicate all the data currently available in standard texts such as the medico-legal aspects of dentistry or details of operative techniques. Thus the text includes practical aspects of oral medicine and pathology, and oral and maxillofacial surgery, including surgery in relation to prosthetics, implantology, and orthodontics, traumatology, and relevant aspects of sedation, anaesthetics and therapeutics.

Dentistry has advanced so rapidly, that it is now recognized that the undergraduate course no longer equips the graduate for independent practice, and mandatory vocational training is now required at least in the UK and some other countries. Specialization is now with us though the need for a period of general professional training is accepted. Continuing Education is now thankfully accepted and may well become mandatory in many more countries.

All the information required by postgraduates is, however, difficult to gather into a assimable form. This book is designed to be such a pocket text for both hospital, general practice, and community dental postgraduate trainees, in North America, the Antipodes, Europe and elsewhere. It should be used in conjunction with the *Oxford Handbook of Clinical Dentistry* and should prove valuable to those on hospital or masters programmes, especially when working for higher clinical examinations, and also to senior students and auxiliary staff.

# Contributors and acknowledgements

## Contributor to Special care, and Being a professional

Dr Zoe Marshman BDS, MPH, MFDS RCS (Glas), DDPH RSC (Eng)
Lecturer, Department of Oral Health and Development, School of Clinical Dentistry, Sheffield, UK

## Advisors to the second edition

### Special care

Professor Joel Epstein DMD, MSD
Professor of Oral Medicine, College of Dentistry, Chicago, Illinois, USA

### Oral and maxillofacial surgery

Mr David Wiesenfeld MDSc, FDSRCPS, FRACDS (OMS)
Senior Oral and Maxillofacial Surgeon, Head of Dental Unit, The Royal Melbourne Hospital, Australia

## Acknowledgements

We are particularly grateful to Mr Steven Layton for his comments on Chapter 12; to Dr Richard Thornton for his comments on Chapters 9 and 10; and to Dr Craig Gordon and Dr Alet Jacobs for their constructive comments.

## Acknowledgements to the first edition

We are particularly grateful to Margaret Seward and Sue Silver who during their time with the *British Dental Journal* encouraged the predecessor of the present text. We are grateful to Dr Joel Epstein of the University of British Columbia, and to Dr David Wiesenfeld of the Royal Melbourne Hospital for their contributions to the earlier edition. We are also grateful to Drs Derek Goodison and St John Crean, of the Eastman Dental Institute, and Dr Tim Probert of the Royal Melbourne Hospital, for their helpful comments on an earlier edition.

# Contents

# History taking

# Introduction

The main aim of a medical consultation is to reach a diagnosis. The purpose of making a diagnosis is to be able to offer the most effective and safe treatment, and an accurate prognosis.

Diagnosis means 'through knowledge' and entails acquisition of data about the patient through an elaborate clinical examination, which comprises a history and physical examination, supplemented in some cases by investigations. By far the most important of these is the history.

▶A detailed history alone can provide the diagnosis in ~80% of cases.

The success of a consultation depends on the use of some well-tested principles and the implementation of several steps that begin before the clinician meets the patient. The importance of establishing a comfortable and friendly environment in which the patient can relax should not be underestimated. Ideally the interviewer should be seated about 1 metre away from the patient, positioned in a way that allows the patients to look away at any time.

It is important to adopt a professional appearance and manner, and introduce oneself clearly and courteously. Cultural and ethnic factors should be considered: a handshake is usually helpful in putting a patient at ease, but there can be cultural bars (e.g. some muslim women may wish to avoid physical contact with a male who is not their relative).

The patient should be asked to confirm their name. It is especially important to be conscious of the way the patient wishes to be addressed as some are conscious of status, and cultures also have an effect.

Adopt a methodical routine, which will allow you to gain the patient's trust and establish good communication and rapport. This makes the interview more pleasant and effective for both and is by far the most important determinant of the outcome of any treatment approach.

## Good interview skills include:

- A confident, but gentle, friendly and empathetic approach
- Attentive listening
- Good use of non-verbal communication
- Appropriate use of open and closed questions
- Clarifying terms and any ambiguities
- Making use of silences
- Reflecting back statements for confirmation or correction
- Ensuring the patient actually fully understands your words

Use open questions as much as possible, as these invariably allow more information to be elicited, especially about the patient's real concerns and expectations. Examples of such questions are:

- 'What started all this?'
- 'Tell me more about your pain'
- 'How does this affect you?'

Once the clinician has identified the complaint(s), it is appropriate to move to targeted closed (but not leading) questions that will clarify details and establish important facts. Some examples are:

- 'Where does it hurt?'
- 'When did it start?'
- 'Did you use pain-killers?'

### A full history should include:

- Presenting complaint (PC) or complaining of (CO)
- History of the present complaint (HPC)
- Relevant or past medical history (RMH or PMH)
- Past dental history (PDH)
- Drug history (DH) and allergies
- Systemic enquiry (SE)
- Family history (FH)
- Social history (SH)
- Habits (e.g. use of drugs of misuse, tobacco, alcohol, betel)

It is helpful (especially for new patients) to use a standard medical questionnaire, which the patient fills in themselves prior to the interview. This allows them more time to think about their relevant medical history and gives them the opportunity to reveal facts they might be embarrassed to admit in a conversation. It also helps patients to document their medication. However, each question must still be checked by the clinician.

Some clinicians write notes while the patient is speaking (which runs the risk of being translated as non-attentiveness), while others will only start writing after the patient has left the room. The authors suggest either employing some calculated breaks during the interview for writing in the case notes, or listening for a while and then saying to the patient ' Let me write all this down', so patients become aware of the need for careful note-keeping. This should ensure that nothing is forgotten, while both parties get a chance to think about what has been established so far and what further issues should be discussed.  It is good practice to share the information elicited  with the patient.

At the end of the interview the clinician should be able to draw up a problem list and a diagnosis, which may be provisional or differential or final. At this point it is useful to invite the patient to provide any further information that may be relevant, or emphasize a point that may have been understated or overlooked. The clinician should then summarize the relevant information gathered, provide the opportunity for the patient to expand or make corrections and explain what could be done next.

The remainder of this chapter, gives details of the successive steps of history taking. This should be completed before the clinician moves further to the physical examination or any form of treatment, even if this means on some occasions that delays may be incurred, as for instance when an interpreter is needed.

📖 For examples of history recording see full clerking samples (Tables 10.6 and 10.7).

# Presenting complaint (PC, or complaining of [CO])

The first thing you should record, following the patient's demographic details (name, age, etc.) is what they are actually complaining of (CO). This might not always agree with what you think the main problem actually is. It should nevertheless be addressed and analysed first and recorded, if possible, in the patient's own words.

The dentist's opening question can put the patient at ease and prompt them to start expressing their main concern or conversely become a source of misinterpretation and embarrassment for both parties. Although it is important to keep some flexibility, well-tested opening questions include:

- 'What can I do for you today?'
- 'What seems to be the problem?'
- 'How have you been since the last time I saw you?'
- 'I have this letter from your dentist/physician, who refers to…. Can you tell me a bit more about this problem?'

The most common presenting complaint, in any specialty, is pain. If there is another complaint, then a list should be drawn with the most important one coming first.

## History of the presenting complaint (HPC)

Starting with open questions, the patient should be asked to elaborate on their presenting complaint and give as much detail as they can. Usually further (closed) questioning is needed to establish all the relevant characteristics. Such characteristics may include:

- Date of onset (and duration)
- Mode of onset (speed and circumstances)
- Course (continuous, periodic or following a pattern)
- Site (main location, or area if diffuse, including any extraoral sites involved)
- Radiation of pain to other areas
- Severity of pain (1–10; where 1 stands for no pain and 10 for worse possible pain one can imagine)
- Character of pain (sharp, shooting, stabbing, crushing, dull, boring, burning)
- Aggravating and relieving factors
- Associated problems
- Any previous management and its effects

# Relevant medical history (RMH)

Aspects of the medical history may have already been revealed, especially if relevant to the presenting complaint. However, the clinician must probe further to reveal all relevant past and present medical problems. The depth to which one should probe depends on the setting, the seriousness of the current problem and the implications of the condition, its management or any relevant medical problem. To state the obvious, one does not need to spend the same amount of time taking a medical history from a patient presenting in general practice for a simple check-up, as they would for a cardiac patient awaiting major head and neck surgery.

## Enquiries on RMH

- Serious past and present illnesses
- Hospitalizations
- Operations
- Specific relevant conditions, especially cardiorespiratory and bleeding problems
- Medications (often guide to answers to the above)

It is best to start with open enquiries such as: 'Are you suffering from a serious condition now?' or 'Have you had any serious illnesses in the past?' Following any positive responses, encourage the patient to expand on any conditions that may be particularly relevant. Having read the completed medical questionnaire, you should already have an idea of the patient's main problems; any contradictions with the verbal history need to be clarified carefully and tactfully.

Other questions that are likely to help the patient recall certain aspects of their past medical history are: 'Have you been admitted to hospital before?' or 'Have you seen a specialist about a specific problem?' or 'Have you had any operations'. Answers to these may reveal serious conditions that the patient may have omitted or forgotten, or decided were irrelevant. Enquiries about perioperative problems such as bleeding, and complications with anaesthetics or other drugs, may also prove important.

One would anticipate that, by this point, all the relevant medical history should have been revealed. However, introduce some closed enquiries ('Have you ever suffered from…?') and you will often be surprised with the amount of relevant information that patients forget or believe is irrelevant or embarrassing. It is the dentist's responsibility to reveal all the relevant information and record it in the notes. Illnesses that are most relevant vary between cases, so it is important to keep some flexibility (and with that, your mind working!). For the patient attending for operative care, the following conditions deserve a specific enquiry:

- **A**naemia
- **B**leeding tendency
- **C**ardiovascular disease, such as myocardial infarction (MI), angina, hypertension, heart valve defects and history of infective endocarditis, rheumatic carditis or cardiac surgery
- **D**iabetes or other endocrine disease
- **E**pilepsy

- Jaundice and liver disease
- Lung disease, such as asthma, chronic obstructive airways disease or tuberculosis
- Mental health
- Neurological disease, including cerebrovascular accidents (CVAs)
- Oral diseases
- Pregnancy

Some of these can be considered particularly relevant in some instances. In such cases, even negative answers are important and should be recorded in the case notes, for example: °diabetes (nil diabetes), or better, as *not diabetic* (Table 1.1).

**Table 1.1** Relevant medical history

| | No: if YES, details of relevant medical history | |
|---|---|---|
| CVS | **Heart disease,** hypertension, angina, syncope | |
| | **Cardiac surgery, rheumatic fever,** chorea | |
| | **Bleeding** disorder, **anticoagulants,** anaemia | |
| RS | Asthma, bronchitis, TB, other chest disease, smoker | |
| GU | Renal, urinary tract or sexually transmitted disease | |
| | **Pregnancy,** menstrual problems | |
| GI/Liver | Coeliac disease, Crohn's disease, hepatitis, jaundice | |
| CNS | CVA, multiple sclerosis, other neurological disease | |
| | Psychiatric problems, drug or alcohol abuse | |
| | Sight or hearing problems | |
| LMS | Bone, muscle or joint disease | |
| Other | **Diabetes,** thyroid, other endocrine disease | |
| | **Allergies:** e.g. penicillin, aspirin, plaster | |
| | Recent or current **drugs**/medical treatment | |
| | **Steroids** | |
| | Skin disease, use of cream or ointments | |
| | Previous **operations,** GA or serious illnesses | |
| | Other conditions (incl. congenital abnormalities) | |
| | Family RHM | |
| | Born, residence or travel abroad | |
| | Relevant questionnaire | |

## Relevant dental history (RDH)

A dental history should be taken, but the depth to which one should go depends greatly on the nature of the complaint. The clinician's questions should be directed toward establishing an accurate concept of:

- Past and present oral care
- Trauma to the oro-facial structures
- Recent dental and oral disease, treatment, attitude and expectations
- Regularity of oral hygiene and attendance at the GDP
- Expectations of the referring dentist

Aetiological connections between any positive findings and the presenting complaint may guide the subsequent examination and investigations, while further management may be affected by the patient's attitudes and expectations. These can be influenced by culture, religion and education.

# Drug history (DH)

Before patients attend a clinic for the first time, they should be asked to bring with them all their medicines and/or their prescription scripts. All prescription-only medicines (POMs) and over-the-counter (OTC) drugs and medicines, and any herbal remedies, should be recorded with their exact name, dose, route, regimen, duration and indication.
For example:

Propranolol  80 mg  PO, bd for 1 year  (hypertension) (see Appendix 1)

If the patient is unable to provide a full account of their drug history, a further appointment may have to be organized. In the case of an emergency, the patient's GMP should be contacted in order to obtain any missing information.
The drug history is likely to provide further information about the presence and significance of medical conditions that the patient has forgotten to mention during the earlier parts of the interview or simply does not fully understand or appreciate.
Another issue that needs to be investigated is the patient's compliance with their drug regimen.
▶ Compliance can be notoriously difficult to establish, but it must be borne in mind that up to 50% of patients are not compliant with treatment. This may have significant implications on their current medical status and may indicate difficulties with the administration of treatment regimens provided by the dentist.
A detailed account of drugs, their uses, interactions, adverse effects and contraindications can be found in Chapter 8, but drugs of special importance include:

- Antimicrobials—as they may
  - enhance effects of anticoagulants
  - predispose to oral candidosis
  - affect choice of further antimicrobial therapy, especially for prophylaxis from infective endocarditis
- Corticosteroids—as they may
  - produce the risk of an adrenal crisis and collapse following a stress such as infection, trauma or an operation
  - predispose to diabetes, hypertension, osteoporosis and infections
- Anticoagulants—predispose to bleeding postoperatively
- A seemingly endless list of drugs can be the cause of oral diseases such as
  - lichenoid reactions
  - ulceration
  - dry mouth
  - disturbed taste
  - hyperpigmentation.

## Drug allergies

Allergies are serious adverse effects of drugs with potentially lethal consequences, and should always be recorded clearly and prominently in the patient notes (including on the cover), drug and other treatment forms as well as in all correspondence. Considering the weight and implications of the diagnosis of an allergy, it should always be made with serious thought and consideration.

▶ True allergy to local anaesthetics (LA) is very rare, but you are likely to hear it claimed surprisingly frequently, in relation to intravascular injections of LA, or even in cases where the patient has misinterpreted a simple faint that occurred before the actual injection! It is much simpler and preferable to admit to the patient the common occurrence of intravascular injection of LA, than label them forever as allergic to LA.

The commonest culprits in true allergies are:
• Latex
• Penicillin
• Aspirin

## Drug misuse

The misuse of common and illicit drugs is increasingly common. If you suspect that the patient is misusing drugs or other substances then you should ask tactfully, but confidently. There are many reasons why truthful or complete responses are not always provided, but you should do your best to obtain them, especially if this is of relevance to the patient's condition or possible management. All responses should be recorded in the notes, but confidentiality should be protected within the treating team. Possible problems with drug addicts include:
• Behavioural problems, including violence
• Drug (and staff) abuse
• Falsely complaining of a painful condition
• Drug withdrawal effects
• Suffering from (and risk of transmission of) HIV or hepatitis viruses.

The advice or help of a psychiatrist is often needed in such cases.

# Systemic enquiry (SE)

As much as you may have tried to use lay terms in your history taking so far, the patient, especially if elderly or of a different culture, may have not fully understood the nature and content of all questions referring to diseases and drugs. At the same time, they may be suffering from symptoms of an illness that is thus far undiagnosed. The purpose of the systemic enquiry is to uncover these symptoms, see if they fit with the patient's medical history and the signs that you will later elicit during the examination, and to help you understand your patient's overall health status.

The time needed for this part of the history depends greatly on the presenting complaint, the medical history (occasionally, even the findings of the physical examination may necessitate a return to the systemic enquiry) and the co-operation of the patient. For example, when admitting an elderly patient for major surgery, it is important to go through all the systems in detail. On the other hand, reviewing the genito-urinary system of a healthy young patient attending an outpatient clinic for the extraction of a wisdom tooth is not only a waste of time but likely to be seen at the very least as inappropriate.

Try to keep in mind the relevance between various symptoms and direct your questions accordingly. The mouth is part of the digestive tract, so someone presenting with a mouth ulcer needs the gastro-intestinal system reviewed in some detail. Similarly if your patient says: 'I've had some heart trouble in the past, can't remember what the specialist called it, but I am certainly much better now', it would be negligent not to review the cardiovascular system in some detail.

In the beginning, it can be hard to remember all the cardinal symptoms of all the systems. These are usually listed in some hospital notes (occasionally a nurse will have gone through them before you). Alternatively, keep a sheet of paper in your pocket for this purpose. It is better to explain to the patient that you are going to read a list of symptoms out of a form, than stand there embarrassingly scratching your head, trying to remember the fifth cardinal respiratory symptom (being too proud to quit at this stage!).

Here, we will only mention these symptoms, but they will be better appreciated after reading Chapter 4. Appendix 1 outlines medical jargon and abbreviations. It is unlikely that the patient will know what 'orthopnoea' means, so it is best to use lay terms during the interview, unless it is the admiration of the patient you are after and not the answer! Such suggested terms are used in brackets in the box that follows.

▶ Remember that not all these need to be enquired in every situation, but, at least in the beginning, it is better to ask and record too much in the notes than too little. Important negative answers should also be recorded.

## Systemic Enquiry (SE) or Systems Review (SR)

*General*

- Feeling unwell or fatigued
- Energy levels and sleep patterns
- Loss of appetite and/or weight
- Fever

*Cardiovascular system (CVS)*

- Chest pain or dyspnoea (shortness of breath) after exertion
- Orthopnoea or paroxysmal nocturnal dyspnoea (breathlessness when lying flat, or suddenly waking the patient at night)
- Palpitations (awareness of one's own heartbeat)
- Ankle swelling
- Leg pain during exertion
- Dizziness or black-outs

*Respiratory system (RS)*

- Dyspnoea
- Wheeze
- Cough: dry or productive
- Sputum: colour, consistency and amount—blood (haemoptysis)
- Chest pain when breathing or coughing

*Gastro-intestinal system (GIS)*

- Dysphagia (difficulty swallowing)
- Indigestion or heartburn
- Nausea or vomiting
- Abdominal pain and its characteristics
- Bowel habit changes: diarrhoea or constipation
- Motion: colour, consistency and presence of slime or blood.
- Jaundice: yellow skin or sclerae, dark urine and pale stools

*Genito-urinary system (GUS)*

- General: frequency (passing urine too often), polyuria (passing large amounts), nocturia (passing at night), dysuria (painful micturition) and haematuria (blood in the urine)
- Males: hesitancy (difficulty starting urination), poor stream and terminal dribbling
- Females: urge or stress incontinence (leakage of urine), heavy or irregular periods or amenorrhoea

*Nervous system (NS)*

- Headaches
- Fits
- Faints (or funny turns)
- Ataxia (imbalance)
- Tremors
- Sensory disturbances (visual, auditory, hypoaesthesia (numbness) or paraesthesiae ('pins and needles')
- Muscle weakness

*Endocrine system*

- Symptoms suggesting diabetes: tiredness, polyuria and polydipsia
- Symptoms suggesting thyroid disease: heat or cold intolerance, etc.

*Musculoskeletal system (MSS)*

- Pain, swelling or stiffness of the muscles or joints

# Family history (FH)

If a condition with a genetic influence is suspected, it is useful to go through a family history. The pattern of inheritance of some diseases is very clearly defined, and in these cases the diseases are referred to as genetic. They can be inherited in an autosomal dominant (e.g. cleidocranial dysplasia), autosomal recessive (sickle cell disease) or X-linked (haemophilia) pattern. It is useful in such patients to draw a family tree (Fig. 1.1).

| | | | |
|---|---|---|---|
| Normal male | □ | Affected male | ■ |
| Normal female | ○ | Affected female | ● |
| Mating | □—○ | | |
| Propositus | ↗■ | | |
| Dead | ⊘ | | |
| Abortion or stillbirth of unspecified sex | ◂ | | |

**Fig. 1.1** Annotation of family trees

Many illnesses have at least some genetic component mixing with environmental factors to produce the final presentation (phenotype). These diseases are called multifactorial or familial, as they have the tendency to crop up in families (without a clear pattern). The list of diseases for which scientific evidence for their genetic component has been found is constantly increasing, particularly since the completion of the Human Genome Project, and this is playing an increasing role in diagnostic and therapeutic methods.

---

**Multifactorial disorders**

Cleft palate and other developmental abnormalities
Cardiovascular disorders (hypertension and ischaemic heart disease)
Diabetes
Asthma
Mental disorders
Some types of cancer

---

These disorders, when relevant, must be enquired upon at the level of first-degree relatives, i.e. parents, siblings and children. Start by asking if these relatives are alive and well, and continue with details as necessary. For those deceased, age and reason of death should be recorded.

## Social history (SH)

The importance of treating the whole patient rather than the disease is increasingly evident. The patient's social circumstances may explain their presenting condition and will often affect their management. The social history is therefore important. However, simply stating only that the patient lives with a partner and is a non-smoker may not suffice. A discussion about the patient's social life may give a good indication of their level of stress and state of mind, and how they are coping with their illness.

Support mechanisms have a prominent position when considering the rehabilitation of a patient likely to need major surgery. The anticipated emotional support must also be considered, as must the patient's concept of quality of life. For example, the decision to perform a radical neck dissection that will sacrifice the accessory nerve should never be taken lightly in an artist devoted to painting.

The following may prove to be important aspects of the social history:

### Use of tobacco, alcohol or betel, or other drugs of abuse
These are always relevant and will be discussed separately.

### Partners, friends and family
The patient's relationships may give an indication of the anticipated level of emotional support. Their domestic circumstances may also dictate practical decisions, such as whether they can be discharged immediately following a procedure under GA or need to be kept in hospital.

### Residence
The type of housing can play a significant role during the rehabilitation period of a patient who is seriously ill.

### Community support
Regular assistance from community health services may already be in place. Conversely, it might be that such services are scarce in the area, and may have to be arranged before a patient is committed to a certain treatment plan. This can be difficult in the care of some elderly patients.

### Financial circumstances
The patient's ability or willingness to pay for part of their treatment (such as complex dental restorative work) may offer more options for a treatment plan.

### Education and occupation
These may suggest the patient's intellectual status or liability to some occupational diseases. In addition, it is wise to know early on if you are treating, for example, a nurse, doctor, dentist or lawyer!

### Hobbies
When asking the patient how their condition is affecting every day life, it is worth making special mention of leisure activities, as these are extremely important for some people.

### Diet
Diet is a major factor in some oral disease. For example, carbonated beverages can cause tooth erosion, certain diets are cariogenic, and dietary deficiencies can cause angular cheilitis, ulcers and/or glossitis.

### Contact with animals
This may be relevant for some allergies (e.g. asthma) or infections (e.g. cat-scratch disease).

### Travel (or migration from) overseas
This can be relevant, mainly in terms of infectious diseases, such as hepatitis viruses, TB, HIV and tropical infections.

### Sexual history
This may be relevant to infectious diseases such as hepatitis viruses, HIV disease, syphilis and gonorrhoea.

### Culture and religion
People from certain cultural backgrounds and religious beliefs can have habits (not least dietary such as veganism) that predispose them to diseases. Their management may also be seriously affected by these beliefs (for instance the refusal of Jehovah's witnesses to accept blood transfusion). Culturally sensitive care is increasingly important.

### Illicit drug use
If the history suggests this and may be relevant to care, then it should be enquired about directly though sensitively.

# Tobacco

Tobacco is a major health hazard implicated in a wide range of disease, from oral cancer to ischaemic heart disease. Tobacco contains nicotine, which is highly addictive, and numerous other substances released during its chewing or combustion that are carcinogens. It is the duty of all health professionals to inform the patient of the adverse effects of tobacco use within their area of expertise, and give cessation advice.

Withdrawal from tobacco often leads to nausea, headache, insomnia, poor concentration, irritability, diarrhoea or constipation and increased appetite and thus, without support, even smokers who wish to quit can have difficulty succeeding. Most health authorities run specialist smokers' clinics and the preferred method is a combination of behavioural support and drug therapy that consists of nicotine replacement and bupropion.

Unfortunately, smoking cessation may lead to weight gain, and aggravation of recurrent aphthous ulcers. Ex-smokers may also take up habits such as eating sweets, that not only make them gain weight, but also increase dental caries.

## Quantifying the effects of smoking

The effects of smoking on health depend on the form of tobacco used, the amount used and the duration. Tobacco can be used as cigarettes, cigars, in a pipe, as well as snuff and chewing tobacco. Cigarette smoking is the commonest habit in the developed world, with well-recognized effects on the aero-digestive tract, especially the lungs. Cigars, pipe and smokeless tobacco have a much more significant effect in the mouth than anywhere else in the body, and their use should alert the oral specialist and prompt them to a detailed history and examination.

It is useful to measure the quantity and duration of a smoking habit in the form of 'packet-years', a measure that represents the number of years a patient has been smoking multiplied by the number of packets they smoke on average in a day (assuming a normal packet contains 20 cigarettes). For example, someone who has smoked 20 cigarettes (1 packet) a day for 20 years and then 10 cigarettes (0.5 packet) for a further 8 years, is calculated to have smoked: $1 \times 20 + 0.5 \times 8 = 24$ packet-years. If the patient is an ex-smoker, this should be noted, as should the packet-years they have had and the length of time since the habit ceased.

## Diseases associated with tobacco

Tobacco-related disorders include:
- Oral problems
  - Cancer
  - Potentially malignant lesions (keratosis; erythroplasia)
  - Acute necrotizing gingivitis
  - Periodontitis
  - Infected extraction socket
  - Xerostomia
  - Candidosis
  - Halitosis
  - Extrinsic tooth staining

- - Hairy tongue
  - Implant failure
- Cardiovascular disease
  - Ischaemic heart disease
  - Cerebrovascular disease
  - Peripheral vascular disease
- Respiratory disease
  - Chronic obstructive airways disease
  - Cancer (e.g. larynx, lungs)
- Gastro-intestinal disease
  - Peptic ulceration
  - Cancer
- Other cancers
  - Pancreas
  - Bladder
  - Breast
- Alzheimer's disease
- Fetal abnormalities

The clinician may also face other problems with patients that are tobacco users, such as resistance to sedation and other types of addiction, not least alcoholism.

# Alcohol

Alcohol misuse is increasingly prevalent and, despite its serious effects on health, excessive drinking is socially acceptable and this is one of the reasons why it is now epidemic, especially in the young (binge drinking). The problem is found across the social classes, and the availability and high disposable income in some, predisposes to it.

## Taking an alcohol history

Start with a general and open question. In most patients' case-notes the term 'drinking socially' is recorded but this is meaningless (unless you know how sociable the patient is, as some people are sociable every hour of every day!). The amount of alcohol should be quantified by going through a typical week's drinking and carefully calculating the consumption in units, where 1 unit is the equivalent of 10 mL of clear ethanol.

> *1 Unit of alcohol is contained in:*
> - Half pint (284 mL) of beer (4% strength)
> - One glass (125 mL) of wine (8% strength)
> - A single measure (25 mL) of spirit (40% strength)

People drinking at home, however, rarely use measures. In these cases, it is better to calculate the number of units from the volume of the beverage in litres and its strength (% alcohol). All you have to do is multiply them. For example, half a bottle of whiskey (or whisky) contains 0.35(Lt) × 40(%) = 14 units.

Consumption of alcohol up to a certain level is considered safe, as long as it is not taken in a single binge. Drinking within 'safe' levels requires no further questioning unless complicated by other risk factors. These levels are different for men and women:

> *'Safe' drinking*
> - ♂ up to 21 units/week
> - ♀ up to 14 units/week
>
> *Hazardous drinking*
> - ♂ 22–50 units/week
> - ♀ 15–35 units/week
>
> *Harmful drinking*
> - ♂ >50 units/week
> - ♀ >35 units/week

If the patient's drinking is regarded as hazardous or harmful, further questioning is justified to establish if there is an addictive pattern, and the examination should try to elicit any signs of alcohol-related disease.

## Patterns of alcohol dependence

*Stage 1*
- Narrowing of repertoire and stereotype drinking
- Uncontrolled desire to drink (including first thing in the morning)
- Primacy (neglect of all other interests and possibly work and health)

*Stage 2*
- Tolerance
- Withdrawal symptoms (only relieved by drinking)

*Stage 3*
- Awareness of the damaging effects of alcohol and feelings of guilt
- Abstinence and re-instatement of the habit

## Alcohol-related problems

- Behavioural, social, occupational and forensic problems
  - Uncooperative and aggressive
  - Abuse of other drugs
  - Sexually transmitted diseases
  - Health neglect
  - Psychiatric disorders (mainly depression and anxiety)
  - Encephalopathies (mostly because of thiamine deficiency)
    — Alcoholic dementia
    — Wernicke's encephalopathy (disorientation and ataxia)
    — Korsakoff's psychosis (amnesic state)
- Trauma, including maxillofacial (from accidents, fights or assaults)
- Malnutrition
  - General malnutrition (calories from alcohol)
  - Folate deficiency
  - Vitamin B deficiency
- Liver disease, resulting in:
  - Liver cirrhosis
  - Liver carcinoma
  - Bleeding tendency
  - Impaired drug metabolism (includes GA)
- Cardiovascular disease
  - Hypertension
  - Cardiomyopathy
- Gastro-intestinal disease
  - Alcoholic gastritis
  - Peptic gastritis
  - Infective gastroenteritis
  - Pancreatitis
- Oral disease
  - Dental and periodontal disease (from neglect)
  - Dental erosion (from regurgitation)
  - Glossitis, ulcers and angular cheilitis (deficiency state)
  - Sialosis (enlargement of salivary glands)
  - Mouth cancer (in association with smoking)
- Other malignancies (pharynx, oesophagus, etc.)
- Fetal damage (fetal alcohol syndrome)
- Others
  - Direct potentiation, inhibition or interaction with drugs (e.g. GA)
  - Myopathy
  - Peripheral neuropathy
  - Disulfiram (Antabuse) reaction if given metronidazole
  - Withdrawal (from simple 'shakes' to delirium tremens)
  - Delayed healing

USEFUL WEBSITES
http://medinfo.ufl.edu/year1/bcs96/slides/history/

# Examination

# Introduction

A full medical examination requires considerable time, but is rarely needed. The system that should most carefully be examined will be dictated by the history of the presenting complaint. Depending on the setting and the situation, systems that have been highlighted during the systemic review or relevant medical history should also be examined.

For most routine cases, you should develop a basic system of examination, likely to give clues about underlying problems in all body systems and which will indicate whether more thorough examination and investigations are needed.

A routine ensures that there are no important omissions. After practice, clinicians should be able to perform the core clinical examination almost automatically. It takes skill to perform a meaningful, relevant, organized and brief examination; repeated practice is essential.

A good clinical examination is based on the principle of using all the senses in order to register every sign the patient presents.

## Methods of examination

- Inspection
- Palpation
- Percussion
- Auscultation

It is better in a clinician's early career to include more, rather than risk omitting a finding that may eventually prove significant. With experience, many able clinicians manage to shorten the time needed for examination, but this does not mean that they regard this as acceptable practice by less experienced colleagues!

Before starting an examination, it is important to explain to the patient what you are intending to do, and why. Ensure you have their full informed consent, and try and have a chaperone present; this is crucial when examining a child or someone of the opposite sex. In the case of some cultures, a person of the same sex should conduct the examination, or the spouse must be present.

A space that maintains the patient's privacy, a comfortable examination chair or bed and good lighting and exposure of the area to be examined are essential. Start by observing the patient's general features and demeanour and then proceed with examination of the systems as appropriate. Remember to keep telling the patient what you are about to do next, and explain clearly what you want them to do, as some of the examination is likely to make very little sense to them, especially because most patients are a little surprised having more than a mouth examination conducted in a dental setting.

A summary of the examination technique of each system is presented in this chapter. Although it is useful to keep the systems in mind, you do not have to take them in turn while performing your examination, as this would inevitably cause some duplication. It is preferable to develop a routine that moves gradually through the various body parts, starting with the hands, moving up towards the face, then down towards the neck, chest, abdomen and finishing with the feet. This integrated approach will be presented last; an example can be seen in Table 10.7.

# General examination

Examination starts as soon as the patient walks into the room, or the clinician arrives at their bedside. Some diagnoses are immediately evident. The experienced clinician will use all possible clues.

### General appearance

What is your impression of the patient? Look at their clothes and their level of personal hygiene. Does the patient look calm and alert, or are they anxious, in distress, uncomfortable, breathless or is consciousness impaired? Are they ill or well?

▶ If you think that the patient looks ill, they probably are.

### Facies

Certain disorders give a unique facial characteristics: these include chromosomal (e.g. Down's syndrome), hormonal (e.g. thyrotoxicosis, acromegaly) and other (e.g. scleroderma, Parkinson's disease) conditions.

### Complexion

Under good lighting conditions, any jaundice, pallor (anaemia), cyanosis, erythema or hyperpigmentation should become evident.

### Facial expression

This says a lot about the patient's well being and their state of mind. Do they look happy to see you, or does their face give away feelings of fear, anger, frustration or antagonism?

### Gait, posture and movements

Is the patient able to walk comfortably? Are they intoxicated, or have they got a gait indicating hemiparesis, cerebellar deficit or Parkinson's disease? Are they exhibiting any abnormal movements, such as tremor, rigidity, fasciculation or facial dyskinesias? Are they lying in bed unable to move? Are they using several pillows (sign of cardiac failure)? Are they bending forward with their arms holding on the sides of the bed or chair, to assist their breathing (using the accessory muscles of respiration)?

### Surroundings

Is the patient attached to drains and catheters? Are they connected to an oxygen delivery apparatus or a nebulizer? Do they have asthma inhalers, GTN spray or other drugs in reach? Is their food lying untouched on the table? There are a number of clues you can collect just by having a good look around, including at the patient's partner, family and friends.

### Height and weight

The patient's height and weight should be recorded. If the patient's weight looks abnormal you should also calculate their 'body mass index' (BMI), which is their weight in kilograms divided by their squared height in metres (BMI = $kg/m^2$). A normal BMI is usually between 20 and 25, while obesity is characterized by a BMI >30. More important, however, is the waist–hip ratio (WHR—normally 0.8). Individuals with fat distributed around the abdomen (WHR >1—typically males) are at higher risk of cardiovascular disease.

## Hydration
The most sensitive measure of hydration is the patient's body weight. Daily measurements are useful and significant changes in short time periods are more likely to be due to dehydration or oedema than to the nutritional status. Oedema caused by cardiac failure is characterized by pitting, which is evident in dependent areas of the body (usually the feet and legs or, in bed-bound patients, the sacral area). Oedema is demonstrated by pressing the fingers into the skin for several seconds, when an impression (pitting) will persist for several minutes.

## Skin and hair
Any skin lesions or abnormalities should be described by their morphology and distribution (for terminology, see page 50). Scalp and body hair quality and distribution may also give some clinical clues regarding certain abnormalities (e.g. hormonal).

## Odours
Halitosis, tobacco or alcohol breath, ketoacidotic breath (hyperglycaemia), hepatic fetor (liver failure), suppurative or anaerobic infection and urine smell of a neglected person are all characteristic.

## Sounds
Dysarthria and dysphonia can have a local or neurological aetiology. Note any cough, wheeze or other abnormal breathing sounds, which are sometimes evident without a stethoscope.

## Hands and nails
Starting from the handshake, you should already be getting clues from a part of the body that can give an impressive amount of information. Signs to look for include:

- *Tremor*, caused usually by anxiety, thyrotoxicosis or drug withdrawal
- *Nicotine stains* indicating a smoking habit
- *Cyanosed hands* that are cold (cardiovascular pathology or Raynauds) or warm (pulmonary pathology)
- *Abnormally large hand size or shape* (arthritis, acromegaly, Marfan's syndrome,)
- *Palmar erythema* seen for example, in liver cirrhosis, rheumatoid arthritis and polycythaemia
- *Dupuytren's contracture* (contracture of the palmar fascia pulling on the fourth and fifth fingers) seeing mainly in alcoholic liver disease
- *Finger distortions* seen, for example, in rheumatoid arthritis
- *Painful finger swelling (dactylitis)* seen in sickle cell disease
- *Muscle wasting* associated with rheumatoid arthritis or a neuropathy
- *Finger clubbing* (thickening of the distal phalanges and increased longitudinal curvature of the nails, resulting in drumstick-like fingers), which can be hereditary or more often associated with some serious disorders:
  - Respiratory (lung cancer, chronic lung suppuration)
  - Cardiovascular (cyanotic congenital heart disease, endocarditis)
  - Gastro-intestinal (inflammatory bowel disease, liver cirrhosis)
- *Nail-biting,* in anxious patients
- *Koilonychia* (spoon-shaped nails) in iron deficiency
- *Nail splinter haemorrhages* from trauma, endocarditis or vasculitis
- *Raynaud's phenomenon* (cold or stress induce digital ischaemia, followed by reactive hyperaemia) seen in 1° Raynaud's disease or 2° to connective tissue disease (systemic sclerosis) or vibration injury, and may cause ulceration, or necrosis of the terminal phalanges.

# Vital signs (1)

The vital signs include the temperature, pulse, BP and respiratory rate and, as the name suggests, are good indicators of the patient's wellbeing. Failure to recognize and record significant abnormalities in the vital signs may have serious consequences for the patient's health. They are routinely recorded by nursing staff in hospital patients.

The dentist should also be prepared to record vital signs and recognize and interpret the significance of changes. The level of consciousness and urine output also become relevant in some settings.

## Temperature

The temperature is traditionally taken using a thermometer. Digital thermometers are now often used, because of speed and practicality.

Skin temperature is variable, depends on the response of the peripheral circulation to the air temperature and is therefore usually of limited diagnostic value. More important is the body core temperature, which is well reflected in the temperature in the mouth, rectum, axilla or ear. The latter is now the commonest site to measure because of its practicality.

Core body temperature may vary slightly between these different sites, as well as between different times of the day (usually slightly higher in the evening). The normal range is 36.5°C ±1°C. Temperatures above this range signify fever (pyrexia; hyperthermia). Temperatures below this indicate hypothermia, and may be due to several different causes.

---

**Causes of fever**
- Recent hot bath, hot drinks or strenuous exercise
- Inflammation (e.g. infection, connective tissue disease, chronic granulomatous disorder, transfusion reaction)
- Haematological malignancy (e.g. Hodgkin's disease)
- Dehydration
- Some drugs (e.g. ecstasy, methyldopa)
- Endocrine and metabolic disorders (e.g. thyroiditis, luteal phase of menstrual cycle, malignant hyperpyrexia)
- Other (e.g. brain damage of thermoregulatory sites, factitious [self-induced] fever)

**Causes of hypothermia**
- Near-drowning or prolonged water or cold exposure
- Patients who have lain for hours unconscious or unable to react (e.g. after head injury, alcohol or drug intoxication, hip fracture)
- Hypothyroidism
- Patient's bed next to an open window!

---

▶ A patient suffering from hypothermia cannot be fully assessed (and certainly not declared dead) until warmed up.

## Pulse

Though the pulse can be measured and recorded from any artery, the radial artery is most frequently used. The examiner's index and middle fingers should press on the radial side of the flexor surface of the wrist, counting the beats for 15 s and then multiplying that figure by four to establish the pulse rate in beats per minute (bpm). The pulse rhythm, volume and character should also be noted.

### Rate

Normal pulse rate is 60–80 bpm for a resting adult and 110–150 bpm for an infant. Some variation is normal but gross changes should be recorded and investigated.

- Tachycardia (>100 bpm) may be caused by:
  - Anxiety, exercise or pain
  - Fever
  - Haemorrhage
  - Hyperthyroidism
  - Drugs (e.g. ecstasy, cocaine, sympathomimetics)
  - Cardiac disorders causing tachyarrhythmias (e.g. atrial fibrillation)
- Bradycardia (<50 bpm) may be seen in:
  - Sleep
  - Athletes
  - Elderly
  - Raised intracranial pressure
  - Hypothyroidism
  - Drugs (e.g. digoxin, beta-blockers, calcium channel-blockers)
  - Cardiac disorders causing bradyarrhythmias (e.g. heart block)

**❶** The pulse rate is occasionally slower than the actual heart rate. This is because when peripheral arteries are used, small volume pulses (such as those of atrial fibrillation and extrasystoles) cannot be felt.

### Rhythm

The rhythm may be:

- Regular (allow for the 'sinus arrhythmia' caused during the normal breathing cycle)
- Irregular
  - Regularly irregular (certain extrasystoles and heart blocks)
  - Irregularly irregular (atrial fibrillation: random rhythm and volume)

### Volume

- Low volume pulse is associated with low cardiac output (e.g. shock)
- Large volume pulse is associated with increased cardiac output (e.g. exercise, fever, thyrotoxicosis, pregnancy, anaemia, drugs, $CO_2$ retention)

### Character

Aortic valve abnormalities usually cause abnormal pulse character, such as slow rising or a collapsing pulse. Assessment of such abnormalities requires certain expertise and usually necessitates a physician's advice.

# Vital signs (2)

## Blood pressure

BP is measured with a sphygmomanometer and a stethoscope, or by machine.

*Technique*
- Seat the patient comfortably, with the upper arm at heart level.
- Wrap the cuff around the upper arm, leaving 3 cm of visible skin above the antecubital fossa.
- Palpate the radial pulse and inflate the cuff up to at least 10 mmHg over the pressure that makes the pulse disappear.
- Deflate the cuff slowly with the stethoscope over the brachial artery (below the cuff and above and medially to the antecubital fossa).
- Record the systolic pressure (1$^{st}$ appearance of Korotkoff sounds).
- Record the diastolic pressure (disappearance of Korotkoff sounds).

Normal adult BP is about 120/80 mmHg. Higher readings should be interpreted with caution and the diagnosis of hypertension must be made only after careful consideration, usually involving re-measurement of the BP 20 min later (after the patient has relaxed) and again on another date.

*Hypertension*
Hypertension has in the past been defined by a persistent BP >160/100 mmHg, although there is an increasing tendency to lower this threshold to 140/90 mmHg, particularly when other risk factors of cardiovascular disease (especially diabetes) coexist.

Causes of high BP include:
- Pain and anxiety (temporary rise in BP)
- Urine retention or fluid overload (temporary rise in BP)
- Primary or essential hypertension (idiopathic; familial; the commonest)
- Secondary hypertension (caused by renal disease, pregnancy, steroid therapy, or rare endocrine problems such as Cushing's syndrome, Cohn's syndrome, or phaeochromocytoma)
- Raised intracranial pressure (rising BP with falling pulse rate)

*Hypotension*
Causes of low BP include:
- Excessive blood or fluid loss (hypovolaemic shock)
- Anaphylactic shock
- Septicaemia
- Drugs (e.g. antihypertensives, general anaesthetics, etc.)
- Addison's disease or steroid withdrawal
- Vagal stimulation (e.g. during abdominal surgery)

## Respiratory rate

Respiration is very much under voluntary control and, if the patient is aware the clinician is measuring it, the reading will almost certainly be affected. The best way to avoid this is by measuring the respiratory cycles following the examination of the radial pulse, keeping the patient's (and the clinician's) arm against the patient's chest throughout. The normal respiratory rate is 12–15 respirations per minute.

Causes of ↑ respiratory rate include:
- Anxiety
- Hysteria (hyperventilation)
- Fever
- Pulmonary pathology (e.g. emphysema or fibrosis)
- Metabolic acidosis (e.g. diabetic)
- Brainstem lesions affecting the respiratory centres
- Anaemia (cardiac rate also increased)
- Cardiac failure

▶ An increased respiratory rate is one of the most sensitive signs of a critically ill patient.

Causes of ↓ respiratory rate include:
- Drugs (e.g. opiates, muscle relaxants, sedatives, and general anaesthetics)
- Metabolic alkalosis (e.g. from excessive vomiting)
- Brainstem lesions (affecting the respiratory centres)
- $O_2$ administration to a patient with COPD (chronic obstructive pulmonary disease).

### Level of consciousness
This is discussed in Chapter 11.

### Urine output
Urine output is recorded postoperatively, and whenever circulatory volume and fluid balance are challenged (e.g. excessive blood loss). The most common reason for ↓ urine output in non-catheterized patients is urinary retention caused by local causes (e.g. urethral obstruction). True reduction in urine output (oliguria) is a significant sign of dehydration or renal failure. Increased urination (polyuria) in contrast can be caused by excessive fluid intake, diuretic drugs, diabetes (mellitus or insipidus) and hyperparathyroidism.

# Cardiovascular examination

This is performed with the patient lying at 45°.

## General features

Observe the facial expression (does the patient look anxious, breathless or in pain?), the patient's colour and state of hydration, and the surroundings (monitors attached, GTN spray, etc.). Look at the face for signs of central cyanosis (blue lips and tongue because of pulmonary oedema or congenital right to left shunts), hyperlipidaemia (xanthelasma, corneal arcus), or anaemia (pale conjunctivae, angular cheilitis). Look carefully at the hands for cyanosis, abnormal temperature, sweating, splinter haemorrhages, finger clubbing, xanthomata (lipid deposits in hypercholesterolaemia), and koilonychia.

## Pulse, blood pressure and respiratory rate

Examine and interpret these as described earlier in this chapter.

## Jugular venous pressure (JVP)

The distension of the internal jugular vein, which lies just anterior and deep to the sternomastoid muscle, depends on the right atrial pressure. This pressure changes slightly during the cardiac cycle, but should not rise over 8 mmHg (9 cm $H_2O$). The pulsation of the internal jugular should therefore be reaching up to 9 cm above the level of the right atrium. When the patient lies at 45°, this should be just over the clavicle. Objectively, the JVP is measured in cm of vertical height from the manubriosternal angle (with the patient lying at 45°, this is 5 cm above the right atrium, therefore normal JVP should be <4 cm). Right heart failure will cause an ↑JVP, which will be obvious as a pulsation reaching high up the neck, as observed on the right side, with the patient's head relaxed and tilted to the left.

❶ Do not confuse raised JVP with the carotid pulsation. Venous pulsation is not palpable, disappears by pressing on the base of the neck and has a complex waveform.

## The precordium

Inspect the chest for deformities or surgical scars. Palpate for the heart apex beat, in the area below the left nipple. The apex beat is the furthest inferolateral point where the cardiac impulse can be felt, and is normally located in the 5th left intercostal space (LICS) in the midclavicular line (MCL). The apex beat may be difficult to locate in obese patients, and it may be displaced in cardiomegaly or following a mediastinal shift.

Now place the flat of the hand gently over the apex area and feel for a heave (forceful pulsation: sign of ventricular hypertrophy) or thrill (fine vibration: a palpable murmur). Do the same along the left side of the sternum and then the upper right parasternal area.

## Auscultation

When listening for the heart sounds, it is important to bear in mind heart physiology. We shall only consider the left side of the heart, as the pressures there are much higher and valvular pathology more common.

Imagine the left ventricle during diastole with blood running from the left atrium through an open mitral valve. When the ventricle is full, it contracts (systole), and this initially causes a backflow of blood, which closes the mitral valve producing the 1st heart sound (HS). As the pressure increases, the aortic valve will open allowing the ventricle to almost empty. The ventricle will then start relaxing (diastole), and when its pressure drops bellow that of the aorta, blood will backflow, closing the aortic valve (2nd HS). Shortly after, and as the pressure keeps dropping, the mitral valve will open (fast initial flow at this stage may produce a 3rd HS) and the cycle is repeated. The cycle lasts for less than one second, and the only way to differentiate between the 1st and 2nd HS (as well as recognize the timing of any added sounds and murmurs) is to feel the carotid pulse at all times while listening to the heart. The 1st HS is heard at the beginning of the pulse-wave and the 2nd HS is heard when the pulse disappears. In other words, the heart is in systole between the 1st and the 2nd HS, and in diastole between the 2nd and the next 1st HS.

## Murmurs

Murmurs are produced by turbulent blood flow through valves and thus can arise either if blood is flowing rapidly (increased cardiac output) or if there are valve irregularities. Only the left heart valves (mitral and aortic) will be considered here, but the same principles apply for the equivalent right heart valves (tricuspid and pulmonary). Left heart murmurs are accentuated in expiration, so ask the patient to hold their breath for a few seconds after a full expiration (remind them to breath after you have finished!). High-pitched murmurs are best heard using the stethoscope diaphragm, while low-pitched murmurs (mitral stenosis) are best heard using the bell.

*Systolic murmurs*
- Mitral regurgitation (incompetence): is best heard with the diaphragm at the apex (and the axilla).
- Aortic stenosis (ejection systolic murmur): is best heard with the diaphragm at the upper right sternal edge (usually radiates all over the precordium, the apex and the carotids).

*Diastolic murmurs*
- Aortic regurgitation (incompetence): is best heard with the diaphragm at the lower left sternal edge and with the patient leaning forward.
- Mitral stenosis: is best heard with the bell at the apex and with the patient in the left lateral position.

## Other features
- Listen at the lung bases for crackles (crepitations) suggesting pulmonary oedema (a result of left heart failure).
- Look for signs of right heart failure—ankle oedema, sacral oedema (in recumbent patients) and ascites (fluid in the peritoneal cavity).
- Feel the peripheral pulses (femoral, popliteal, posterior tibial and dorsalis pedis). Impalpable pulses along with cold and ulcerated feet strongly suggest peripheral vascular disease.
- Assess the vital signs not thus far examined (temperature, respiratory rate and level of consciousness).

# Respiratory examination

This is also performed with the patient lying at 45°.

## General features

First inspect the patient from the end of the bed. Are they breathless, cachectic or confused (respiratory failure)? Are they using the accessory muscles of respiration (holding on to the sides of the bed) and breathing through pursed lips (signs of COPD)? Are they cyanotic or using supplementary oxygen? Are they coughing and keeping a sputum pot next to them (remember to check the sputum)?

Look at the face for central cyanosis (hypoxia: type I respiratory failure), anaemia or polycythaemia. Inspect the hands for nicotine stains or finger clubbing (e.g. bronchial carcinoma or pulmonary suppuration). Look for hand tremor, dilated veins and a bounding pulse indicating $CO_2$ retention (hypercapnia: type II respiratory failure). Briefly examine the upper respiratory tract.

Look for signs of pulmonary hypertension causing right-sided heart failure (cor pulmonale). These include oedema of dependent areas (sacrum or ankles) and raised JVP. Oedema of the upper body usually indicates superior vena cava (SVC) syndrome, from a lung cancer occluding the SVC. Lung cancer may also metastasize and first become evident at the lower deep cervical lymph nodes, which must always be examined carefully. A lung apex tumour may invade the cervical sympathetic plexus, causing ipsilateral Horner's syndrome (ptosis, myosis, hypohydrosis and enophthalmos).

## Chest inspection and palpation

Inspect the chest from the front, the sides and the back. Look for scars or obvious deformities such as kyphoscoliosis (restricting lung capacity) or barrel chest (chest overinflation due to emphysema). Palpate the trachea in the suprasternal notch (warn the patient before!) and record whether it is central or deviated. Tracheal deviation may be caused most frequently by lung fibrosis or collapse pulling the trachea towards the affected side, or by pressure from a tumour, pneumothorax or effusion.

Examine the respiratory rate, depth and pattern. If the patient is dyspnoeic try to establish whether their difficulty is mainly on inspiration (laryngeal or tracheal stridor), on expiration (asthma or COPD) or is non-specific. Observe the exposed chest carefully and establish if expansion is adequate. If in doubt, lightly place one hand on either side of the chest, just under the clavicles and note elevation. Alternatively, extend your fingers laterally around the chest with the thumbs meeting in the midline at full expiration and note separation of thumbs during deep inspiration (normally ~5 cm). Reduced expansion of one side indicates localized pathology (infection, effusion, collapse or consolidation).

## Percussion

Firmly place the middle phalanx of the left middle finger on the patient's chest, and sharply strike it with the middle finger of the right hand, listening for the sound it elicits. Aim for intercostals spaces on various positions along the anterior and posterior chest wall, comparing equivalent positions of the two sides. The percussion note of a healthy lung is resonant (hollow). If the lung contains more air than normal (pneumothorax, emphysema), the resonance will be increased (hyperresonant). If an area of the lung is consolidated (e.g. fluid accumulation due to pulmonary oedema or infection), collapsed (due to blockage of a main bronchus) or fibrosed, the resonance decreases (percussion note is dull). It can even become stony dull in cases of pleural effusion.

## Auscultation

The breath sounds are best heard using the stethoscope bell placed lightly on the top, middle and bottom of the anterior and posterior chest wall as well as the axilla, comparing the two sides. Ask the patient to cough up any sputum first, before starting to breath deeply through their mouth.

Normal breath sounds are termed vesicular and are more prominent during inspiration and early expiration. If these sounds are increased and heard throughout expiration as well as inspiration, they are called 'bronchial', and are due to loss of the normal spongy consistency of the lungs (consolidation, collapse or fibrosis). On the other hand, the sounds may be diminished if conduction through the chest wall is prevented (pneumothorax or effusion), or if there is reduced air movement (emphysema or bronchial obstruction and collapse).

*Added sounds*

- Wheezing (rhonchi)—tubular expiratory sounds caused by narrowed air passages (obstruction, asthma or chronic bronchitis).
- Crackles (crepitations)—bubbling inspiratory sounds caused by fluid in the bronchioles or the alveoli (pulmonary oedema or infection).
- Pleural rub—rubbing sounds caused by friction of the pleural surfaces in pleurisy (fluid in the pleural space due to inflammation [pleurisy] or pulmonary embolism).

## Other features

- Assess the vital signs.
- Check the oxygen saturation (by pulse oximetry).
- Measure 'peak expiratory flow rate' (PEFR), maximum rate of air expiration (using a simple plastic spirometer). If PEFR is <300 L/min, airway obstruction is present (asthma or chronic bronchitis).
- Vocal resonance and tactile vocal fremitus are often examined, but these rarely have anything more to add to the findings collected so far.

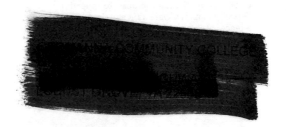

# Abdominal examination

This is best performed with the patient lying supine.

## General features

Note if the patient is in pain or looks cachectic. Inspect the hands for palmar erythema, Dupuytren's contracture, koilonychia, leuconychia or finger clubbing. Check for 'liver flap', which indicates liver failure (patient stretches their arms out with hands extended upwards at the wrists; watch for flapping of the hands downwards after a while). Inspect the eyes for jaundice or anaemia. Examine the mouth for ulcers (may be a feature of inflammatory bowel disease) and for signs of anaemia and iron, $B_{12}$ or folate deficiency (ulcers, glossitis [smooth tongue], and angular cheilitis). Smell for hepatic fetor (liver failure), check for sialosis (bilateral painless parotid swelling in e.g. alcoholism or bulimia) and look for telangiectasia (e.g. liver disease). Finally, palpate the neck for enlarged lymph nodes (a left supraclavicular node may represent metastatic disease from an abdominal tumour).

## Inspection

Inspect the abdomen for any obvious scars, dilated veins (may indicate inferior vena cava obstruction, while veins radiating from the umbilicus [caput Medusa] are a sign of portal hypertension). Obvious swellings of the abdomen can be due to one of the '5 Fs' (fat, fluid, faeces, flatus or fetus) or an intra-abdominal mass.

Record diagrammatically the location of what you see or feel, or describe locality using the terminology suggested in Appendix 4.

## General palpation

Question the patient about any abdominal pain or tender spots, reassure them and proceed to palpate the abdomen gently, starting away from any known tenderness and constantly looking at the patient's face for signs of discomfort. Use the flat of the hand and cover the whole abdomen in a systematic way regardless of where you start or finish. After the initial light palpation, proceed with a deeper palpation, following the same principles.

Some normal structures (liver edge, aorta, distended bladder, parts of the colon and faeces) may be palpated in healthy patients and can cause undue concern. Any localized inflammation will usually be revealed by tenderness. A characteristic sign of deep-seated inflammation is 'rebound tenderness' (apply pressure on the abdominal wall and then suddenly release it; this causes sudden movement and pain of the inflamed organ). A common site of such tenderness is McBurney's point (a third of the way along the line that connects the anterior superior iliac spine with the umbilicus) and this is a sign of acute appendicitis.

Guarding (spasm of voluntary muscle detected during palpation) indicates a tender area or may be due to anxiety. Generalized rigidity (continuous muscle spasm) is an ominous sign, usually indicating peritonitis.

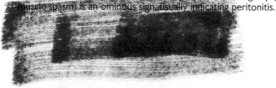

## Palpation of the abdominal organs

*Liver and gallbladder*

Place the flat of the hand on the right side of the abdomen, pressing with the side of the index finger deeply and upwards. Ask the patient to take a deep breath while the deep pressure is released to allow the liver edge to slide under the fingers. You may have to repeat more superiorly depending on the position and the size of the liver (usually felt just below the rib cage). The liver may be enlarged in hepatitis, cirrhosis, fatty infiltration (alcoholism), liver carcinoma or right heart failure. If the patient suddenly stops breathing in, because of pain elicited while pressure is applied, cholecystitis is the most likely cause.

*Spleen*

Place the flat of the hand in the middle of the abdomen with the tips of the fingers pointing towards the left hypochondriac region and pressing towards it. Try to feel for an enlarged spleen using the same technique as for the liver. The spleen should not be palpable unless infiltrated by diseases such as haemolytic anaemia, connective tissue disease, amyloidosis, leukaemia or lymphoma or enlarged in glandular fever.

*Kidneys*

Use one hand just under the rib cage posteriorly to push the kidney while the patient is breathing in (diaphragm is pushing intra-abdominal structures inferiorly) and feel the kidney anteriorly with the other hand. Enlargement may be due to a tumour, amyloidosis or polycystic disease.

## Percussion

This can be used to confirm the position and size of the liver and spleen (dull note over the organs, resonant superiorly and tympanitic inferiorly over the bowel), the consistency of any masses palpated, and the presence of ascites (free fluid in the abdomen) confirmed by testing for shifting dullness. To do this, percuss in the umbilical region (this should normally sound hollow even in the presence of ascites, as air floats) and continue laterally towards the flanks until you get a dull note. Then turn the patient towards the opposite side, keeping your finger at the same point. A few seconds later percuss again. If that point is not dull any more (redistribution of free fluid), ascites is confirmed.

## Auscultation

Listen for bowel sounds. These are absent (a situation termed 'ileus') immediately following GI surgery, but in other circumstances consider whether this could be due to drugs, neuropathy, obstruction (tumour) or an infection (which can also cause increased sounds ['borborygmi'], especially in the early stages).

## Other features

- Check the vital signs.
- Inspect and palpate the inguinal area for enlarged lymph nodes and hernias. Hernias can be femoral, umbilical or incisional, are best examined with the patient standing, and may be revealed by coughing.
- A digital rectal examination (DRE) is also an integral part of the abdominal examination and is indicated in all cases where abdominal or prostatic pathology is suspected. It should not be done before taking blood for prostate specific antigen (PSA), and is best left to an experienced clinician, as it can be unpleasant to repeat!

# Neurological examination

This examination is essential when the history or examination suggest a defect in the central or peripheral nervous system.

## General features

- Check the vital signs.
- Assess the mental state (page 38).
- Assess the level of consciousness (see Glasgow Coma Scale, page 558).
- Assess speech, abnormalities of which may be due to:
  - dysarthria (localized oral, oropharyngeal, neurological or muscle pathology),
  - dysphonia (upper or lower respiratory pathology), or
  - dysphasia (abnormalities in the content of speech due to damage in one of the language areas of the brain).
- Examine the cranial nerves (page 48).
- Examine for neck stiffness (meningeal inflammation).
- Examine posture and gait (broad-based ataxia in cerebellar deficit, shuffling in Parkinsonism, high stepping in peripheral leg neuropathy, swinging leg in hemiparesis, etc.).

## Motor system

### Appearance

Examine muscles for wasting (motor neurone disease or myopathy), fasciculation (involuntary twitches of groups of fibres [e.g. due to motor neurone disease; also a benign form of fasciculation in eyelids may be due to tiredness]), tremor (anxiety, drugs, coffee, alcohol or drug withdrawal, CVA, hyperthyroidism, Parkinsonism), dystonia (e.g. torticolis), myoclonus (sudden jerky muscle movements), tics (partially controlled repetitive movements [e.g. Tourette's syndrome]), orofacial dyskinesias (involuntary tic-like movements involving the lips and the tongue—a long term side-effect of antipsychotics), facial myokymia (fine worm-like contractions of periorbital or perioral muscles [e.g. in multiple sclerosis or brain stem lesions]), etc.

### Tone

Ask the patient to lie and relax. Rock the legs gently (do they appear to be stiff or too floppy?). Move the patient's limbs at the various joints and in various random directions, noting any abnormal resistance.

- ↓ tone can be a sign of a lower motor neurone (LMN) lesion or a recent upper motor neurone (UMN) lesion (e.g. CVA).
- ↑ tone is due to an established UMN lesion (loss of upper centre negative feedback) or Parkinson's disease.

### Power

Test muscle power by asking the patient to flex and extend at the various joints of the arms and legs, while you are exerting resistance. Try to isolate muscle groups responsible by providing appropriate support. Muscle power is usually given a score between 0 (poor) and 5 (good). Any neuropathy or myopathy may ↓ muscle strength.

*Coordination*

Loss of movement coordination is usually due to cerebellar dysfunction (well demonstrated in alcohol intoxication), and can be revealed by examining the following:

- Speech (dysarthria)
- Posture (difficulty in standing may also be due to visual, vestibular or proprioceptive defects)
- Gait (ataxic)
- Eye movements (nystagmus)
- Finger–nose test (look for intention tremor and past pointing)
- Heel–toe walk
- Heel–shin test

*Reflexes* (Appendix 2)

The spinal reflexes (biceps, triceps, supinator, knee and ankle jerks) test the integrity of the LMN (reflexes ↓ in LMN disease), the cerebellum and the UMN (reflexes ↓ initially, but ↑ later—hyperreflexia follows the pattern of hypertonia in UMN disease, as a result of loss of upper centre negative feedback).

Another important reflex is the plantar reflex, where scratching the lateral aspect of the sole induces flexion and adduction of the toes in the normal subject. If the toes extend and abduct (Babinski response), an UMN lesion is diagnosed.

## Sensory system

Different pathways in the posterior and lateral spinal cord convey different sensory modalities:

- *Dorsal columns* consist of large fast-conducting axons that have not yet decussated, and serve:
  - Touch (tested with cotton wool)
  - Vibration (tested with a tuning fork)
  - Proprioception (move a joint slightly with the patient's eyes closed and ask them to recognize the direction of the movement)
- *Spinothalamic tracts* in the lateral spinal cord, consist of small slow-conducting axons that have decussated at their entry into the cord and serve the following sensory modalities:
  - Pain (tested with a pin-prick)
  - Temperature (tested with a warm object)

*Sensory defects*

- Peripheral neuropathies (e.g. diabetes) can cause a characteristic 'glove or stocking' pattern of sensory loss (all modalities affected) starting from the periphery and extending proximally.
- Nerve root injuries cause pain or hypoaesthesia in a dermatomal pattern.
- A lesion of the posterior spinal cord will cause ipsilateral loss of touch, vibration and proprioception in the area of the body served beyond the level of the lesion.
- A lesion of the lateral spinal cord will cause a contralateral loss of pain and temperature sensation.
- Higher lesions of the spinal cord can cause a wide variety of sensory deficits.

# Mental state examination

Mental state examination is important in any patient with a suspected psychiatric disease, including acute organic disorders (delirium: caused by drug or alcohol overdose or withdrawal, systemic infection, electrolyte imbalance, hypoglycaemia, hypoxia or head injury), chronic organic disorders (Alzheimer's disease or multi-infarct dementia), mood disorders and neuroses (anxiety). Even if you think that the patient needs to be referred to a psychiatrist, you will still be expected to be able to give an outline of the patient's mental state that justifies your referral.

If your patient looks confused or disorientated, or is behaving inappropriately or not making perfect sense, proceed without delay with this examination.

Approach tactfully and explain what you need to do, reassuring the patient that you know some questions may sound silly or not applicable to them in anyway. Examination of the mental state consists of interviewing and observing the patient, and involves collecting data in a systematic manner as below.

❶ The most important point to assess is whether the patient poses a risk to themselves or to others.

### Appearance and behaviour

Inspect the patient's clothing and appearance, and look for signs of care or neglect. Are they clean and well kempt? Look at their facial expression and their manners. Are they appropriate? Do they look anxious? Are they restless or exhibiting some abnormal movements? Are they overactive, hypoactive or completely non-responsive? Do they maintain eye contact? Is rapport established easily, or are they suspicious and uncooperative?

### Speech

- Assess the speech volume, rate and quantity. For example:
  - pressured speech (impossible to interrupt) or flight of ideas ('butterfly speech') may indicate mania
  - poverty of speech may suggest depression
  - new words (neologism) may indicate schizophrenia.
- Note any abnormalities in the form of speech (e.g. flight of ideas, derailment, talking past the point, etc.) on any slurring (e.g. drug abuse)

### Mood (affect)

Record the subjective (ask the patient) and the objective (clinical impression) mood. Is the patient elated, euphoric, depressed, anxious or irritable? Is their affect blunted, labile (changeable) or inappropriate?

### Thoughts and beliefs

Ask about any:
- obsessions (repeated annoying thoughts that the patient recognizes, but cannot cast off) that may lead to compulsions (repetitive acts),
- preoccupations (worrying thoughts that take disproportionate significance in the patient's mind) including hypochondriasis,

- phobias (specific fears, for example of dentists),
- overvalued ideas (make sure these are not cultural or religious beliefs),
- delusions (false beliefs that the patient holds with conviction despite overwhelming evidence to the contrary),
- suicidal thoughts (there is no evidence that you may put such an idea in the patient's mind if it was not there before, so do not hesitate to ask).

## Perceptions

Ask about any perceptual (sensory) deceptions, such as:
- illusions (misinterpretations of existing external stimuli) or
- hallucinations (false perceptions in the absence of any appropriate external stimuli).

## Cognition

The patient's cognitive state is assessed by examining the following:
- *Orientation.* The patient may be disorientated
  - in person ('Please tell me your name?' or 'Who am I?'),
  - in time ('What time is it?' or 'Tell me what date it is'—the year is usually the first to go) or
  - in place ('Where are we now?').

Be careful, as patients who confabulate (e.g. chronic alcoholism) can be adept at avoiding answering clearly and, for example, when asked 'Where are we?' may reply 'don't be silly', but cannot state the name of the clinic or hospital.
- *Memory.* Check for:
  - immediate recall or registration (ask them to repeat the names of three objects after you),
  - short-term memory (ask for the same three objects 5 min later),
  - recent long-term memory (ask about important recent news items), and
  - remote long-term memory (do they remember their date of birth?).
- *Attention and concentration.* Ask the patient to start from 100 and serially subtract 7 (consider the patient's intellectual level and adjust accordingly, e.g. start from 20 and subtract 3).
- *Intelligence.* This should be evident by this stage.

Most hospitals have a standardized list of questions that take account of all the above-mentioned elements that define the patient's cognitive state. These can be used to get an objective and reproducible 'Mini Mental State' score, and to follow the patient's progress.

## Insight

Does the patient appreciate their condition? Do they recognize their symptoms as part of their illness?

# Musculoskeletal examination

Musculoskeletal examination requires an expertise that would not normally be required from a dentist. However, it is useful to have a basic idea of the approach required.

The aim of the examination is to identify the site of any pathology (joint, bone, muscle, tendon or ligament) and its nature (inflammation, degeneration or injury), as well as to recognize any loss of function (disability) or complications (deformity, muscle wasting, nerve compression or calluses).

A simple approach is to localize the problem, inspect the area, palpate it, check for integrity of function (movement) that it serves, and finally think of and examine for any other complications.

The usual musculoskeletal screening examination involves inspecting and examining the gait, arms, legs and spine (GALS) systematically. Here, only a few important and potentially relevant parts of this will be described.

## Gait

Ask the patient to walk slowly away and then towards you. Note the smoothness of movements, symmetry and any pelvic tilt or pattern that might suggest pain.

## Arms

- **Shoulders:** Ask the patient to put their hands behind their neck with the elbows as far back as possible, then drop the arms down and reach behind their back as high as they can.
- **Elbows, forearms and wrists:** Check for flexion, extension, pronation and supination.
- **Hands:** Check for swellings, deformity, muscle wasting or skin changes. Palpate the tendon sheaths and squeeze across the metacarpals or the knuckles to see if this elicits any tenderness (e.g. rheumatoid arthritis). Check for fine pinch (lift a coin of the table) and grip (ask the patient to grasp one of your fingers), to assess if there is disability.

## Legs

- **Hips:** Check posture and gait. Lie the patient and passively flex, and rotate the hip laterally and medially by gently manipulating the leg.
- **Knees:** Note any lateral or medial deviation or hyperextension with the patient standing. Perform the patellar tap to check for effusion (press above the patella to push any fluid into the retropatellar space and then press/tap on the patella with a finger of the other hand to feel for any fluctuation).
- **Feet:** Look for deformities, calluses or ulcers, and squeeze across the metatarsals for any tenderness.

## Spine

Inspect the spine from the front, the back and the sides. Note any abnormal curvatures (forwards [kyphosis], laterally [scoliosis] or backwards [lordosis]). Palpate for tenderness over the bony processes and in the trapezius. Check the lateral flexion of the cervical spine (ask the patient to tilt their head to each side) and the flexion of the lumbar spine (ask them to bend forward reaching for their toes and note for separation of two lumbar vertebrae by keeping two fingers over them or by marking them with a pen). Test for nerve root compression (ask the patient to lie in bed supine and raise their leg up straight; this stretches the sciatic nerve and elicits pain if this is compressed by a prolapsed [slipped] intervertebral disc).

# Head (1)

## Face

- *Morphology:* characteristic in some genetic conditions (Down syndrome), endocrine and other conditions (e.g. 'moon face' in steroid therapy or Cushing's syndrome).
- *Symmetry:* as possible variations are limitless, it is comparing with the opposite side that makes it easier to recognize localized abnormalities.
- *Colour:* racial variance; blue in cyanosis; pale in anaemia; erythematous in polycythaemia, fever or inflammation; or yellow in jaundice.
- *Skin lesions:* angiomas, telangiectasias, pigmentation, cysts or lumps, rashes (as in the malar 'butterfly rash' of systemic lupus erythematosus).

## Cranial vault

The size and shape of the cranium may indicate a congenital abnormality such as microcephaly, hydrocephaly, Down syndrome, Crouzon's syndrome, Apert's syndrome, Treacher–Collin's syndrome or cleidocranial dysplasia. The circumference sometimes needs to be measured in children. In older people the cranium may enlarge in Paget's disease and that can become obvious by a suddenly ill-fitting hat.

The cranial vault needs to be inspected and palpated carefully if an injury is possible.

## Nose and sinuses

The nose and the frontal sinuses may be enlarged and prominent in acromegaly. A large and red nose covered with a sebaceous secretion is characteristic of rhinophyma, associated with alcoholism. It may be narrow (asthma), deformed (injury or surgical trauma) or saddle-shaped due to a septal defect (congenital syphilis, cocaine-sniffing or post-traumatic). Following a nasal injury, a good inspection through the nares is necessary to exclude the formation of a haematoma on the septum, as this can result in necrosis of the cartilage and perforation of the septum. This inspection can also assess the presence of other pathology such as polyps, discharge from the maxillary sinus or obstruction of its opening. Maxillary or frontal sinus inflammation may be confirmed by palpating for tenderness over these structures.

## Eyes

Full examination of the eyes needs expertise and involves several steps.

- *Eyeball position:* enophthalmos, exophthalmos (thyroiditis) or hypophthalmos (blow-out fracture of the orbit).
- *Sclerae:* normally white, these may become yellow (jaundice), red (inflammation or trauma) or blue (osteogenesis imperfecta).
- *Conjunctivae:* evert the eyelids and look for pallor (anaemia), redness (inflammation), dryness (Sjögren's syndrome) or scarring (e.g. pemphigoid).
- *Eyelids:* oedema, inflammation, bruising (nasal or zygomatic fracture), ptosis (oculomotor nerve injury), lumps (basal cell carcinomas), ectropion (scar pulling eyelid outwards), xanthelasma (hyperlipidaemia) or abnormal shape of palpebral fissures (Down syndrome).

- *Extraocular muscles:* are examined by asking the patient to follow with their eyes the examiner's finger, while it is moving upward, downward and then laterally. Observe the eye movements and ask about double vision. Restricted ocular movements, strabismus, nystagmus and diplopia may be signs of trauma or neurological disease.
- *Pupillary reflexes:* with the patient's eyes looking into the distance, shine a pen torch at each eye in turn. Check for direct (pupil constriction in same eye) and consensual (pupil constriction in the opposite eye) responses. If you do not get the normal response of constriction of both pupils, try to work out whether it is the afferent (optic nerve) or the efferent (parasympathetic fibres in oculomotor nerve) pathway that is affected and in which eye (see cranial nerves, page 48).
- *Visual acuity:* is normally examined using a Snellen chart, which gives each eye a score (for example, a score of 6/9 means that the smaller characters the patient can read at 6 metres, can be seen at 9 metres by a normally sighted person). Simpler methods, such as reading a sign or counting the examiner's fingers, may usually be adequate as a crude assessment. Visual acuity tests may reveal pathology of the eye itself or the optic nerve.
- *Visual fields:* are usually examined by slowly bringing a moving finger in front of the patient, coming from different directions. This checks whether there are particular defects of the visual field (temporal, nasal, central) and therefore traces defects at specific points in the optic pathway.
- *Fundoscopy:* should concentrate mainly on the optic disk (papilloedema may indicate raised intracranial pressure) and the retina and its vessels (for signs of diabetes, hypertension or trauma).

### Ears

Certain ear malformations are characteristic of syndromes such as Treacher–Collin's and Down syndromes, or may be the result of chronic trauma (e.g. the boxer's cauliflower ear). The pinna should be examined for signs of sun damage; and the external auditory canal for signs of inflammation. The tympanic membrane should be examined with an auroscope for signs of inflammation or perforation. Middle ear infection may explain a non-specific facial pain or headache.

Rinne's and Weber's tests use a tuning fork in various positions to try and differentiate between nerve and conduction defects. In conduction defects, hearing is improved when placing the fork on the forehead or mastoid process (as it bypasses the conducting part of the ear) and this differentiates it from nerve defects.

### Zygomas

These are examined mainly when a fracture is suspected. All sutures of the zygoma should be palpated for tenderness or a step deformity (at the infraorbital rim, the lateral orbital rim, the zygomatic arch and the zygomatic buttress intraorally). Any depression deformities will become more evident when studying the patient's face from above.

# Head (2)

### Temporomandibular joints (TMJ)

The degree and direction of opening of the mandible, and mandibular excursions, should be assessed and recorded. Normal interincisal distance at maximum opening is about 40 mm. This can be reduced (trismus) in TMJ pathology, caused by local infection, or jaw fracture. A closed lock of the jaws may be caused by anterior displacement of the articular disk. Subluxation of the joint may present with recurrent open lock (usually the dramatic presentation of a patient who cannot close their mouth). Lateral excursions may be restricted by a zygomatic arch fracture.

Examination of the TMJ may elicit tenderness, clicking or crepitus on movement. Both TMJs should be palpated simultaneously while asking the patient to perform the full range of mandibular movements. Tenderness and abnormal sounds of the TMJs may be produced by trauma (including condylar neck fracture), inflammation (including the temporomandibular pain-dysfunction syndrome [TMJ pain-dysfunction]) and, rarely, degenerative joint disorders (e.g. osteoarthritis).

### Muscles of mastication

The masticatory muscles should be palpated because spasm, as in TMJ pain-dysfunction, may cause them to be tender.

- Palpate the masseter bimanually by placing a finger of one hand intraorally and the index and middle fingers of the other hand on the cheek over the masseter at the lower mandibular ramus.
- Palpate the temporal origin of the temporalis muscle by asking the patient to clench their teeth. Palpate the insertion of the temporalis tendon intraorally along the anterior border of the ascending mandibular ramus and the coronoid process.
- Palpate the medial pterygoid muscle intraorally lingual to the mandibular ramus.
- Examine the lateral pterygoid muscle indirectly, as it cannot readily be palpated: ask the patient to open the jaw against resistance and to move the jaw to one side while applying a gentle resistance force.

### Salivary glands

Inspect and palpate the major salivary glands (parotids and submandibular glands), noting any swelling or tenderness, and the character and volume of saliva exuding from their ducts.

Early enlargement of the parotid gland is characterized by outward deflection of the lower part of the ear lobe, which is best observed by inspecting the patient from behind. This simple sign may allow distinction of parotid enlargement from simple obesity. Swelling of the parotid sometimes causes trismus. The parotid duct (Stensen's duct) is most readily palpated with the jaws clenched firmly as it runs horizontally across the upper masseter where it can be gently rolled. The duct opens at a papilla on the buccal mucosa opposite the upper molars. Any exudate obtained by milking the duct should be noted.

The submandibular gland is best palpated bimanually with a finger of one hand in the floor of the mouth lingual to the lower molar teeth, and a finger of the other hand placed over the submandibular triangle. The submandibular duct (Wharton's duct) runs anteromedially across the floor of the mouth to open at the side of the lingual fraenum.

Examine intraorally for signs of xerostomia (a mirror placed in contact with he buccal mucosa draws a string of thick saliva as it is slowly moved away).

# Neck

The neck contains important structures that may cause significant pathology. Swellings are often due to enlarged cervical lymph nodes, but may be caused by lesions affecting salivary glands, thyroid gland or other tissues. Keeping in mind the anatomy, the patient's age and other finding of the history and examination, it is important to establish the anatomical origin of neck swellings, as well as their nature.

- In children neck swellings are most likely to be of infective nature or represent developmental anomalies.
- In young adults, infections (usually viral) or leukaemia/lymphoma are more common.
- In an elderly patient, malignancy becomes more likely.

Swellings of the neck should be described according to their:

- Position (midline, lateral, deep, superficial, etc.)
- Size (cm diameter is preferable to comparisons with fruits!)
- Shape
- Consistency (fluctuant, soft, rubbery or hard)
- Fixation (can it be moved independently, with the skin or the trachea, or is it fixed?)
- Tenderness (not very specific, but more indicative of infection)
- Auscultation (may reveal vascular lesions)

The **lymph nodes** are mostly deep and small, and should not normally be palpable. Any lymph nodes felt therefore, are usually abnormal and should be described carefully. The anatomy of the lymphatic system of the head and neck is rather complicated, but it is important for the dentist to have knowledge.

## Lymphatic regions of the neck

### Waldeyer's ring

- Pharyngeal tonsil (adenoids)
- Palatine tonsils (the 'tonsils')
- Lingual tonsil (lymphoid tissue in the posterior [pharyngeal] tongue)

### Transitional lymph nodes (between the head and the neck)

- Sublingual
- Submental
- Submandibular
- Preauricular (parotid)
- Retroauricular
- Suboccipital
- Retropharyngeal
- Facial

***Cervical lymph nodes***
- Nodes in the anterior triangle of the neck
  Lateral
  - Superficial (along the external jugular vein)
  - Deep (1. along the internal jugular vein including the jugulo-digastric and the jugulo-omohyoid nodes, 2. along the accessory nerve and 3. supraclavicular lymph node chain)
  Anterior
  - Superficial (along the anterior jugular vein)
  - Deep (prelaryngeal, prethyroidal, pretracheal, paratracheal)
- Nodes in the posterior triangle of the neck (termed 'posterior')

Palpate for the lymph nodes in a systematic fashion, starting from the head and working down the neck. Most areas are examined easier if the clinician stands behind the patient and asks them to relax their head, letting it drop slightly forward. It is helpful to use all the fingers (except the thumb), moving them in a circular pattern and trying to press any nodes against hard surfaces like the lower border of the mandible. Then the posterior groups can be palpated from the front.

❶ It is a common pitfall to confuse the carotid body with a lymph node.

When one or more of the lymph nodes are enlarged, it is important to describe them carefully. Start thinking whether they could represent 1° pathology of the lymphatic system or a 2° reaction or metastasis from an infection or malignancy in the drainage area of the nodes in question. Enlargement of certain lymph nodes can be characteristic for the area drained: for example, the jugulo-digastric nodes react mainly to pathology of the palatine tonsils, while enlarged supraclavicular nodes may be due to lung or upper digestive tract tumours.

*Infective* lymph nodes tend to be tender or painful in the early stages and are more commonly found in children and young people. They usually follow dental, tonsillar or ear infections but other causes include glandular fever (Epstein–Barr virus or cytomegalovirus), HIV infection, brucellosis, tuberculosis, syphilis, cat scratch fever and toxoplasmosis.

Enlarged lymph nodes from *metastatic disease* are hard, fixed, and may or may not be tender. They are seen mainly in older people and it is imperative to search carefully for a 1° site of malignancy. The usual culprits are the floor of mouth, the lateral borders of the tongue, the retromolar region, the palatine tonsils, the pharynx, the larynx and the skin of the head.

1° *malignancies* of the lymphatic system (lymphoma and lymphocytic leukaemia) can affect patients of any age.

Lesions arising from the ***skin*** (e.g. superficial infections, sebaceous or epidermoid cysts) can usually be moved with the skin and are generally easily recognizable.

The ***salivary glands*** are important structures of the upper neck and their examination has already been discussed.

The ***thyroid gland*** is attached to the anterior aspect of the upper trachea and moves characteristically with it during swallowing. This should be observed from the front but palpated from behind the patient.

# Cranial nerves

The dental surgeon should be adept in examining the cranial nerves. Their main functions, the technique of their examination, possible causes and sites of damage and abnormal findings are listed below.

### Olfactory (I)
*Function:* Smell.
*Examination:* Substances such as coffee or peppermint are passed before each nostril in turn.
*Lesions:* Obstruction; tumours; fracture of cribriform plate (head injury).
*Abnormal finding:* Anosmia.

### Optic (II)
*Function:* Vision.
*Examination:* Visual acuity; pupillary reflexes; visual fields; fundoscopy
*Lesions:* Trauma to the orbit; brain tumours; vascular accidents.
*Abnormal findings:* Impaired visual acuity; loss of the direct and consensual pupillary responses (when shining a light at the affected eye, neither eye will react); visual field defects; abnormalities on fundoscopy.

### Oculomotor (III)
*Function:* Motor for most extraocular muscles (medial, superior and inferior recti, inferior oblique, and levator palpebrae superioris); visceral motor (parasympathetic fibres) for pupillary sphincter and ciliary muscle (lens accommodation).
*Examination:* Check eye movements (page 43); test focusing of lens.
*Lesions:* Any neuropathy (although muscle trauma or disease is usually the culprit of eye movement abnormalities).
*Abnormal findings:* Eye looks down and out (from IV and VI nerve action); impaired eye movements; diplopia; ptosis (of upper eyelid); dilated pupils; loss of direct pupillary response (consensual response is preserved, i.e. the opposite eye will react while shining light at the affected eye).

### Trochlear (IV)
*Function:* Motor for superior oblique muscle.
*Examination:* Check inferolateral eye movement.
*Lesions:* As for III.
*Abnormal findings:* Difficulty looking down (particularly from the adducted position); strabismus; diplopia.

### Trigeminal (V)
*Function:* Sensation from head; motor (muscles of mastication, mylohyoid, anterior belly of digastric, tensor veli palatini and tensor tympani).
*Examination:* Test light touch (with cotton wool) ± pain (with pin prick); corneal reflex (touch the cornea with a wisp of cotton wool); open and close jaw against resistance; jaw jerk.
*Lesions:* Brain lesions; facial bone fractures (orbital floor, mandible, etc.).
*Abnormal findings:* Facial hypoaesthesia or paraesthesia; abnormal reflexes; weakness and wasting of masticatory muscles.

## Abducens (VI)

*Function:* Motor for lateral rectus muscle.
*Examination:* Check lateral eye movement.
*Lesions:* As for III.
*Abnormal findings:* Impaired eye movement to affected side; diplopia.

## Facial (VII)

*Function:* Motor (muscles of facial expression, stylohyoid, posterior belly of digastric and stapedius); secretomotor (parasympathetic fibres to lacrimal, submandibular and sublingual salivary, nasal and palatine glands); taste (from anterior two-thirds of tongue through chorda tympani).
*Examination:* Test facial movements (eye shutting, smiling, etc.); Schirmer's test (lacrimation); check for xerostomia; test taste sensation (applying salty, sweet, sour and bitter substances on the tongue).
*Lesions:* UMN lesions (brain lesions); LMN lesions (e.g. Bell's palsy, parotid surgery, etc.).
*Abnormal findings:* Contralateral facial weakness with partial sparing of the upper face (bilateral innervation) in UMN lesions; ipsilateral facial weakness ± impaired lacrimation, salivation and taste in LMN lesions.

## Vestibulo-cochlear (VIII)

*Function:* Balance and hearing.
*Examination:* Nystagmus tests; Rinne's and Webber's tests (page 43).
*Lesions:* Acoustic neuroma.
*Abnormal findings:* Impaired balance; nystagmus; impaired hearing (tests will differentiate from conduction deficit); tinnitus.

## Glossopharyngeal (IX) and Vagus (X)

*Function:* IX serves motor (stylopharyngeus); secretomotor (parasympathetic fibres to parotid gland); sensory (pharynx); taste (posterior third of tongue). X serves motor (pharynx, palate and larynx); taste (palate and epiglottis) autonomic innervation of heart, lungs and intestines.
*Examination:* Inspect the palate while patient says 'aah'; gag reflex.
*Lesions:* Brainstem lesions or injury (bulbar palsy).
*Abnormal findings:* Deviation of uvula to unaffected side; impairment of gag reflex, taste, speech and cough.

## Accessory (XI)

*Function:* Motor (sternocleidomastoid and trapezius).
*Examination:* Test head flexion/rotation and shoulder elevation.
*Lesions:* Neck lacerations; radical neck dissection.
*Abnormal findings:* Weakness and wasting of muscles; shoulder drop.

## Hypoglossal (XII)

*Function:* Motor (intrinsic and extrinsic muscles of tongue).
*Examination:* Test tongue protrusion.
*Lesions:* Neck lacerations; other neurological disorders.
*Abnormal findings:* Wasting; fasciculation; dysarthria; deviation of protruded tongue towards affected side.

# Describing lesions

When examining the patient it is important to record the signs using recognized terminology. Lay terms should be avoided, as they can have ambiguous meaning and may not help accurate diagnosis. This is especially true where more than one clinician is likely to be involved in the patient's care, and when communication between professionals becomes necessary. The use of correct terminology is particularly significant when describing lesions of the mouth or skin, although not all clinicians fully understand the terms! Some descriptive terms for lesions are listed below; Fig. 2.1 shows a chart for outlining their site, size and shape.

*Flat lesions*
- *Macule:* circumscribed area with altered colour or texture.
- *Petechia:* small (<2 mm) haemorrhagic macule.
- *Ecchymosis:* large (>2 mm) haemorrhagic macule.

*Raised lesions*
- *Papule:* elevation <5 mm in diameter.
- *Papilloma:* nipple-like projection, often pedunculated.
- *Plaque:* slightly elevated area >5 mm in diameter.
- *Scale:* dry and flat flake of keratin.
- *Stria:* linear elevation. May be an aggregation of papules.
- *Nodule:* a solid mass in, or under the skin/mucosa, >5 mm in diameter.
- *Tumour:* any tissue enlargement. Term is generally avoided as it commonly suggest malignancy to patients. The terms 'nodule', 'mass' or even 'swelling' are thus preferable.
- *Haematoma:* an area consisting of blood extravasated inside a tissue.

*Fluid filled lesions*
- *Vesicle:* fluid filled elevation <5 mm in diameter.
- *Bulla:* fluid filled elevation >5 mm in diameter.
- *Pustule:* accumulation of pus in skin/mucosa.

*Lesions resulting from tissue loss*
- *Atrophy:* thinning of the skin/mucosa and loss of normal markings.
- *Erosion:* loss of epidermis/epithelium. Heals without scar.
- *Ulcer:* loss of epidermis/epithelium and dermis/corium.
- *Fissure:* linear slit, (commonly at mucocutaneous junctions [lips, anus]).
- *Crust (scab):* dried blood, serum and other exudates covering an ulcerated area of skin.
- *Pseudomembrane:* a crust in a moist area (mucosa).
- *Scar:* permanent replacement of lost normal tissue by fibrous tissue.

*Abnormal passages*
- *Fistula:* an abnormal passage between two epithelially lined structures.
- *Sinus:* blind ended track or cavity—some represent normal structures.

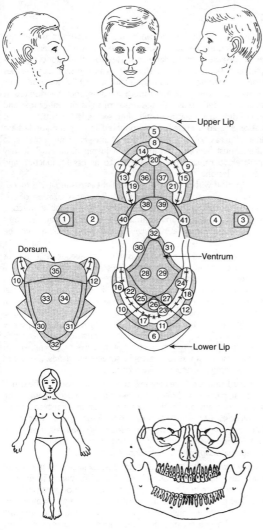

**Fig 2.1** Diagrams for outlining the site, size and shape of lesions

# Mouth

Most oral diseases have a local cause, can be readily recognized and are not very serious. However, some—such as oral cancer—are life-threatening.

Many systemic diseases, particularly diseases of the blood, gastro-intestinal tract and skin, cause oral signs or symptoms. In some cases these symptoms constitute the main complaint as in HIV, leucopenia or leukaemia. However, even now, the mouth is sometimes overlooked at examination, and the delay between the onset of signs of oral cancer and the institution of definitive treatment still often exceeds 6 months.

The examination should therefore be conducted in a systematic fashion to ensure that all areas are included. If the patient wears any removable appliances these must be removed in the first instance, although it may be necessary later to replace the prostheses to assess fit, function and relationship to any lesion.

Complete visualization with a good source of light is essential. All muco-sal surfaces should be examined, starting away from the location of any known lesions. The lips should first be inspected. The labial mucosa, buccal mucosa, floor of mouth and ventrum of tongue, dorsal surface of the tongue, hard and soft palates, gingivae and teeth should then be examined in sequence.

*Lip* examination is facilitated if the mouth is gently closed, so that the lips can be everted to examine the mucosa. Features such as cyanosis (central cyanosis) are seen mainly in cardiac or respiratory disease. Angular cheilitis is seen mainly in oral candidosis or iron or vitamin deficiencies. The labial mucosa normally appears moist with a fairly prominent vascular arcade. In the lower lip, the many minor salivary glands, which are often exuding mucus, are easily visible. The lips therefore feel slightly nodular and the labial arteries are readily palpable. Many adults have a few yellowish pin-head-sized papules in the vermilion border (particularly of the upper lip) and at the commissures; these are ectopic sebaceous glands (Fordyce's spots), and may become numerous as age advances.

The **cheek (buccal) mucosa** is readily inspected if the mouth is held half open. The vascular pattern and minor salivary glands so prominent in the labial mucosa are not obvious in the buccal mucosa but Fordyce's spots may be conspicuous particularly at the commissures and retromolar areas in adults. Faint white striae may be benign leucoedema, not to be confused with lichen planus, one of the commoner diseases of the mouth. Leucoedema disappears if the mucosa is stretched.

The **floor of mouth and ventrum of tongue** are best examined by the patient pushing the tongue into the opposite cheek. This also raises the floor of mouth, an area where tumours commonly start (the coffin or graveyard area of the mouth). The posterior part is the most difficult area to examine well and therefore one where lesions are most easily missed. Lingual veins are prominent and, in the elderly, may be conspicuous (lingual varices). Bony lumps on the alveolar ridge lingual to the premolars are most often tori (torus mandibularis). Occasionally, patients (or even clinicians not famil-iar with the oral anatomy) recognize these, as well as the openings of the submandibular glands as alarming lumps in the mouth.

During this part of the examination the quantity and consistency of saliva should be assessed. Examine for the normal pooling of saliva in the floor of the mouth. Xerostomia is confirmed by placing the surface of a dental mirror against the buccal mucosa: the mirror should normally lift off easily but it adheres to the mucosa if xerostomia is present.

The *dorsum of tongue* is best inspected by protrusion, when it can be held with gauze. The anterior two-thirds are embryologically and anatomically distinct from the posterior third, from which they are separated by a dozen or so large circumvallate papillae. The dorsum of the anterior two-thirds is coated with many filiform but relatively few fungiform papillae. Behind the circumvallate papillae, the tongue contains several large lymphoid masses posteriorly (lingual tonsil) and the foliate papillae lie on the lateral borders posteriorly. These are often mistaken for tumours.

A healthy child's tongue is rarely coated but a mild coating is not uncommon in healthy adults. The tongue may be fissured (scrotal) but this is usually regarded as a developmental anomaly and is often accompanied by geographic tongue (erythema migrans).

The voluntary tongue movements and sense of taste should be formally tested. Abnormalities of tongue movement (neurological or muscular disease) may be obvious from dysarthria, involuntary movements (e.g. fasciculations) or wasting.

Testing of taste sensation with salt, sweet, sour and bitter should be carried out by applying solutions of salt, sugar, dilute acetic acid and 5% citric acid to the tongue on a cotton swab or cotton bud.

The *hard palate* mucosa is firmly bound down as a mucoperiosteum (similar to the gingivae) and with no obvious vascular arcades. Rugae are present anteriorly on either side of the antero-central incisive papilla that overlies the incisive foramen. Bony lumps in the posterior centre of the vault of the hard palate are usually tori (torus palatinus). Patients may complain of lumps distal to the upper molars that they think are unerupted teeth but the pterygoid hamulus is usually responsible for this complaint.

The *soft palate and fauces* may show a faint vascular arcade. Just posterior to the junction with the hard palate is a conglomeration of minor salivary glands. This region is often also yellowish. The palate should be inspected and movements examined while the patient says 'Aah'. Using a mirror, this also permits inspection of the posterior tongue, pharynx, and even sometimes offers a glimpse of the larynx.

Healthy *gingivae* are firm, pale pink, with a stippled surface, and form sharp gingival papillae between the teeth. There should be no bleeding on gently probing the gingival margin. The 'keratinised' attached gingivae (pale pink) are clearly demarcated from the non-keratinized alveolar mucosa.

Periodontal disease is mainly evident on the free margins of the gingivae, but the attached gingivae may also present signs of significant pathology (e.g. desquamative gingivitis), which are frequently overlooked or misinterpreted as inflammatory (plaque-related) periodontal disease.

# Teeth

The dentition should be checked to make sure the complement of teeth present is that expected for the patient's age. Abnormalities in the number, size, shape, colour and structure of teeth and their possible causes are outlined in Chapter 7. Deficiency of teeth (oligodontia, hypodontia or anodontia) as well as abnormalities of size, shape, colour or structure may be features of many syndromes, but teeth are far more frequently missing because they are unerupted, or lost as a result of caries or periodontal disease.

Extra teeth (hyperdontia) are supplemental if part of the normal series or supernumerary if of abnormal morphology.

Teeth should be carefully examined and described in the patient's notes. Some abnormalities may on occasions be correlated with other findings from the history and general examination. The clinician should be alert to the possibility of such associations and prepared to go back to the history or adjust further examination and investigations according to such findings.

Detailed description of dental and periodontal examination techniques can be found in standard textbooks. Even a non-dentally trained clinician though should be prepared to perform a basic dental examination using the general principles of inspection, palpation and percussion.

---

**Basic dental examination** (see Table 2.1)

*Inspection:* Look for carious, mobile, heavily or poorly restored teeth, retained roots or other signs that could explain extensive local (e.g. facial abscess) or systemic (e.g. infective endocarditis) pathology.

*Palpation:* Feel for tenderness or swelling of the alveolar process adjacent to apical areas of suspicious teeth (feel the buccal/labial and lingual/palatal sides of the alveolus)

*Percussion:* Use a long metal instrument (like the handle of a dental mirror) to tap on suspicious teeth (warn the patient and start gently, or rapport may be lost in a second!). Any tenderness elicited may signify pulpal or periodontal/periapical inflammation.

*Vitality testing:* Non-vital teeth are primary suspects of local pain and infections, occasionally even when they are root-treated. In such cases, the patient should report no sensation of hot (melting gutta percha), cold (ethyl chloride on a cotton bud) or electric (special apparatus; pulp vitality tester) stimuli.

---

All findings should be charted using one of various systems of tooth notations (Table 2.2). The system most widely used worldwide is the Federation Dentaire Internationale (FDI) system.

Finally, the occlusion of the teeth should be checked, as it may be disturbed in some jaw fractures, or dislocation of the mandibular condyles.

**Table 2.1** Investigative procedures in diseases of teeth

| Procedure | Advantages | Disadvantages | Remarks |
|---|---|---|---|
| Percussion (tapping and pressure) | Simple. May reveal periostitic teeth | Crude | Teeth may be periostitic due to abscess formation. Maxillary teeth may be periostitic if there is sinusitis |
| Application of hot or cold stimuli to teeth | Simple | Crude. Heat or cold may be transferred to adjacent teeth | Cold stimuli may be useful to locate pulpitic teeth or exposed dentine |
| Electric pulp test | Simple | Unpleasant May give false positives or negatives. Requires special apparatus | May be useful to locate pulpitic teeth |
| Radiography | Simple. Can reveal caries, fractures and much pathology in jaws | Pulp exposures may be missed as view is only two-dimensional. Caries does not show well on extra-oral films | Simple periapical films are valuable. Bitewing films do not show the periapical bone (see page 82) |

**Table 2.2** The more commonly used tooth notations

| | |
|---|---|
| **Palmer** | |
| Permanent dentition | Upper |
| | 87654321 \| 12345678 |
| | Right                            Left |
| | 87654321 \| 12345678 |
| | Lower |
| Deciduous dentition (anonymous classification) | EDCBA \| ABCDE |
| | EDCBA \| ABCDE |

**Haderup**

Permanent dentition

$$(8+)(7+)(6+)(5+)(4+)(3+)(2+)(1+) \mid (+1)(+2)(+3)(+4)(+5)(+6)(+7)(+8)$$
$$(8-)(7-)(6-)(5-)(4-)(3-)(2-)(1-) \mid (-1)(-2)(-3)(-4)(-5)(-6)(-7)(-8)$$

Deciduous dentition

$$(50+)(40+)(30+)(20+)(10+) \mid (+01)(+02)(+03)(+04)(+05)$$
$$(50-)(40-)(30-)(20-)(10-) \mid (-01)(-02)(-03)(-04)(-05)$$

**Universal**

Permanent dentition

| 1 | 2 | 3 | 4 | 5 | 6 | 7 | 8 \| 9 | 10 | 11 | 12 | 13 | 14 | 15 | 16 |
| 32 | 31 | 30 | 29 | 28 | 27 | 26 | 25 \| 24 | 23 | 22 | 21 | 20 | 19 | 18 | 17 |

Deciduous dentition

A B C D E \| F G H I J
T S R Q P \| O N M L K

**Fédération Dentaire Internationale (two-digit)**

Permanent dentition

| 18 | 17 | 16 | 15 | 14 | 13 | 12 | 11 \| 21 | 22 | 23 | 24 | 25 | 26 | 27 | 28 |
| 48 | 47 | 46 | 45 | 44 | 43 | 42 | 41 \| 31 | 32 | 33 | 34 | 35 | 36 | 37 | 38 |

Deciduous dentition

55 54 53 52 51 \| 61 62 63 64 65
85 84 83 82 81 \| 71 72 73 74 75

# Integrated examination

A routine examination should be flowing smoothly from one body part to the next. In some cases, you may have to concentrate on one system and examine it exhaustively, as described in this chapter. In most instances, however, you need only to integrate the most important aspects of the examination of these systems into a unified approach that avoids duplication and saves time.

The basic features you need to examine and record are listed below.

*General*
- General physical appearance (body size, hydration, colour, any cyanosis or breathlessness)
- Mental state and level of consciousness  (alert, anxious, depressed, confused)
- Surroundings (oxygen, drains, catheters, several pillows in bed)
- Speech (volume, content, form, articulation, associated discomfort)
- Vital signs (temperature, pulse rate, BP, respiratory rate)

*Arms*
- Hands (temperature, colour, deformities, nails, skin, muscle wasting, tenderness)
- Radial pulse (rate, rhythm, volume, character)
- Neurological and musculoskeletal examination (if necessary)

*Head*
- Eyes (anaemia, jaundice, pupillary reflexes, eye movements)
- Face (skin, parotids, TMJs, lumps, deformities, muscle weakness or tenderness)
- Mouth (oral hygiene, state of dentition, mucosa, amount of saliva, lumps, ulcers, infections)
- Cranial nerves (ones that may be most relevant)

*Neck*
- Lymph nodes
- Thyroid
- Jugular venous pressure and carotid pulse
- Trachea (central or deviated?)

*Chest (cardiorespiratory),* lying at 45°
- Inspection (scars, deformities)
- Palpation of precordium (apex beat, any heaves or thrills)
- Auscultation of the heart (heart sounds, any murmurs)
- Chest expansion (inspect and feel for adequacy and symmetry)
- Percussion of the chest (map out any abnormalities)
- Auscultation of the lungs (breath sounds, any added sounds)
- Back of chest (inspection, percussion, auscultation of lungs, any sacral oedema)

*Abdomen,* lying flat
- Inspection (scars, distension)
- Palpation: gently, firmly and during inspiration (tenderness, guarding, rigidity, masses, hernias, enlargement of liver, spleen or kidneys)
- Percussion (liver, spleen, masses, shifting dullness)
- Auscultation (bowel sounds)
- Digital rectal examination (record if not necessary)

*Legs*
- Peripheral pulses
- Calves (tenderness indicating a deep vein thrombosis [DVT])
- Ankle oedema
- Feet (ulcers, calluses, temperature)
- Neurological and musculoskeletal examination (if necessary)

USEFUL WEBSITES
http://www.meddean.luc.edu/lumen/MedEd/MEDICINE/PULMONAR/PD/Pdmenu.htm

# Investigations

# Introduction

Following the history and examination, investigations may be required to help make or confirm the diagnosis. Sometimes investigations are simply needed to exclude some diagnoses in order to reassure the patient (and/or the clinician).

Inadequate investigation could lead to a:
- misdiagnosis,
- missed diagnosis,
- complaint of bad practice, or
- legal action.

When planning investigations, it is important to consider carefully what you expect to learn from them and how the results may affect your patient's management. Too often, investigations are carried out with a 'shotgun' approach, without adequate thought or planning. If investigations are unlikely really to make any difference to the diagnosis, prognosis or treatment, reconsider your decision to perform them. Superfluous investigations can be:
- time-consuming,
- expensive,
- occasionally dangerous,
- liable to engender undue anxiety on the part of the patient, partner, relatives or clinician, and
- the cause of subsequent unnecessary interventions.

It is the duty of dental staff to ensure that the patient understands the relevance of any suggested investigations and the advantages and disadvantages of carrying them out. Patients not uncommonly complain that they have been ill-informed about their diagnosis, investigations and the results of these.

For most investigations there is a range within which results are considered to be 'normal'. However, 'normality' is a relative term, its range usually including 95% of the population—which means that 5% of healthy individuals will be outside this range. Thus an 'abnormal' result may not necessarily signify disease and, in any event, should always be checked, as it could also be a technical error, or even the result from someone else's sample! Performing tests that are not clearly indicated increases the chance of getting abnormal results that are clinically insignificant and potentially harmful.

---

### When ordering an investigation

- Check that it has not already been performed or ordered!
- Consider first getting in touch with the person performing it or analysing it. This may give you an earlier and more thorough report.
- Fill in the request form fully and correctly, and label any samples properly, with the patient's full name, hospital number, etc.
- Give all relevant clinical information (the importance of this is frequently underestimated).
- State what you expect to learn from the investigation and how urgent the result is.

---

To state the obvious, it is important that you remember to check the results of the investigations that you have ordered. Interpret these results with caution and always in the light of your clinical impression. If the results are very different from what you expected, or they are grossly abnormal, question their validity. There are many factors that can influence the results of an investigation, not least human error, investigation technique, technical fault, food and drugs.

## Points to remember when performing an investigation

- The first principle must be to do no harm.
- Informed consent is required.
- Only an operator adequately skilled in a procedure should perform it.
- All surgery is invasive and an oral biopsy is often an unpleasant procedure, as the mouth is very sensitive.
- All body fluids and tissues are potentially infectious. Barrier precautions must therefore always be employed in order to prevent transmission of infection to patients and clinical or laboratory staff.
- Many investigations can be carried out in general practice, but, for several reasons, the dental surgeon may elect to refer to a specialist.

## Informed consent

Consent is implied for taking a history and performing relevant clinical examinations. Investigations are another matter, and the dentist must get informed consent, clearly explaining their:
- nature,
- potential benefit,
- possible adverse effects,
- problems and advantages of NOT carrying them out.

These points must be explained to the patient in a way that can be readily understood. If the patient agrees to the investigation or procedure, then informed verbal consent has been obtained but, if any invasive or hazardous procedure is involved, consent should be obtained in writing. Routine urinalysis is usually accepted as an integral part of medical and insurance examinations. For other procedures, informed consent should always first be obtained, particularly where there are sensitive issues such as HIV infection, when the patient must be professionally counselled before testing. Remember that patients are free to decline any or all investigations should they so wish, but it is wise for the clinician to clearly record any such decision in writing in the case records.

# Urinalysis

Urinalysis is simple, cheap, non-invasive and widely available (Table 3.1).

## Inspection

*Colour.* The urine may be clear-yellow (normal urine), brown (concentrated urine or bilirubinuria), red (beetroot eating, blood, myoglobin, rifampicin or porphyria) or cloudy (infection).

*Volume.* This is mainly monitored in catheterized patients (urine output is one of the vital signs).

## Dipstick analyses

A combination urinalysis stick is dipped into the patient's fresh urine for a second. Excess urine is shaken off and, holding the stick in a horizontal position, the colour of each reactant is compared with the key on the dipstick container at the times specified.

*Specific gravity.* This is a measure of the concentration of urine.

*pH.* Urine is usually acid (pH ~5), but this may vary depending on the kidney function in maintaining acid–base balance.

*Glucose.* Glycosuria may indicate pregnancy, diabetes mellitus or other endocrinopathies, sepsis, renal damage or head injury.

*Ketones.* Ketonuria may be a sign of diabetic ketoacidosis or starvation. Febrile or traumatized patients may also have ketones in their urine.

*Protein.* Traces of protein in the urine can be normal, especially in young people and in pregnancy. It may also be due to exercise, prolonged standing, fever, drugs, menstruation or contamination of the container with disinfectants. On the other hand, proteinuria may indicate UTI, renal or cardiac failure, ↑ BP, endocarditis, diabetes mellitus, multiple myeloma or amyloidosis.

*Nitrites.* Nitrite is a product of bacterial metabolism and its presence in the urine is a strong indicator of a UTI. However, not all bacteria produce nitrite, and even when they do, it may be undetected if the urine is too fresh.

*Blood.* Haematuria may be caused by renal or urinary tract disease (inflammation, cancer, trauma, calculi, etc.), catheterization, ↑ BP, bleeding tendencies, endocarditis or drugs. False positive results may be due to menstruation, specimen pot contamination with detergents, or stale urine.

*Bilirubin.* Bilirubinuria may be due to drugs (e.g. phenothiazines) or jaundice (hepatocellular or obstructive).

*Urobilinogen.* Some urobilinogen is normally excreted in the urine, but ↑ amounts are due to drugs (sulphonamides, ascorbic acid, etc.), prolonged antibiotic therapy or jaundice (usually haemolytic).

## Urine microscopy

A drop of fresh urine can be examined under the microscope for:
- red blood cells (haematuria),
- white blood cells (infection),
- epithelial cells (infection),
- bacteria (infection),
- hyaline or granular casts (proteinuria),

- red cell casts (haematuria),
- white cell casts (infection) and
- cystine or urate crystals (↑ risk of calculi).

## Microbiological examination

A midstream urine (MSU) sample can be collected for culture and sensitivity (C&S) tests (see page 92). Detection of UTI depends on the assessment of numbers of bacteria present. Normal urine should not contain more than 10 000 bacteria/mL (usually much fewer), which are contaminants from the urethra and skin. Infected urine generally has more than 100 000 bacteria/mL. The nature of the bacteria isolated may be important; commensals (such as lactobacilli) are usually of no significance. For these criteria to hold, urine must be cleanly collected, after a small initial amount has been passed (MSU). It should also be received in the laboratory within 2 h of being passed. Urinary organisms multiply at room temperature and cells may undergo lysis. If further delay is inevitable, the urine must be kept in a refrigerator at 4°C.

If neither of these courses is possible, a dip inoculum technique may be used. A special slide bearing culture medium obtained from the laboratory is dipped into the urine as soon as it has been passed into a sterile vessel. The excess is drained off, and the slide is returned to its container and sent to the laboratory with the urine specimen.

For tubercle bacilli, three early morning urines (EMU; complete specimen rather than mid-stream) are required.

## 24-h urine collection

This allows examination of renal function, by measuring the excretion of various substances. Simultaneous collection of a blood sample allows calculation of renal clearance of creatinine (creatinine clearance: a measure of glomerular filtration rate).

**Table 3.1** Urinalysis: interpretation of results[a]

| | Protein | Glucose[b] | Ketones | Bilirubin[c] | Urobilinogen[c] | Blood[d] |
|---|---|---|---|---|---|---|
| Health | Usually no protein, but a trace can be normal in young people | Usually no glucose, but a trace can be normal in 'renal glycosuria' and pregnancy | Usually no ketones, but ketonuria may occur in vomiting, fasting or starved patients | Usually no bilirubin | Usually present in normal healthy patients, particularly in concentrated urine | Usually no blood |
| False positives | Alkaline urine. Container contaminated with disinfectant, e.g. chlorhexidine. Blood or pus in urine. Polyvinyl pyrrolidone infusions | Cephamandole. Container contaminated with hypochlorite | Patients on L-dopa or any phthalein compound | Chlorpromazine and other phenothiazines | Infected urine. Patients taking ascorbic acid, sulphonamides or paraminosalicylate | Menstruation. Container contaminated with some detergents |
| Disease | Renal diseases. Also cardiac failure, diabetes, endocarditis, myeloma, amyloid, some drugs, some chemicals | Diabetes mellitus. Also in pancreatitis, hyperthyroidism, Fanconi syndrome, sometimes after a head injury, other endocrinopathies | Diabetes mellitus. Also in febrile or traumatized patients on low carbohydrate diets | Jaundice. Hepatocellular and obstructive | Jaundice. Haemolytic, hepatocellular and obstructive. Prolonged antibiotic therapy | Genito-urinary diseases. Also in bleeding tendency, some drugs, endocarditis |

[a] Using test strips. Normal or non-fresh urine may be alkaline; normal urine may be acid.
[b] Dopa, ascorbate or salicylates may give false negatives.
[c] May be false negative if urine not fresh.
[d] Ascorbic acid may give false negative.

# Venepuncture (phlebotomy)

## Sites
- ❶ A vein you can feel is preferable to a vein you can see. If there is an option, the lateral aspect of the antecubital fossa is safest, as the brachial artery runs deep to the medial aspect.
- The antecubital fossa is the most commonly used site, as veins there are usually large and easily seen.
- The forearm is an easy but painful alternative (the radial side of the wrist is probably the easiest site).
- The dorsum of the hand is also painful, usually more difficult, and prone to haematoma formation.
- The femoral vein should be used only as a last resort. The femoral artery runs midway between the anterior superior iliac spine and the symphysis pubis and it can be palpated just below this point.
  The femoral vein is just medial to the artery.
- Do NOT be tempted to use an arteriovenous fistula for access.

## Equipment
- Gloves
- Tourniquet
- Skin cleansing swab (e.g. isopropyl alcohol)
- Gauze swab or cotton wool
- Syringe (large enough to contain the amount of blood needed)
- Needle (size: 19 or 20 gauge for adults, 21 or 23 gauge for children)
- Containers for sample
- Band Aid or elastoplast (or alternative adhesive bandage if allergic)
- Yellow sharps container.

## Procedure
- For children, use EMLA cream (a mixture of lidocaine [2.5%] and prilocaine [3.5%]) 1 h before, to minimize discomfort.
- Wear disposable gloves.
- Clean skin with alcohol swab.
- Place tourniquet >5 cm above the venepuncture site, tight enough to obstruct superficial venous return (if this is too tight it may also reduce the arterial supply). A BP cuff inflated up to a maximum of 80 mmHg is a good alternative.
- Use gravity (lower the arm) to make veins more prominent. If necessary ask the patient to clench and unclench their fist repeatedly (muscle pump) or gently tap the skin with your finger.
- Use the thumb of your non-dominant hand just below the selected entry point to stretch the skin.
- Insert the needle obliquely through the skin in the line of the vein and with the bevel facing upwards. A decrease in resistance is felt when the vein wall is penetrated.
- Keep holding the syringe steadily and with your non-dominant hand withdraw the plunger slowly (too rapid removal of blood may cause haemolysis).
- If blood is not drawn, withdraw the needle slightly or redirect it.

- When sufficient blood has been obtained, release the tourniquet.
- Place a cotton wool roll over the site while the needle is removed, but only press on it AFTER the needle has been fully removed.
- Ask the patient to hold this in place for 1–2 min then inspect and apply a small plaster.
- Carefully dispose of the needle in a sharps container and fill up the appropriate specimen tubes with the right amount of blood. Great care should be taken to avoid spillage of blood and needle pricks.
- If the specimen tube contains anticoagulant, ensure mixing by gently rolling the tube.
- Label the blood collection tubes with the patient's full details.
- Complete fully and sign the appropriate request forms.

*Vacutainer system*
The technique here is basically the same as above, but the equipment is slightly different. A special double-ended needle is fitted in one end of a special plastic cylinder. At the other end of the cylinder several vacutainer bottles can be pressed until their rubber cover is pierced by the proximal end of the needle. These bottles are colour-coded for each test and they automatically draw the correct amount of blood needed.

This technique is easier in every way, except for the fact that you do not know whether you are within a vein until after the vacutainer bottle is connected, and by the time you correct your position, the vacuum may have been lost. For difficult veins therefore, the syringe is still the preferred method.

## Precautions

- Blood samples for platelet counts and blood calcium estimation require that the tourniquet should be loosened after insertion of the needle and before taking blood.
- If the patient is on a drip, take blood samples from the arm that does not have the drip.
- Muscle pump is a very useful technique to aid distention of veins, but it can significantly increase the serum potassium level and it should only be used if absolutely necessary.

## Complications

- Failure (especially likely if you are a beginner or anxious, or the patient is elderly, shocked or an IV drug user)
- Anxiety (the patient may worry about the result)
- Pain, haematoma or infection (usually due to poor technique)

---

### Ask a physician, a phlebotomist or the laboratory to take the sample if

- it is a 'renal' patient (their veins are valuable),
- the patient usually has had difficulty having venepuncture,
- you have doubt as to the success of your venepuncture or
- you fail twice to obtain the sample.

---

# Blood tests

Normal values and interpretation of the various haematological and biochemical tests are listed in Tables 3.2 and 3.3.

## Haematological tests

Samples must be sent to the haematology laboratory or the blood bank (blood grouping and cross-matching).

*Full blood count (FBC)* (4 mL purple top container with EDTA)

This is one of the laboratory investigations most frequently requested because anaemia and changes in the white blood cell count occur so commonly in a wide variety of diseases. Blood is anticoagulated with dry potassium edetate and should be received in the haematology laboratory within 24 h. Blood cells are usually counted and sized in automatic blood cell counters. Folate can also be assayed (corrected whole blood folate).

*Blood film*

This is prepared from the same sample as FBC, if indicated by the history or by the blood count results, for visual inspection of blood cells.

*Erythrocyte sedimentation rate (ESR) or plasma viscosity*

These tests are global measurements of non-specific plasma protein changes in disease (principally, ↑ concentration of certain globulins, and ↓ albumin level). Both are ↑ mainly in inflammatory diseases and in anaemia. They can usually be performed on the same sample as FBC.

*Coagulation screen* (3.5 mL blue top container with citrate)

This is required to diagnose coagulation disorders. Blood should be received in the haematology laboratory within 4 h.

*Serum iron, ferritin, transferrin, and vitamin B$_{12}$* (plain tube)

Levels of these are useful in the diagnosis of anaemias due to deficiencies. Ten millilitres of blood is added to a plain tube, and should be received in the haematology laboratory within 24 h.

*Blood group and cross-match* (6 mL pink top container with EDTA)

These are required prior to blood cell transfusion. Blood should be received in the haematology laboratory within 4 h.

## Biochemistry tests

Blood samples should be sent to the biochemistry laboratory. If special or unusual tests are required, it is best to contact the lab first.

*Urea, creatinine and electrolytes (U&Es)* (4 mL gold top container)

These assays require a plain tube (no anticoagulant), and are used to diagnose renal failure (↑ urea and creatinine levels), and electrolyte disturbances.

*Liver function tests (LFTs)*

These can be carried out on the same sample as U&Es and include measurement of bilirubin, liver enzymes (aspartate transaminase [AST], alanine transaminase [ALT], alkaline phosphatase [AlkPase], gamma glutamyl transpeptidase [GGT]) and albumin, which are useful in the diagnosis of jaundice, liver and biliary tract disorders.

*Serum calcium, phosphate and alkaline phosphatase*
These can be carried out on the same sample as U&Es and are useful in the diagnosis of bone disease.

*Cardiac enzymes*
These can be carried out on the same sample as U&Es and include measurement of Troponin (a specific marker of cardiac damage), creatine kinase (CK), aspartate transaminase (AST) and lactate dehydrogenase (LDH), which are all useful in the diagnosis of acute MI.

*Lipids* (cholesterol, triglycerides and lipoproteins)
These require a plain tube and are used to diagnose hyperlipidaemias.

*Hormones*
These require a plain tube and are assayed in the diagnosis of endocrine disorders.

*Blood glucose* (2 mL grey top container with sodium fluoride)
Random or fasting serum glucose measurements are important for the diagnosis and management of diabetes mellitus.

*Autoantibodies*
These require a plain tube and include rheumatoid factor, antinuclear factor and organ-specific autoantibodies.

## Arterial blood gases

These require arterial puncture, usually of the radial or brachial artery, and a heparinized syringe (see page 97). Measurements are made by special machines usually available in Intensive Care and A&E departments.

**Table 3.2** Interpretation of haematological results

| Blood | Normal range[a] | Level ↑ | Level ↓ |
|---|---|---|---|
| Haemoglobin | Male 13.0–18.0 g/dL<br>Female 11.5–16.5 g/dL | Polycythaemia (vera or physiological) myeloproliferative disease | Anaemia |
| Haematocrit (packed cell volume or PCV) | Male 40–54%;<br>Female 37–47% | Polycythaemia; dehydration | Anaemia |
| Mean cell volume (MCV) | 78–99 fL<br>$MCV = \frac{PCV}{RBC}$ | Macrocytosis in vitamin $B_{12}$ or folate deficiency; liver disease; alcoholism; hypothyroidism; myelodysplasia; myeloproliferative disorders; aplastic anaemia; cytotoxic agents | Microcytosis in iron deficiency; thalassaemia; chronic disease |
| Mean cell haemoglobin (MCH) | 27–31 pg<br>$MCH = \frac{Hb}{RBC}$ | Pernicious anaemia | Iron deficiency; thalassaemia; sideroblastic anaemia |
| Mean cell haemoglobin concentration (MCHC) | 32–36 g/dL<br>$MCHC = \frac{Hb}{PCV}$ | | Iron deficiency; thalassaemia; sideroblastic anaemia; anaemia in chronic disease |
| Red cell count (RBC) | Male $4.2–6.1 \times 10^{12}/L$<br>Female $4.2–5.4 \times 10^{12}/L$ | Polycythaemia | Anaemia; fluid overload |
| White cell count | $4–10 \times 10^9/L$ | Pregnancy; exercise; infection; trauma; leukaemia | Early leukaemia; some infections; bone marrow disease; drugs; idiopathic |

| | | | |
|---|---|---|---|
| Total Neutrophils | Average $3 \times 10^9$/L | Pregnancy; exercise; infection; bleeding; trauma; malignancy; leukaemia | Some infections; drugs; endocrinopathies; bone marrow disease; idiopathic |
| Lymphocytes | Average $2.5 \times 10^9$/L | Physiological; some infections; leukaemia; bowel disease | Some infections; some immune defects (e.g. AIDS) |
| Eosinophils | Average $0.15 \times 10^9$/L | Allergic disease; parasitic infestations; skin disease; lymphoma | Some immune defects |
| Platelets | $150–400 \times 10^9$/L | Thrombocytosis in bleeding; myeloproliferative disease | Thrombocytopenia related to leukaemia; drugs; infections; idiopathic; autoimmune |
| Reticulocytes | 0.5–1.5% of RBC | Haemolytic states; during treatment of anaemia | — |
| Erythrocyte sedimentation rate (ESR) | 0–15 mm/h | Pregnancy; infections; anaemia; connective tissue disease; myelomatosis; malignancy; temporal arteritis | — |
| Plasma viscosity | 1.4–1.8 cp | As ESR | — |

[a] Adults unless otherwise stated. Check values with your laboratory.

**Table 3.3** Interpretation of biochemical results

| Biochemistry[a] | Normal range[b] | Level ↑ | Level ↓ |
|---|---|---|---|
| Acid phosphatase | 0–13 IU/L | Prostatic malignancy; renal disease; acute myeloid leukaemia | — |
| Alanine transaminase (ALT)[c] | 3–60 IU/L | Liver disease; infectious mononucleosis | — |
| Alkaline phosphatase | 30–110 IU/L (3–13 KA units) | Puberty; pregnancy; Paget's disease; osteomalacia; fibrous dysplasia; malignancy in bone, liver disease; hyperparathyroidism (some); hyperphosphatasia | Hypothyroidism; hypophosphatasia; malnutrition |
| α₁-antitrypsin | 200–400 mg% | Cirrhosis | Congenital emphysema |
| α-fetoprotein | <12 microgram/L | Pregnancy; gonadal tumour; liver disease | Drop in pregnancy indicates fetal distress |
| Amylase | 70–300 IU/L | Pancreatic disease; mumps; some other salivary diseases | — |
| Antistreptolysin O titre (ASOT) | 0–300 Todd units/mL | Streptococcal infections; rheumatic fever | — |
| Aspartate transaminase (AST)[d] | 3–40 IU/L | Liver disease; biliary disease; MI; trauma | — |
| Bilirubin (total) | 1–17 μmol/L | Liver or biliary disease; haemolysis | — |
| Caeruloplasmin | 1.3–3.0 μmol/L | Pregnancy; cirrhosis; hyperthyroidism; leukaemia | Wilson's disease |

| | | | |
|---|---|---|---|
| Calcium | 2.3–2.6 mmol/L (total calcium) | Hyperparathyroidism (some); malignancy in bone; renal tubular acidosis; sarcoidosis; thiazides | Hypoparathyroidism; renal failure; rickets; nephrotic syndrome |
| Cholesterol | 3.9–7.8 mmol/L | Hypercholesterolaemia; pregnancy; hypothyroidism; diabetes; nephrotic syndrome; liver or biliary disease | Malnutrition; hyperthyroidism |
| Complement (C3) | 0.79–1.60 g/L | Trauma; surgery; infection | Liver disease; immune complex diseases: e.g. lupus erythematosus |
| (C4) | 0.2–0.4 g/L | — | Liver disease; immune complex diseases; HANE |
| Cortisol (see steroids) | | | |
| Creatine phosphokinase (CPK) | 50–100 IU/L (<130) | MI; trauma; muscle disease | — |
| Creatinine | 0.06–0.11 mmol/L | Renal failure; urinary obstruction | Pregnancy |
| C reactive protein (CRP) | <10 microgram/ml | Inflammation; trauma; MI; malignant disease | — |
| C1 esterase inhibitor | 0.1–0.3 g/L | — | Hereditary angioedema |
| Ferritin | Adult male 25–190 ng/mL Adult female 15–99 ng/mL Child mean 21 ng/mL | Liver disease; haemochromatosis; leukaemia; lymphoma; other malignancies; thalassaemia | Iron deficiency |

**Table 3.3** Contd.

| Biochemistry[a] | Normal range[b] | Level ↑ | Level ↓ |
|---|---|---|---|
| Fibrinogen | 200–400 mg% | Pulmonary embolism; nephrotic syndrome; lymphoma | Disseminated intravascular coagulopathy (DIC) |
| Folic acid | 3–20 microgram/L (red cell folate 120–650 microgram/L) | Folic acid therapy | Alcoholism; dietary deficiency; haemolytic anaemias;malabsorption; myelodysplasia; phenytoin; methotrexate; trimethoprim; pyrimethamine; sulphasalazine; cycloserine; oral contraceptive |
| Free thyroxine index (FTI) (serum $T_4 \times T_3$ uptake) | 1.3–5.1 U | Hyperthyroidism | Hypothyroidism |
| γ glutamyl transpeptidase (GGT) | (5–42 IU/L) | Liver disease; MI; pancreatitis, diabetes; renal diseases; tricyclics | — |
| Globulins (total) (see also under protein) | 22–36 g/L | Liver disease; myelomatosis; autoimmune disease; chronic infections | Chronic lymphatic leukaemia; malnutrition; protein-losing states |
| Glucose | 2.8–5.0 mmol/L | Diabetes mellitus; pancreatitis; hyperthyroidism; hyperpituitarism; Cushing's disease; liver disease; after head injury | Hypoglycaemic drugs; Addison's disease; hypopituitarism; hyper-insulinism; severe liver disease |

| Test | Reference range | | |
|---|---|---|---|
| Hydroxybutyrate dehydrogenase (HBD) | 100–250 IU/L | MI | — |
| Immunoglobulins Total | 7–22 | Liver disease; infection; sarcoidosis; connective tissue disease | Immunodeficiency; nephrotic syndrome; enteropathy |
| IgG | 5–6 g/L | Myelomatosis; connective tissue diseases | Immunodeficiency; nephrotic syndrome |
| IgA | 1.25–4.25 g/L | Alcoholic cirrhosis; Buerger's disease | Immunodeficiency |
| IgM | 0.5–1.75 g/L | Primary biliary cirrhosis; nephrotic syndrome; parasites; infections | Immunodeficiency |
| IgE | <0.007 mg% | Allergies; parasites | — |
| Lactic dehydrogenase (LDH) | 90–300 IU/L | MI; trauma; liver disease; haemolytic anaemias; lymphoproliferative diseases | Radiotherapy |
| Lipase | 0.2–1.5 IU/L | Pancreatic disease | — |
| Lipids | 50–150 mg% (triglycerides) | Hyperlipidaemia; diabetes mellitus; hypothyroidism | — |
| Magnesium | 0.7–0.9 mmol/L | Renal failure | Cirrhosis; malabsorption; diuretics; Conn's syndrome; renal tubular defects |
| Nucleotidase | 1–15 IU/L | Liver disease | — |

**Table 3.3** Contd.

| Biochemistry[a] | Normal range[b] | Level ↑ | Level ↓ |
|---|---|---|---|
| Phosphate | 0.8–1.5 mmol/L | Renal failure; bone disease; hypoparathyroidism; hyperparathyroidism | Hyperparathyroidism; rickets; malabsorption syndrome; insulin |
| Potassium | 3.5–5.0 mmol/L | Renal failure; Addison's disease | Vomiting; diabetes; diarrhoea; Conn's syndrome; diuretics; Cushing's disease; malabsorption |
| Protein (total) | 62–80 g/L | Liver disease; myelomatosis; sarcoid; connective tissue diseases | Nephrotic syndrome; lymphomas; enteropathy; renal failure |
| Albumin | 35–55 g/L | Dehydration | Liver disease:malabsorption; nephrotic syndrome; myelomatosis; connective tissue disorders |
| α₁-globulin | 2–4 g/L | Oestrogens | Nephrotic syndrome |
| α₂-globulin | 4–8 g/L | Infections; trauma | Nephrotic syndrome |
| β globulin | 6–10 g/L | Hypercholesterolaemia; liver disease; pregnancy | Chronic disease |
| γ globulin | 6–15 g/L | (see Immunoglobulins) | Nephrotic syndrome; immunodeficiency |

| | | |
|---|---|---|
| SGGT (see GGT) | | |
| SGOT (see AST) | | |
| SGPT (see ALT) | | |
| Sodium | 130–145 nmol/L | Dehydration; Cushing's disease | Oedema; renal failure; Addison's disease |
| Steroids (corticosteroids) | 110–525 mol/L (14 ± 6 microgram%) | Cushing's disease; some tumours | Addison's disease; hypopituitarism |
| Thyroxine (T4) | 50–138 nmol/L | Hyperthyroidism: pregnancy; contraceptive pill | Hypothyroidism; nephrotic syndrome; phenytoin |
| Urea | 3.3–6.7 mmol/L | Renal failure; dehydration | Liver disease; nephrotic syndrome; pregnancy |
| Uric acid | 0.15–0.48 mmol/L | Gout; leukaemia; renal failure; myelomatosis | Liver disease; probenecid; allopurinol; salicylates; other drugs |
| Vitamin B12 | 150–800 ng/L | Liver disease; leukaemia | Pernicious anaemia; gastrectomy; Crohn's disease; ileal resection; vegans; metformin |

Note: Values may differ from laboratory to laboratory. There are many more causes of abnormal results than are outlined here.
[a] Serum or plasma.
[b] Adult levels; always consult your own laboratory.
[c] ALT = SGPT (serum glutamate-pyruvate transaminase).
[d] AST = SGOT (serum glutamate–oxaloacetic transaminase).
SI values: $10^{-1}$ = deci (d); $10^{-2}$ = centi (c); $10^{-3}$ = milli (m); $10^{-6}$ = micro ($\mu$); $10^{-9}$ = nano (n); $10^{-12}$ = pico (p); $10^{-15}$ = femto (f).

# Radiology

Radiological and other imaging tests (apart from ultrasound and MRI) involve ionizing radiation exposure, which, even if not serious, often worries the patient. Pregnancy should always be excluded (risk of foetal irradiation) before performing procedures that involve radiation exposure, especially to the abdomen and pelvis.

Dental radiography in the UK is subject to 2 main pieces of legislation:
- The Ionizing Radiation Regulations 1999, and
- The Ionizing Radiation (Medical Exposure) Regulations 2000 (IR[ME]R).

These set the framework for practising radiography, and classify dental professionals involved in radiography, into 'Referrers', 'Practitioners' and 'Operators'. It is entirely feasible that all three are one and the same person, i.e. the dentist. The 'Operator' can also be a 'Professional Complementary to Dentistry' (PCD) with appropriate training.

## Request form

The request form for radiography should be completed and signed by the dentist and must include:
- Vital patient data (full name, address, date of birth, unit number, ward or outpatient department and specialist in charge)
- Details that facilitate correct investigations and accurate opinion
  - investigations required (region to be examined and, where relevant, special investigation needed)
  - diagnostic problem
  - relevant clinical features
  - known diagnoses
  - previous relevant operations
- Other information (i.e. whether patient is a walking or trolley case, whether an urgent or routine report is required, date, place and type of previous radiographs, etc.)

## Radiation effects

Because of the cumulative effect of radiation hazard, all investigations must be justified as benefiting the patient. The clinician requesting the examination or investigation, as well as the patient and, when relevant, the radiologist, must be satisfied that each investigation is necessary, and that the benefit outweighs the risk. Hospital radiology departments will justifiably question investigations that appear not to be clearly indicated.

Some authorities suggest that a protective lead apron and neck shield should be worn by the patient. Another school of thought would claim that the radiation exposure following routine oral radiography is almost negligible compared with the natural radiation one receives on a daily basis. Current evidence does not support the use of lead apron in dental radiography: 'There is no justification for the routine use of lead aprons for patients in dental radiography. Their use during panoramic radiography is positively discouraged'.

A particular problem arises during pregnancy, because of the hazard to the fetus. The clinician should always ascertain whether a woman is pregnant before requesting a radiograph. All investigations required on pregnant patients should first be discussed with the patient and radiologist. Restricting X-ray investigations on women of child-bearing age to the 10 days following the start of a menstrual period (the 10-day rule) should be considered for those examinations with a relatively high gonad radiation risk, though even this rule has now fallen into disfavour.

## Portable X-rays

The quality of portable films is rarely as good as that of corresponding films taken using non-portable equipment. Portable radiography therefore should only be used if there is an absolute contraindication to the patient being brought to the radiography department. If there is any doubt, consult a radiologist. Theatre radiography is done only when results are needed during the operation.

## Digital radiography

For many years, film has been used to acquire radiographic images. However, electronic sensors are now available to produce radiographic images. Advantages of these sensors are the immediate availability of the images, the lower radiation dose, the possibility of image enhancement, image reconstruction and computer-aided image analysis, transmission of images by Internet, and storage of large numbers of images in image-databases.

USEFUL WEBSITES
Guidelines on Radiology Standards for Primary Dental Care: Report by the Royal College of Radiologists and the National Radiological Protection Board (http://www.nrpb.org/publications/documents_of_nrpb/abstracts/absd5-3.htm#synopsis)

# Imaging techniques: simple

Diagnosis of dental disorders often requires detailed radiographic investigation. A panoramic view is useful as a general survey, but cannot be used to diagnose caries or lesions in the midline. Often two or three intra-oral views of the lesion in question are needed, to give detail (Table 3.4).

### Intra-oral radiography

*Periapical radiographs* are useful for demonstrating pathology in the periapical region (abscess, granuloma, cyst, etc.), the tooth root and the adjacent bone. The paralleling technique using a film holder is considered to have many advantages over the bisecting angle technique.

*Bitewing radiographs* show both upper and lower premolar and molar teeth on one film but do not show the tooth apex. They are useful for revealing proximal caries and demonstrating the alveolar bone crest.

*Occlusal films* may be useful in assessing the facial and lingual cortices, the submandibular glands, the position of impacted upper canines, etc.

### Panoramic radiography (dental panoramic tomography [DPT], orthopantomography [OPTG; OPT; OPG])

The OPTG radiation dose is considerably lower than a full mouth survey using periapical films, and it is a very simple, quick and convenient technique. Nevertheless, it has certain disadvantages; namely, it:

- lacks the detail and clarity obtained by plain radiographs,
- is particularly poor in showing the anterior jaws,
- does not show caries until this is advanced,
- can result in ghost shadows and blurring, and
- examines only a slice of tissue.

OPTG is mainly used in the evaluation of dental development, third molars, mandibular fractures, TMJs and large lesions of the jaws.

### Plain extraoral radiography

Useful in the diagnosis of fractures, dislocations, bone and tooth disorders, joint disease and foreign bodies. Several projections of skull and facial bones may be useful to the dentist.

*Posteroanterior (PA)*—good visualization of both skull and facial bones for the diagnosis of trauma (e.g. mandibular fractures) and developmental abnormalities.

*Lateral skull*—useful for assessing trauma (e.g. skull and nasal fractures) and developmental abnormalities. When the projection concentrates on the hard and soft tissues of the face rather than the skull, it is called a **lateral cephalometric**, which is useful in orthodontics and in orthognathic surgery.

*Mandibular lateral oblique (or oblique lateral)*—useful for visualizing the lateral mandibular body or the ramus and condyle, to reveal pathology (fractures, third molar pathology or other lesions). Largely superceded by the OPTG, it is still used when greater clarity is required or when there is no panoramic machine available.

**Reverse Towne's**—similar to PA, but taken at a different angle and with the mouth open. Useful in assessment of condylar fractures.

**Occipitomental (OM)**—good visualization of the mid-face, especially the maxillary sinuses and orbits, and therefore very useful in assessment of zygomatic and infraorbital fractures (OM views at 10° and 30° are generally preferred for this).

**Submentovertex (SMV)**—useful for evaluation of the zygomatic arch (e.g. in fractures). However, a high radiation dose is usually needed, and so radiology departments will often perform this only when specifically requested. When taken specifically for the zygomatic arches alone, the exposure can be significantly reduced.

**Table 3.4** Radiographs recommended for demonstrating lesions at various sites[a]

| Region required | Views | |
|---|---|---|
| | **Standard** | **Additional** |
| Skull[b] | Postero-anterior (PA) 20<br>Lateral<br>Townes (1/2 axial view) | Submentovertex (SMV)<br>Tangential |
| Facial bones | OM<br>OM 30<br>Lateral | Zygoma<br>Reduced exposure SMV |
| Paranasal sinuses | OM for maxillary antra | Upper occlusal or<br>lateral SMV<br>OPTG, tomography |
| Orthodontics | OPTG<br>Cephalometric lateral skull | |
| Pre- and<br>post-osteotomy | OPTG<br>Cephalometric lateral skull<br>Cephalometric PA skull | |
| Nasal bones | OM 30<br>Lateral<br>Soft tissue lateral | |
| Mandible | OPTG | Lateral obliques<br>PA mandible<br>Mandibular occlusal |
| TMJs | Transcranial lateral obliques<br>or OPTG (mouth open and<br>closed) | Transpharyngeal<br>Arthrography<br>Reverse Townes<br>Reverse OPTG<br>Consider CT scan/MRI |

[a] **Radiography requests:** to enable the radiographic staff to give you the best or most appropriate radiographs for the region under investigation: (1) Fill in the request form as fully as possible with full, relevant clinical findings. (2) Request the region required rather than specific views, except for panoral tomography, when OPTG will suffice.
[b] CT scanning is valuable in craniofacial injuries.

# Imaging techniques: advanced

## Digital radiography

Digital imaging has the advantages of versatility, speed and practicality but, most importantly it significantly reduces the radiation exposure to the patient, which is useful particularly where repeated films are needed, such as in endodontics. It also eliminates the need for film processing, and in a limited-space highly-computerized world it is projected to totally replace film-based radiography, despite a high initial set-up cost.

## Tomography

The OPTG is the most commonly used dental tomographic technique. Tomography, or sectional radiography, examines only 'slices' of tissues and is therefore useful when the clinician wants to isolate and view a specific plane. Film-based tomography has now been largely superseded by CT, but is still useful in implant site and TMJ assessment.

## Computerized tomography

CT integrates information from multiple radiographic 'slices' into images of internal tissues (e.g. brain, orbit, sinuses and neck). CT has considerable advantages in visualizing complex anatomical areas inaccessible to conventional radiographs, as it not only avoids superimposition of structures, but also offers a high-contrast resolution, allowing visualization of minor differences in tissue density.

CT is useful in the assessment of almost any hard or soft structure and is used in the head and neck for assessing pathology (especially tumour spread), and planning surgery. Its latest advancements, especially in 3D reconstruction, make CT an increasingly powerful diagnostic tool. In 3D CT, data acquired by axial CT scans (CAT scans) are integrated and reproduced into a 3D image, with applications in facial trauma management and reconstructive surgery. It is superior to MRI (below) for visualizing hard tissues.

Disadvantages are the fairly high radiation exposure and cost.

## Magnetic resonance imaging

MRI is not an X-ray technique but utilizes electromagnetic waves created by a large magnet to produce a sectional image. The great advantage therefore is that MRI does not involve ionizing radiation and therefore is much safer than CT. Nevertheless, MRI has a limitation in that it cannot be used in the presence of metal (e.g. pacemakers, surgical clips and orthodontic fixed or removable appliances or prostheses). It is also expensive and patients may find it claustrophobic.

MRI produces an impressively high contrast resolution, which makes it very sensitive at visualizing soft tissue differential densities. MRI is therefore superior to CT for soft tissue imaging, but is of limited use in hard tissues. It is therefore used mainly to image internal organs, such as brain and spine.

In the maxillofacial region, MRI is useful in diagnosing soft tissue, TMJ and salivary gland disease.

## Ultrasonography (ultrasound [US])

Ultrasonography employs a transducer to produce US waves and receive their reflection from tissues, allowing recording of the relative position and density of tissues and live display on a monitor. US is simple, rapid, inexpensive, and does not involve radiation exposure.

Nevertheless US images are not especially clear, and thus limited to the visualization of internal organs, especially of the abdomen where radiography is not very informative. It may be useful for imaging of soft tissue pathology of the neck and salivary glands, including cysts, lymph nodes, neoplasms and inflammatory lesions.

*Doppler US* allows the study of blood flow through vessels and is thus useful for assessing vascular lesions, and blood vessels used in microvascular free flap surgery.

## Radionuclide imaging (isotope scanning)

Isotope scanning involves the intravenous injection of radioactive compounds that are taken up preferentially by certain diseased organs, and visualization with a gamma camera. This allows identification of tissues undergoing biochemical processes, even if there are no structural changes. It is, most commonly used in the diagnosis of bone, thyroid, lymph node and salivary gland disorders (e.g. Sjögren's syndrome).

## Contrast-media radiography

This involves the infusion of radiopaque contrast media within fluid-filled body cavities and subsequent imaging of these by plain radiography, tomography, CT scanning or MRI. It should not be used in patients with a known allergy to contrast media. Examples include:

*Sialography*—the infusion of contrast media into the salivary ductal system, to reveal ductal pathology (e.g. calculi) or inflammatory disorders of the parenchyma (e.g. Sjögren's syndrome). It should not be used in infected glands.

*Arthrography*—the injection of contrast media in the lower (and occasionally the upper) TMJ spaces, followed by imaging. This allows the indirect study of disc anatomy and function.

*Angiography*—injection of radiopaque contrast agents into arteries (arteriography) or veins (venography).

# Histopathology

Histopathology is the microscopic examination of a tissue sample taken from a patient, usually during a biopsy. It is mainly indicated in order to confirm or make a precise diagnosis, but it must be remembered that histopathology is only an adjunct in the diagnostic process of oral diseases. If adequate specimens and clinical data are provided by the surgeon, the pathologist can perform optimally. Certain conditions cannot be 100% confirmed by a histopathological examination, which may then only suggest that the appearance is 'consistent with' and not 'diagnostic of' the suspected pathological process. A common example is in the differential diagnosis between lichen planus and lichenoid reaction, where a definitive diagnosis is hard to reach, unless clinical data (such as the patient's medication) are provided. Even then, pathologists can err.

## Indications for biopsy

- Lesions of uncertain aetiology (soft or hard tissue) persisting 3 or more weeks.
- Enlarging lesions or lesions with neoplastic or potentially malignant features
  - Erythroplakia
  - Leucoplakia
  - Focal hyperpigmented lesions
  - Lumps
- Persistent lesions failing to respond to treatment
  - Ulcers
  - Lumps
  - White or coloured lesions
  - Periapical lesions
  - Gingival lesions
  - Non-healing extraction sockets
- Confirmation of clinical diagnosis, e.g.
  - Carcinoma and other malignant neoplasms
  - Vesiculobullous disorders (immunostaining is mandatory)
  - Sjögren's syndrome (labial salivary gland biopsy)
  - Lichen planus
  - Chronic granulomatous lesions (TB, sarcoidosis, Crohn's disease, orofacial granulomatosis [OFG])
  - Some chronic infective lesions (e.g. syphilis, deep mycoses, parasites)
- Lesions causing the patient extreme concern

## Request form

Complete the request form with the:
- patient's details (full name, hospital number, date of birth, etc.)
- date, clinic location and requesting clinician's name
- site of biopsy (diagrams can be useful)
- clinical résumé and
- dates and numbers of all previous biopsies.

The container must be labelled clearly with the:
- patient's full name and hospital number,
- date and time of the procedure, and
- specimen site.

# Biopsy techniques

Informed consent is mandatory for biopsy as for all operative procedures, particularly noting the likelihood of postoperative discomfort, the possibility of bleeding or bruising, and any possible less-transient adverse effects such as postoperative reduction or loss of sensation. Care must be taken not to produce undue anxiety; some patients equate biopsy with a diagnosis of cancer.

## Incision biopsy

In the case of a large lesion, especially if malignancy is suspected, it is advisable to take a sample and confirm diagnosis before definitive treatment is planned.

Perhaps the most difficult and important consideration is which part of the lesion should be included in the biopsy specimen. In the case of a suspected potentially malignant or malignant lesion, any red area should ideally be included in the specimen. In some cases where no obvious site can be chosen, vital staining with 'toluidine blue' may first be indicated. Suspect areas absorb the dye preferentially and stain a deep blue.

As a general rule, the biopsy should include lesional and normal tissue. In the case of ulcerated mucosal lesions, most histopathological information is gleaned from the peri-lesional tissue as, by definition, most epithelium is lost from the ulcer itself. The same usually applies for vesiculobullous conditions, where the epithelium in the area mainly affected will, more often than not, separate before it ends up under the microscope, and results will be compromised.

Another consideration is whether to use a scalpel or a biopsy punch. The punch has the advantage that the incision is controlled, an adequate specimen is obtained (typically 4 mm or 6 mm diameter) and suturing may not be required. However, in vesiculobullous disorders, the punch may split the epithelium or detach it from the lamina propria. When a scalpel is used, a specimen of elliptical shape is usually taken, most commonly from an edge of the lesion. The scalpel should be held vertically against the mucosa or skin, as bevelled edges do not give satisfactory specimens and do not allow optimal closure of the surgical wound.

### Procedure

- A local analgesic should be given, although in some cases (e.g. in children or anxious adults), conscious sedation or a general anaesthetic may be necessary.
- Make a peripheral incision around the desired specimen, using a scalpel with a number 15 blade.
- Do not squeeze the specimen with forceps while trying to dissect the deep margin. A suture is best used for this purpose (and also to protect the specimen from going down the suction tube!).
- A suture may also be used to mark specific areas of the specimen.
- Place tissue on to a small piece of paper before immersing in fixative, to prevent curling.
- Put the specimen into a labelled pot containing fixative, ideally in at least 10 times its own volume of buffered formalin, and leave at room temperature.

- Suture the wound if necessary, intraorally using resorbable sutures (e.g. Vicryl) or, on the skin, non-resorbable sutures (e.g. nylon).

In the laboratory, following appropriate preparation, slices of the specimen are usually stained with haematoxylin and eosin (H&E) prior to examination under the microscope.

### Special considerations

If direct *immunofluorescence* is planned (suspected vesiculobullous disorder), then a further biopsy specimen (or half of a larger biopsy) should be immediately snap-frozen on solid carbon dioxide or liquid nitrogen (or put into Michel's solution if the specimen cannot be taken to the laboratory immediately). The more usual practice is to put the specimen into an empty pot and immediately transfer it to the lab, where someone (informed in advance) can perform the freezing process.

If *bacteriological examination* is required (e.g. suspected TB), send a separate specimen (without fixative) to the microbiology department. It is helpful to contact the laboratory in advance, to obtain advice on specimen sampling and transport (and to get someone interested in your case!).

### Needle core biopsy (needle biopsy)

Needle biopsy is a type of incision biopsy, which provides a simple, minimally invasive and effective way to sample deep structures and organs. Using a special needle, a small piece of tissue is removed, retaining its histological structure. Imaging techniques such as US may be employed to guide the needle.

## Excision biopsy

When the lesion in question is <1 cm or is almost certainly benign in nature, it is reasonable to try and remove the whole lesion (and occasionally a small margin of healthy surrounding tissue). This avoids the need for a second operation, by providing diagnosis and definitive treatment in one procedure.

A scalpel (or laser) excision is necessary and the procedure is similar to that described above, except for the margin size, which may vary depending on the provisional diagnosis. Both peripheral and deep margins must be planned with consideration of the suspected nature of the lesion.

## Frozen sections

Frozen sections are specimens taken for rapid diagnosis during an operation. Usually, the sections include tissues that could not be sampled preoperatively (as often happens with cervical lymph nodes), or from the margins of a large tumour to establish whether resection is complete (i.e. the excision margins are tumour-free), or whether further tissue must be removed before reconstructing the defect.

Communicate with the pathologist no later than the day before the operation. Specimens should be immediately snap-frozen (on solid carbon dioxide or liquid nitrogen) and taken to the laboratory, or collected by the pathology team. Telephone the laboratory when the specimen is on its way. Warn the pathologist about any tissue containing calcified material that could break the microtome.

# Cytology

Cytology is the microscopic study of cells, examination of which may indicate or even confirm the presence of certain pathological processes affecting the tissue of origin. Cells obtained by superficial smears (scrapes) or by deep fine needle aspirates do not carry the same diagnostic value as biopsy tissue samples, but can be strong indicators of disease (e.g. atypical cells obtained from dysplastic or malignant lesions) and in some cases may provide enough information for diagnosis to be established (e.g. large numbers of candidal hyphae in an oral smear).

Smears can be extremely useful in screening for dysplastic cells in some parts of the body (e.g. cervical smears), but their use is limited in the mouth mainly due to the thickness of the oral epithelium. Sampling of superficial oral cells (keratin squames) is of limited diagnostic value, as most of the dysplastic changes occur at or near the basal layer. However, the oral brush biopsy may help overcome this problem.

## Oral smears

- Take smears by 'scraping' the mucosa with a wooden or metal spatula, or dental plastic instrument.
- Spread evenly on the centres of two previously labelled glass slides.
- Fix immediately in industrial methylated spirit. Do not allow the slides to dry in air, as cellular detail is rapidly lost and artefacts develop.
- After 20 min of fixation, the smears can then be left to dry in the air or left in fixative.

Prepared in this way, smears will keep for up to 3 weeks. It usually takes the pathologist a long time to go through the whole slide carefully. Presence of candidal hyphae, atypical cells and their relevant numbers are reported.

## Fine needle aspiration

For FNA, a standard needle and syringe are used for sampling deep-seated lesions such as submucosal oral masses and enlarged lymph nodes. However, adequate sampling requires experienced hands. Aspirates are 'sprayed' over a slide and processed as described above (see 'Oral smears'). Any cells remaining in the needle or syringe can be retrieved by drawing a special solution, which dilutes them, and can then be emptied into a separate pot, which will be centrifuged to isolate the cells for examination.

## Oral brush biopsy

The oral brush biopsy is performed without anaesthetic and using an instrument designed to obtain a transepithelial specimen containing cells from the basal, intermediate, and superficial layers of the epithelium. It is important to ensure that the brush penetrates to the basal cell layer by applying firm pressure when rotating the brush on the lesion.

The laboratory evaluation involves computer-assisted analysis to verify cellular representation from each layer of the epithelium, so that false negatives due to inadequate brush biopsy technique are reduced or eliminated. In these instances, the laboratory informs the dentist that the lesion should be re-tested. A 'negative' result indicates that no epithelial abnormality was detected. Any abnormal cells identified by the computer system are reviewed by pathologists and classified as either 'positive' or 'atypical'. There is controversy about the exact sensitivity and specificity.

# Microbiology

When completing a microbiology request form, ensure correct labelling and provide all relevant clinical data. Highly infectious specimens must be clearly labelled with a warning of biohazard.

In order to recognize pathogens and assist in diagnosis, direct microscopy or culture of specimens may be employed. Infection by certain pathogenic organisms can be detected indirectly by identifying host antibodies specific to the pathogen. However, increasingly, specialized tests that detect specific microbial antigens or nucleic acids are used; these tests are invariably sensitive, specific, and rapid—but expensive!

## Microscopy

Microscopy is a fast and simple method to detect certain organisms, often able to offer a diagnosis within minutes of sampling. Simple *light microscopy* is used for the detection of certain organisms and inflammatory cells. *Staining* can be very useful in the differentiation of organisms based on their cell wall characteristics. Most commonly the Gram stain is used for the classification of bacteria. Ziehl–Neelsen stain will reveal mycobacteria. *Dark-field microscopy* is useful in the identification of thin motile organisms, such as spirochaetes. *Electron microscopy* can be used for the detection of viruses.

## Culture

Culture remains the most reliable universally available method for the accurate diagnosis of many infections, and allows implementation of the right treatment by performing antibiotic sensitivity tests. Most bacteria and fungi can now be cultured in the appropriate media. Viral cultures are also possible, but require tissue culture cells.

Collection of live micro-organisms and quick transport to the laboratory is essential, as delays can result in death of the micro-organisms and therefore a false negative result, or overgrowth and thus overestimation of the numbers of micro-organisms. Certain transport media, however, will preserve viability of the micro-organisms without allowing them to overgrow.

When specimens are collected from non-sterile parts of the body, such as the mouth and the skin, care must be taken to avoid contamination. When sampling an abscess for example, collect a pus aspirate rather than taking a swab after incision. Aspirates can be collected with a syringe and needle and quickly sent (without any transport medium) to the laboratory, where pus will be inoculated into the appropriate culture media and incubated under aerobic and/or anaerobic conditions.

Specimens from superficial mucosal or skin lesions are usually collected with a swab, which should immediately be placed in its transport medium. In these cases, rapid transport is not essential, but sampling should be performed in a way that keeps contamination to a minimum. It is important for the lab to be aware of the particulars of any possible contamination, so that they treat the specimen and interpret the result accordingly. Another way to sample possible pathogens from oral lesions (e.g. Candida) is an oral saline rinse collected in a sterile container.

When a serious systemic infection is suspected (endocarditis, pneumonia, etc.), bacteraemia can be established by performing blood cultures. Blood samples should be collected from two different sites and each one split into two special bottles, one for aerobic culture and one for anaerobic. A total of four bottles must therefore be sent to the laboratory.

Cultured organisms can be identified by their characteristic colonies in the culture plates (usually apparent 24–48 h after inoculation), by their growth requirements or by direct microscopy. Biochemical and other tests can also be performed to help identify the cultured organisms.

Antibiotic disks are usually placed in the culture plates to assess effectiveness of these in restricting microbial growth. These results are also normally available within 24–48 h and can be a useful guide to treatment.

## Detection of microbial products (typing)

Specific commercially available antibodies can attach to certain microbial antigens or toxins, an interaction which can be detected by the formation of visible precipitation or agglutination reactions, or by appropriate labelling of the antibodies. Antibodies can be labelled with fluorescein or enzymes (enzyme-linked immunosorbent assay [ELISA]). The antigen–antibody complexes can be viewed by fluorescence microscopy of the specimen (direct immunofluorescence) or by the effect of the enzyme on an appropriate substrate respectively.

Although false negatives are common, antigen detection is a rapid method of revealing certain micro-organisms that are difficult to culture, and does not even depend on the viability of the micro-organisms.

## Detection of microbial nucleic acids

Certain microbial nucleic acid sequences can be detected by their interaction with appropriately labelled, commercially available, complementary nucleic acids. The sensitivity of this method can be considerably increased if, prior to this interaction, the microbial DNA sequence is multiplied using the polymerase chain reaction (PCR).

Although still expensive, PCR is so sensitive and specific, that it is becoming the most useful tool for the identification of micro-organisms, particularly those that are difficult to culture, especially viruses.

## Serum antibody detection (serology)

Micro-organisms can be identified by the detection of specific antibodies in the patient's serum. This is a two-stage technique, in which commercially available microbial antigens are incubated with the patient's serum. The antigen–antibody complex can be visualized following further addition of fluoresceinated or enzyme-labelled, animal-derived antibodies to human immunoglobulin (indirect immunofluorescence or ELISA). This is a qualitative and also quantitative technique (antibody titre measurement).

Antibodies of different classes of immunoglobulins can be identified and quantified during these tests. Acute infection is established by detection of specific IgM antibodies or a fourfold rise of specific IgG antibodies between the first blood test (acute serum) and one taken at least 10 days later (convalescent serum). Chronic infection and immunity are assessed by IgG antibody measurements. Serology is used mainly for micro-organisms difficult to sample or culture (e.g. hepatitis viruses and HIV).

# Investigations in cardiovascular disease

## Electrocardiography (ECG)

The contraction of the heart depends on depolarization and repolarization of the myocardium. These electrical phenomena can be detected with appropriate electrodes placed on the body surface, and recorded as an ECG. Detailed ECG analysis and interpretation is beyond the scope of this text, but some basic information is provided.

### Performing an ECG

The ECG is a simple and non-invasive procedure. Nevertheless, the patient should be informed of what is involved and verbal consent should be obtained.

A standard 12-lead ECG uses 6 chest and 3 limb electrodes, which are normally clearly labelled as to their attachment sites. Hairy skin should be avoided (shave if necessary). Encourage the patient to keep as still as possible while looking at the trace for a smooth recording. Modern ECG machines will automatically give the rate of the heartbeat and report any abnormalities in the trace (and their possible interpretation), but these are no substitute for clinical judgement.

### ECG interpretation

Examine the ECG (Fig. 3.1) systematically for:

- Rate and rhythm (atrial fibrillation gives a characteristic picture, not least because of the irregularly irregular beat).
- Cardiac axis (estimated from the limb leads [I, II, III, VR, VL, VF]).
- P waves and PR intervals (atrial pathology and conduction problems).
- QRS complexes
  - Wide (bundle branch block or ventricular rhythm)
  - Large Q wave (MI)
  - Large R wave (ventricular hypertrophy)
- ST segment
  - Elevated (acute MI)
  - Depressed (ischaemia)
- T wave (inverted in ischaemia, MI, pulmonary embolism).

### Exercise ECG

In patients with suspected ischaemic heart disease (IHD), diagnosis can usually be confirmed by an ECG recorded while the patient exercises on a treadmill at increasing effort levels. The level of exercise at which symptoms (chest pain or breathlessness) and relevant ECG changes (ST segment depression) develop is important diagnostically and prognostically.

### Ambulatory ECG

Portable devices that record an ECG over a 24 h period are useful for the diagnosis of intermittent arrhythmias.

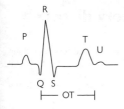

**Fig. 3.1**

## Cardiac enzymes

Enzymes released following cardiac muscle death (see page 71) rise in serum several hours after an MI and can assist in confirming the diagnosis.

## Chest radiograph

A plain posteroanterior (PA) CXR (front of chest nearest to the film) is the preferred projection, as it causes minimal enlargement of the heart shadow. Anteroposterior (AP) projections are only acceptable for bed-ridden patients.

A PA film may reveal several signs of heart failure, such as:

- Cardiomegaly (↑ cardiothoracic ratio [maximum horizontal diameter of the heart >50% of the diameter of the thorax at the same level])
- Pulmonary hypertension (dilated blood vessels)
- Pulmonary oedema (consolidation in parenchyma)
- Pleural effusion (obliteration of costophrenic angles)
- Enlargement of certain compartments (look at the cardiac outline)

## Echocardiography

US is useful for demonstrating heart anatomy and function, and particularly important for the accurate diagnosis of valve anomalies.

*Doppler US* may be used for assessing the blood flow through various parts of the heart and the peripheral vascular system.

## Cardiac catheterization

Cardiac catheterization permits measurement of heart pressures, and enables coronary angiography (and occasionally balloon angioplasty) to be undertaken but is an invasive, high-risk procedure.

## Radionuclide imaging

Radioisotope scanning can assess:

- ventricular function,
- myocardial perfusion and
- MI (when other investigations have proved unsatisfactory).

# Investigations in respiratory disease

## Chest radiograph

A PA film is usually adequate, but occasionally a lateral view may help localize lesions. Comparisons with older CXR films may help interpretation of findings and assessment of disease progress. When examining a CXR, be systematic, starting from the centre and working towards the periphery, specifically examining:

*Heart* See page 95. Additionally, if cardiothoracic ratio ↓ and the heart appears elongated, consider hyperinflation (in COPD).

*Mediastinum* Study the tracheal position (deviated?), the major vessels (aneurysms?), the oesophagus (hiatus hernia?) and any masses.

*Hila* If these appear enlarged, consider lymph nodes (sarcoid? metastases?), dilatation of pulmonary vessels (pulmonary hypertension) or masses.

*Diaphragm* The right hemidiaphragm is normally higher (because of the underlying liver). The diaphragm may be displaced by thoracic or abdominal pathology, pushing or pulling on it.

*Lung parenchyma (lung fields)* The inflated lungs are relatively radiolucent, with characteristic diffuse lung markings. Any densities, especially if not symmetrical, should be investigated. Reticular opacities are characteristic of lung fibrosis; nodular opacities indicate abscesses, granulomas or tumours; while alveolar shadowing (consolidation) is usually due to fluid in the air spaces (pulmonary oedema, pneumonia, etc.).

*Pleura* The pleura are not seen on a CXR, unless the pleural space is filled with fluid (hydrothorax), pus (empyema) or air (pneumothorax—well defined peripheral radiolucency).

*Bony thorax* Look for fractured ribs (history of chest injury), as well as lytic or sclerotic defects of bones (metastatic lesions).

## Advanced chest imaging

*CT* Mediastinal and diffuse interstitial lung disorders are best investigated with CT. Pulmonary embolism (PE) is best diagnosed with spiral CT.

*US* is most useful for diagnosing pleural pathology (effusion, empyema), and guiding needle aspiration or biopsy.

*Pulmonary angiography* is a high-risk technique, occasionally used for the diagnosis of PE and pulmonary hypertension.

*Radionuclide scanning* This may involve:
- Inhalation of a radio-isotope (*ventilation scan*)
- Injection of a radio-isotope (*perfusion scan*)

*Ventilation/perfusion* scans may reveal mismatching that is usually diagnostic for PE and helpful in the investigation of chronic lung disorders.

## Sputum

A sputum sample can be collected for microscopy and culture.

## Blood tests

- *FBC* White blood cell counts are indicated when infection is suspected.
- *Serology* is useful for investigating infections and inflammatory diseases.

## Arterial blood gases

*Technique*

Arterial blood is usually sampled from the radial artery. The skin over the radial flexor surface of the wrist is disinfected and the artery carefully palpated, wearing sterile gloves. A special heparinized syringe is used, the plunger of which withdraws automatically under the pressure of arterial blood. The blood should be immediately taken to a blood gas analyser.

*Interpretation of results*

- ↓ $PaO_2$ (hypoxia) usually signifies ventilation/perfusion mismatch.
- ↑ $PaCO_2$ (hypercapnia) signifies type II respiratory failure.
- ↓ $PaCO_2$ (hypocapnia) is usually due to hyperventilation.
- ↓ pH (acidosis) may indicate hypercapnia.
- ↑ pH (alkalosis) indicates hypocapnia.

## Spirometry

A simple technique for assessing airways patency is the plastic peak-flow meter (page 33). More specialized investigations require a spirometer.

*Forced vital capacity (FVC)* measures the 'usable' lung volume, and is ↓ in restrictive lung diseases such as fibrosis.

*Forced expiratory volume in 1s (FEV1)* measures the air the patient expires in the 1st second of a forced expiration. In healthy individuals FEV1 represents 80% of FVC. FEV1 is markedly ↓ in obstructive pulmonary disease (narrowed bronchi), e.g. asthma or chronic bronchitis. Consequently, the FEV1/FVC ratio is also ↓ (<0.8) in these conditions.

Other tests that measure lung volumes and gas transfer can also be useful in the investigation of lung disorders.

## Bronchoscopy

Fibreoptic bronchoscopy under sedation and local analgesia allows direct visualization of large airways for the investigation of obstructions (e.g. bronchial carcinoma) and may allow biopsy, removal of foreign bodies and collection of lavage fluid for microbiological investigations.

# Investigations in abdominal disease

## Abdominal radiography

Plain radiographs of the abdomen are usually less informative than are CXRs. Abdominal radiographs are usually taken in an AP direction in a supine or erect position. Features to search for include:

- *GI tract*—usually easily distinguishable from the position and the gas contained. The stomach usually has air in the fundus. The small bowel has multiple internal folds (valvulae) that cross the whole lumen. The large bowel is wider, has folds (haustra) that do not cross the lumen and may contain some faeces. Dilatation of the bowel may be due to an obstruction (e.g. bowel cancer).
- *Gas outside the bowel*—is abnormal and may be due to GI perforation. The wall of the bowel can not normally be seen, unless there is gas on either side; so a clearly defined bowel wall is diagnostic of pneumo-peritoneum. On an erect radiograph, abnormal gas will collect under the diaphragm.
- *Calcifications*—stones may show on a plain radiograph (if radiopaque) in gallbladder or kidney/ureter.

## Contrast radiography

*Barium studies.* Barium is radiopaque and coats the mucosa, useful for detailed GI tract imaging. *Barium swallow* images the oesophagus. *Barium meal* may reveal stomach pathology and *barium follow through* shows the small intestine. Optimum imaging of the small bowel is achieved by intro-ducing the barium via duodenal intubation (*small bowel enema*). *Large bowel enema*, where barium is introduced per rectum, is often indicated when there has been persistent constipation, diarrhoea, or rectal bleeding.
*Endoscopic retrograde cholangiopancreatography (ERCP)* is when con-trast medium is injected via an endoscope into the common bile duct, and then radiographs visualize the biliary tree and pancreatic ducts.
*Renal angiography* may diagnose renal stenosis,
*IV urography* (IV injection of contrast medium and imaging while it is cleared by the kidneys) is used to examine the kidneys or urinary tract.

## Other imaging techniques

*CXR*—displacement of the diaphragm may be due to an abdominal mass. Air under the diaphragm may indicate a perforated viscous (do not be confused by the normal air bubble of the stomach, often seen just under the left hemidiaphragm).
*US*—abdominal US is a useful diagnostic tool for abdominal and pelvic pathology (soft tissue masses and cysts). US may help guide needle aspi-rations and biopsies. US is also extensively used in obstetrics.
*CT*—is used widely in GI and GU diagnostics, particularly in assessment of tumours and their spread.
*MRI*—is useful, as most abdominal pathology involves soft tissues.

## Endoscopy

Endoscopy may require the patient to be sedated. A fibreoptic endo-scope is used to directly visualize lesions in the GI tract lumen, and for taking biopsies and introducing contrast media (e.g. in ERCP). Depending on the part of the GI or GU tract investigated, the technique is called gastroscopy, proctoscopy, sigmoidoscopy, colonoscopy or cystoscopy.

*Laparoscopy* is a minimally invasive operation, but which often requires a GA. It involves introducing an endoscope through a small skin incision and inflating the peritoneal cavity with gas to allow visualization of the abdominal and pelvic organs. A second skin incision is used to allow other instruments to be introduced to facilitate biopsy, the excision of tissues (e.g. appendicectomy or cholecystectomy) or the ligation of Fallo-pian tubes (sterilization).

## Blood tests

Check the FBC for anaemia (GI bleed) or leucocytosis (infection). Assess liver function (LFTs), and haemostasis (coagulation screen) and, if neces-sary, infection (hepatitis viruses serology). Renal disease may be assessed using urea, creatine and electrolyte assays.

## Cytology and histopathology

Needle aspiration, needle-core biopsy, endoscopy-guided biopsy or, occasionally, open biopsy (during abdominal surgery) are used.

## Microbiology

Microscopy, culture and sensitivity of stool samples are helpful in the diagnosis of GI infections.

**Urinalysis** is discussed on page 64.

# Investigations in salivary gland disease

(Table 3.5, page 102)

## Sialometry (salivary flow rate)

Sialometry is a simple, fast and non-invasive method, which may confirm or refute xerostomia, but is by no means precise. There is a wide range of normal values.

*Unstimulated whole salivary flow rate* is usually measured (the largest contribution to this is from the submandibular gland). The patient is asked to sit quietly, not to talk, not to swallow their saliva for 10 min, but expectorate it into a small container. Flow rates of less than 1 mL/10 min are low.

*Stimulated salivary flow rate* (the largest contribution to this is from the parotid) can be measured after stimulation with 1 mL of 10% citric acid on the tongue. A special suction cup fitted around the parotid duct opening and connected to a container collects the saliva. Flow rates of less than 1 mL/min may signify reduced salivary function. Alternatively, pilocarpine 2.5 mg IV may be used to stimulate salivation, but is contraindicated in cardiac patients or those with hypotension.

## Sialochemistry

Saliva may be biochemically analysed and this may assist in the diagnosis of Sjögren's syndrome ($\uparrow$ $\beta_2$-microglobulin). It is rarely used, however, except for assay of the levels of some drugs or hormones, or occasionally for HIV or other antibody testing.

## Microbiology

The commonest salivary gland infection is mumps, a clinical diagnosis, occasionally needing confirmation by serology (specific IgM viral antibodies). Cytomegalovirus and Epstein–Barr virus may also need to be investigated for, especially in immunocompromised patients (e.g. AIDS).

Bacterial sialadenitis usually affects patients with reduced salivary flow (dehydration, Sjögren's syndrome, antimuscarinic drugs, duct stone or stenosis, etc.). Investigations should be directed towards revealing these predisposing factors as well as the causative organisms. In most cases it is practically impossible to collect uncontaminated pus, which would require catheterization of the duct. A swab is therefore the usual sampling method, and the causative bacteria are usually staphylococci, streptococci and anaerobes, as revealed by microscopy and culture. Rarely, mycobacteria or actinomyces are involved.

## Salivary gland biopsy

*Major salivary gland biopsy* is rarely performed, as it can be associated with complications, can result in seeding of tumours, and does not often affect management. Needle aspiration or core biopsy are also often avoided, as they can result in seeding of tumours but, if strongly indicated, they should be guided by US.

*Minor (labial) salivary gland biopsy* is simple and may reflect changes in other salivary (and exocrine) glands, such as Sjögren's syndrome. Nevertheless, it often gives a false negative result and can leave some numbness of the lower lip. To avoid damage to the mental nerve and the labial artery, incisions should be made vertically, next to the midline and near the sulcus. At least 3 or 4 salivary gland lobules should be removed.

## Blood tests

FBC may reveal leucocytosis in the case of salivary gland infections. ESR and CRP may be raised in inflammatory, connective tissue or malignant disease. ↑ blood glucose may indicate diabetes mellitus (one cause of xerostomia).

Serology may be helpful as SS-A (anti-Ro) and SS-B (anti-La) autoantibodies are useful diagnostic indicators of Sjögren's syndrome, and RF and ANA may reveal systemic disease (e.g. rheumatoid arthritis or systemic lupus erythematosus) such as can be associated with Sjögren's syndrome.

## Imaging

*Plain radiography* Some calculi may be evident in plain radiographs. Lower occlusal, lateral oblique and panoramic radiographs are appropriate to localize submandibular stones, while soft tissue films are needed for parotid sialoliths.

*Sialography*—is the most useful imaging technique in the investigation of inflammatory salivary gland disorders such as Sjögren's syndrome. Contrast medium is infused into the salivary duct followed by imaging with plain radiographs. Sialography can demonstrate ductal pathology (calculi, stricture and dilatation), as well as parenchymal pathology and space-occupying lesions (ideally combined with CT). However, it temporarily compromises the washing action of salivary flow and can cause infective sialadenitis.

*US* can differentiate between solid and cystic lesions and can be used to guide needle aspiration or biopsy.

*CT and MRI* are employed mainly for the precise localization of tumours. MRI has the advantage of not exposing the patient to irradiation.

*Scintigraphy*—may give information about salivary gland function and vascularity, revealing areas of salivary retention (due to blockage of the ducts) and can highlight tumours (hotspots). Radioisotope imaging is not without hazards, and suffers from relatively poor sensitivity and specificity, especially in the diagnosis of tumours.

**Table 3.5** Investigative procedures in salivary gland disease

| Procedure | Advantages | Disadvantages |
|---|---|---|
| Sialometry[a] (salivary flow rates) | Simple rapid clinical procedure that may confirm or refute xerostomia | Somewhat imprecise. Wide range of normal values |
| Sialochemistry | Laboratory investigation. Useful mainly in Sjögren's syndrome ($\beta_2$-microglobulin raised) | Salivary composition varies with many factors. Far less useful than blood and other tests |
| Blood tests | Simple and can reveal systemic disease (e.g. rheumatoid arthritis) | Will not usually reflect local disease of salivary glands |
| Plain radiography | Lower occlusal and oblique lateral or OPTG may show submandibular calculi. Soft PA film may show parotid calculi | Calculi may not be radio-opaque. Sialography may be needed |
| Sialography | Useful to eliminate gross structural damage, calculi or stenoses | Time-consuming and somewhat crude and insensitive. May cause pain or occasionally sialadenitis[b] |
| Salivary gland biopsy | Labial gland biopsy is simple and may reflect changes in other salivary (and exocrine) glands. Major gland biopsy may be diagnostic in localized gland disease. Needle biopsy may be useful | Invasive. May give false negative in disease of patchy distribution. Major gland biopsy may result in facial palsy or salivary fistula |
| Scintigraphy and radiosialometry | Measures uptake of radionuclide.[c] Radiosialometry more quantitative. High uptake (hotspots) may reveal tumours. Also demonstrates duct function and potency and gland vascularity | Expensive and with hazards associated with use of radionuclides. Taken up by thyroid gland; rare instances of thyroid damage |
| MRI, CT scanning and US | Useful for investigating space occupying lesions | Expensive, and not universally available |

[a] Unstimulated whole salivary flow rates are usually used; flow rates of less than 10 mL/10 min are low. Alternatively, stimulate parotid salivary flow with 1 mL 10% citric acid on to tongue; flow rates of less than 1 mL/min may signify reduced salivary function. Alternatively, pilocarpine 2.5 mg IV may be used but is contraindicated in cardiac patients or those with hypotension. Most centres use citric acid stimulation.
[b] Combined sialography with CT scanning may be useful in diagnosis and localization of salivary gland lesions, particularly parotid neoplasms.
[c] Usually technetium pertechnetate.

# Investigations for bone lesions (Table 3.6)

## Imaging

*Plain radiographs* (intraoral or extraoral) are adequate for the diagnosis of most lesions affecting facial bones. An OPTG and an OM are good projections for general screening of inflammatory or neoplastic lesions and fractures. Specific areas may need more specialized projections, as described on pages 106–107 for facial bone fractures.

*CT* is the gold standard for investigating bone pathology, especially multiple lesions. The extent of the lesions both in the hard and the soft tissues can be clearly outlined and management can be more accurately planned. The decision to use CT rather than plain radiography must be clearly justified, because of the expense and the high radiation dose.

*MRI* is useful mainly to examine extension of lesions into soft tissues.

*Scintigraphy* may be indicated to investigate metabolic and inflammatory bone disorders. A full body bone scan may be useful in revealing generalized or metastatic bone disease.

## Aspiration

Aspiration of radiolucent lesions may reveal pus (osteomyelitis—sample can be sent for microscopy, culture and sensitivity tests), clear fluid (cyst—protein content of cystic fluid may be of diagnostic value [e.g. protein levels <4g% in keratocysts]) or blood (haemangioma). Alternatively, cells collected may be sent for cytology.

## Biopsy

An open bone biopsy should provide definitive diagnosis of a bone lesion.

## Blood tests

- Leucocytosis may indicate bone infection.
- A raised alkaline phosphatase (ALP) indicates increased bone turnover (associated with several bone abnormalities, including Paget's disease and malignancy) or cholestasis.
- ↑ calcium and ↓ phosphate may indicate hyperparathyroidism and explain lytic bone lesions.

**Table 3.6** Investigative procedures in diseases of the jaws and sinuses

| Procedure | Advantages | Disadvantages | Remarks |
|---|---|---|---|
| Radiography (see Table 3.4) | Reveals much data not obvious on clinical examination | Specialized techniques may be difficult | Most useful views are panoramic, oblique lateral, occipitomentals |
| CT scan and MRI | Reveal data often not seen on clinical or conventional radiographic examination | Expensive and not universally available. Interpretation requires additional training | Demonstrate both hard and soft tissues and give spatial relationships |
| Fibre-optic endoscopy | Simple; good visualization | Skill needed | Useful to examine nasal passages, pharynx and larynx |
| Aspiration of cystic lesion | Simple | May introduce infection | May show presence of haemangioma. Protein content of cyst fluid may be of diagnostic value (protein levels below 4 g% in keratocysts) |
| Bone biopsy | Definitive | Invasive | — |
| Bone scan | Surveys all skeleton | Those of any isotope procedure | May reveal pathology (for example) metastases or osteomyelitis |

# Investigations in facial trauma

### General screening
When no fractures are clinically obvious, but other features (mechanism and severity of injury) suggest there is still the possibility of facial bone fractures, a standard set of radiographs usually taken includes:
• PA skull and face
• Lateral skull and face
• 10° OM (occipitomental)

### Dentoalveolar trauma
Intraoral radiographs from different angles are usually adequate:
• Periapicals (combination of different horizontal angles)
  • paralleling and
  • bisecting-angle
• Occlusal
  • midline or
  • lateral

*In extensive trauma, extraoral radiographs may be necessary:*
• OPTG
• Lateral facial

### Mandibular fractures
At least two views at right angles to each other are indicated:
• OPTG (or lateral oblique) and
• PA (or SMV, or lower occlusal)

### Condylar fractures
At least two views at right angles to each other are indicated:
• Lateral projection: OPTG or lateral oblique
• Frontal projection: reverse Towne's or reverse OPTG

### Maxillary fractures
*Plain radiography* (OM 10° and 30°, PA and lateral) may give some information on localized maxillary fractures, such as those involving the orbital floor (blow-out fractures) or another maxillary sinus wall. OM projections, however, will not show the extent of the injury. The isolated sign of a fluid level in the maxillary sinus, seen on OM films, is common and usually suggests a simple 'crack' of one of the lateral sinus walls (this only requires prophylaxis from surgical emphysema, by avoiding nose-blowing).
Plain radiographs are rarely adequate for the assessment of middle third (Le Fort) fractures, as the complex anatomy, soft tissue swelling and superimposition of structures make their interpretation difficult.
*CT* is the investigation of choice for midfacial and orbital fractures, allowing excellent visualization of both hard and soft tissue injuries. 3D reconstruction in particular assists planning of management.

## Zygomatic fractures

Radiographic investigation of the zygomas includes:

- OM 30° (most important; should reveal a fracture at the zygomaticomaxillary [ZM] and zygomaticofrontal [ZF] sutures)
- Reduced exposure SMV (if clinical examination suggests fracture of the zygomatic arch)
- CT (if injury appears to be complex or extensive)

## Nasal fractures

Simple nasal fractures may be viewed with plain films:

- Lateral facial
- Lateral soft-tissue nasal
- OM 30°

Complex naso-ethmoidal fractures require CT scans.

## Skull fractures

Useful projections include:

- 20° PA skull
- Lateral skull
- *Towne's*
- SMV
- CT

## Soft tissue injuries

Foreign bodies (e.g. glass) in soft tissues may be revealed by plain soft-tissue radiographs.

## Other investigations

*FBC* A baseline haemoglobin estimation should be taken as it may be important if severe blood loss has occurred (e.g. in midfacial fractures) or is likely to occur during surgical treatment of extensive facial injuries.

*U&Es* may reveal dehydration following blood loss or high alcohol intake (there is a strong association between alcohol use and facial trauma).

*Biochemical analysis* of blood-stained fluid running from the nose (rhinorrhoea) may confirm CSF (in naso-fronto-ethmoidal fractures). $\beta_2$-transferrin, a protein found in CSF but not in mucus, may assist diferentiation.

*Angiography* may be necessary in serious injuries (e.g. gun-shot wounds), especially those affecting the neck.

# Investigations in oral oncology

## Cytology

The roles of smear (oral brush) and fine-needle aspiration (of enlarged lymph nodes) cytology in the investigation of oral squamous cell carcinoma (SCC) are discussed on page 90.

## Histopathology

*Incisional biopsy* is the most important investigation for oral cancer and, in most cases, will give a definitive diagnosis.

*Needle core biopsy* is useful for deeper masses or lymph node studies.

*Frozen sections* facilitate immediate decisions during major surgery.

## Imaging

Imaging for lesions arising in bone is discussed on page 104. The location, size and extent of lesions in soft tissues can usually be assessed with:
- CT (soft and hard tissue involvement) or
- MRI (mainly in isolated soft tissue lesions).

Jaw involvement by oral SCC may be assessed with plain radiography, such as:
- Occlusal (cortical involvement)
- Lateral oblique of mandible
- OPTG

An OPTG is necessary in patients with oral cancer as a general survey *but cannot reliably detect caries (intraoral films are required).*

## Endoscopy

Fibreoptic endoscopy of the nasal passages, pharynx and larynx are occasionally necessary, when screening for:
- possible recurrence of a treated SCC,
- a second primary tumour or
- the primary site of a histologically proven metastatic SCC in the neck lymph nodes (often inconspicuous in the root of the tongue, the tonsils, nasopharynx or elsewhere).

When the site of the primary tumour can not be found, an *examination under (general) anaesthesia (EUA)* is indicated. Careful endoscopic examination and several 'blind' (i.e. there is no visible lesion) biopsies of the tonsils, the base of tongue and pharynx are usually performed.

## Chest radiography

CXR is almost always performed, as it may reveal not only metastatic disease or a second primary tumour, but it is also excellent for screening respiratory, cardiovascular and even abdominal disorders, that are common in the older age group usually affected by SCC.

## ECG

Even in the absence of cardiac signs or symptoms, many authorities instigate the routine use of ECG for patients >50 years, prior to major surgery, not only because undiagnosed cardiovascular disease is common at this age, but also because the ECG provides a useful baseline should cardiovascular complications (e.g. MI or cardiac failure) follow surgery.

## Blood tests

- FBC will give a baseline haemoglobin prior to major surgery.
- U&Es are also important for assessing baseline renal function.
- LFTs and a coagulation screen are useful if liver damage is suspected (e.g. in alcoholics).
- Alkaline phosphatase may indicate invasion or metastasis in bone or liver.
- All the above blood investigations are important prior to chemotherapy (baseline bone-marrow, renal and hepatic function).
- Detection of disseminated malignant cells is now possible and may become an important tool in prognostication.
- SickleDex test (sickle-cell anaemia screening) may be indicated for some ethnic groups prior to surgery under GA (see page 121).

## Urinalysis

Dipstick urinalysis (page 64) is routine in patients admitted to hospital.

# Investigations for oral mucosal lesions

(Tables 3.7 and 3.8)

## Biopsy

Specimens from incisional or excisional biopsies may be submitted for:
- H&E histopathology,
- Histopathology with special stains or immunohistochemistry (to determine the origin of the tissue in the case of neoplasms),
- Direct immunofluorescence (for dermatoses [e.g. pemphigus] and infections [e.g. viruses]) or
- Gram staining (if bacterial infection is suspected),
- PAS staining (if candidal infection is suspected),
- Other microbiological tests.

## Smear

Cells scraped from the surface of the lesion can be used for:
- direct microscopy (cytology)
- microbiological investigations for detection of
  - bacteria (isolated organisms may be commensals or indicate 2° infection)
  - viruses (electron microscopy or immunostaining of smears may give rapid results)
  - fungi (presence of *Candida* does not necessarily imply a causative relation with the lesion, but should be treated anyway)

## Swab

Culture and sensitivity tests may be performed for:
- bacterial infections
- fungal infections
- viral infections—cultures are indicated in some acute ulcerative or vesiculobullous lesions, and may give a diagnosis earlier than does serology, but nucleic acid studies are more sensitive, specific and speedy.

## Blood tests

Haemoglobin, red and white cell indices and haematinics (iron, $B_{12}$ and folate) often need to be investigated to exclude systemic causes of oral mucosal disease (especially ulcers, glossitis and angular stomatitis).
*Serology:* indirect immunofluorescence, enzyme linked immunosorbent assay (ELISA) or other tests may be performed on the patient's serum, for the diagnosis of:
- Viral and other infections (a rise in titre of specific IgG antibodies must be detected between 'acute' and 'convalescent' [3 weeks later] serum; serology only gives a retrospective diagnosis [but for certain infections, e.g. HIV, hepatitis viruses and syphilis, serology is essential])
- Dermatoses, connective tissue diseases or other immunological disorders (for the detection of autoantibodies [Table 3.12]).

## GI investigations

Certain oral lesions may be associated with GI disorders (e.g. Crohn's disease) and, when this is suspected, referral to a gastroenterologist for investigations (e.g. colonoscopy) may be indicated.

**Table 3.7** Investigative procedures in oral mucosal disease

| Procedure | Advantages | Disadvantages | Remarks |
|---|---|---|---|
| Biopsy | Gives definitive diagnosis in many instances | Invasive | Mucosal biopsies should be submitted for histopathological and often direct immunofluores-cence examinations if a dermatosis is suspected (see Tables 3.8 and 7.4) |
| Exfoliative cytology | Simple, non-invasive procedure | Many false negatives | Biopsy has super-seded cytology |
| Bacteriological smear and culture | Simple clinical procedure | Isolation of organisms does not necessarily imply causal relation with disease under investigation | Anaerobic techniques may be indicated in oral lesions in the immunocompro-mised host |
| Fungal smear | Simple clinical procedure | As above | *Candida* hyphae suggest *Candida* species are pathogenic |
| Viral culture | Simple sensitive clinical procedure. Often gives diagnosis more rapidly than does serology[a] | May require special facilities and may only give retrospective diagnosis. False negatives possible | Indicated in some acute ulcerative or bullous lesions. Serology should also be undertaken |
| Haematological screen; haemo-globin, red cell and white cell indices | Simple clinical procedure | Detection rate may not be high | Essential to exclude systemic causes of oral disease, especially ulcers, glossitis or angular stomatitis (see Chapter 4) |
| Serology | Demonstration of a rise in titre of specific antibodies between acute and convalescent serum may be diag-nostically useful. Specific tests available, e.g. HIV antibodies | Serum auto-antibodies may not mean disease. Serum auto-antibodies may be absent in pemphi goid. Diagnosis of viral infections is retrospective | Essential in suspected HIV, dermatoses, connective tissue disease, auto-immune or other immunological disorders |

[a] Electron microscopy gives the quickest results.

**Table 3.8** Immunostaining in skin and oral mucosal diseases

| Condition | Antibody directed against | Main antigens | Antibody class[b] |
|---|---|---|---|
| Pemphigus vulgaris | Intercellular | Desmoglein | IgG |
| Paraneoplastic pemphigus | Intercellular | Desmoplakin | IgG |
| IgA pemphigus | Intercellular | Desmocollin | IgA |
| Bullous pemphigoid | Basement membrane area | BP1 | IgG |
| Mucous membrane pemphigoid | Basement membrane area | BP2, epiligrin, integrin, laminin, or uncein | IgG[a] |
| Angina bullosa haemorrhagica | None | — | — |
| Dermatitis herpetiformis | Basement membrane area | Transglutaminase | IgA |
| Linear IgA disease | Basement membrane area | Ladinin | IgA[a] |
| Lichen planus | Basement membrane area | ? | Fibrin |
| Chronic ulcerative stomatitis | Basal cell layer[b] | ANA | IgG |

[a] Usually with complement deposits.
[b] Of transitional epithelium.
ANA, antinuclear antibody; NR, not relevant;. BP, bullous pemphigoid.

# Investigations of the paranasal sinuses

## Plain radiography

*Maxillary sinus*
- OM
- periapicals
- lateral upper occlusal
- OPTG

*Frontal sinus*
- OM
- lateral skull

*Sphenoid sinus*
- lateral skull
- SMV

*Ethmoidal air cells*
- lateral skull

## CT

CT provides optimal visualization of all paranasal sinuses and the adjacent structures.

## MRI

MRI can give good images of tumours extending from or towards the sinuses. It is unsurpassed in differentiating between soft tissue masses and fluids within the sinuses.

## Sinusoscopy

Endoscopy of the maxillary sinus requires skill, but can offer direct visualization of its lining and contents. It may also assist in the collection of a biopsy specimen or the removal of a foreign body (e.g. root fragment).

# Investigations in TMJ disorders (Table 3.9)

TMJ investigations are indicated if there is a background of severe dysfunction and/or worsening symptomatology.

## Imaging

*Plain radiographs*
- transpharyngeal
- transcranial
- transorbital

*OPTG* with mouth open and closed

*Reverse OPTG*

*Plain tomography*

*CT*

*MRI* gives excellent soft tissue visualization (articular fluid, capsule and disc)

*Arthrography* can assist in demonstrating the disc indirectly, by injecting a contrast agent in the lower articular space prior to imaging.

## Arthroscopy

Arthroscopy is widely used in other joints (e.g. knee) and utilizes methods similar to those described for laparoscopy. A small incision on the preauricular skin allows an arthroscope to be inserted into the joint space giving direct visualization of the internal structures. A further incision facilitates the insertion of a further instrument, allowing therapeutic applications during the same procedure.

Arthroscopy is an invasive technique that requires a GA. However, as benefits have not been unequivocal, many surgeons have abandoned it.

**Table 3.9** Investigative procedures in TMJ disease

| Procedure | Advantages | Disadvantages |
|---|---|---|
| Radiography | Simple. Can reveal much pathology | — |
| | CT scan can provide excellent information | Expensive |
| Arthrography (double contrast) | Provides excellent information | Danger of introducing infection. Painful |
| MRI | Provides excellent information without exposure to ionizing radiation Non-invasive | Expensive and not universally available |
| Arthroscopy | Minimally invasive, good visualization | Requires anaesthesia Technically demanding |

# Investigations in orthodontics

## Imaging

*OPTG* is excellent to survey the dentition, the position and stage of development of unerupted teeth, the TMJs, etc.

*Lateral cephalometry* is often the most important investigation, particularly when fixed appliances are planned. This projection is then hand or digitally traced (*cephalometry*).

*Upper occlusal* films facilitate assessment of the position of upper anterior teeth, especially canines.

*Periapicals* can assist in the localization of impacted teeth (parallax views) and give good detail of dental and periodontal pathology.

*Bitewings* may reveal dental caries and therefore assist in treatment planning.

## Clinical photographs

*Extraoral*
- Full frontal at rest
- Full frontal smiling
- ¾ profile
- Side profile

*Intraoral*
- Frontal
- Buccal left
- Buccal right
- Upper arch
- Lower arch
- Tongue
- Palate

## Study models

Cast models of the upper and lower dentition can be used to allow the study of the dental occlusion and assist treatment planning. Along with photographs, they represent good records for assessing treatment progress.

# Investigations for anaemia

If the history and clinical examination suggest anaemia, a haemoglobin (Hb) assay is indicated (↓ Hb is the definition of anaemia). Anaemia is not a diagnosis in itself and the cause must always be investigated.

## Standard investigations

*Hb*—value will depend on age, sex and other physiological variables (e.g. pregnancy), and assay is needed to define the presence and severity of anaemia. Results must be interpreted with caution: following acute blood loss (e.g. trauma or surgery), declining Hb levels will not become evident until the blood fluid volume is replaced, and this can take days.

*Haematocrit (packed cell volume [PCV])*—the percentage of cells in the blood volume. Changes usually reflect those of Hb.

*Red blood cell count (RBC)*—↓ levels can indicate anaemia or fluid overload.

*Mean cell volume (MCV)* (the ratio of PCV/RBC)—indicates the red cell size.

Anaemias are classified on MCV values into microcytic, macrocytic or normocytic:

- microcytosis (↓ MCV [small cells])
  - iron deficiency (chronic bleeding)
  - thalassaemia
  - chronic disease
- macrocytosis (↑ MCV [large cells])
  - alcoholism (commonest cause of ↑ MCV with normal Hb)
  - vitamin $B_{12}$ deficiency (also produces megaloblastic bone marrow)
  - folate deficiency (also produces megaloblastic bone marrow)
  - liver disease
  - hypothyroidism
  - myelodysplasia or myeloproliferative disorders
  - cytotoxic drugs
- normocytosis (normal MCV)
  - haemorrhage
  - chronic disease
  - haemolytic anaemia
  - endocrinopathies
  - concurrence of microcytic and macrocytic anaemia (small and large cells [anisocytosis]), as in coeliac disease

*Mean cell haemoglobin (MCH) and mean cell haemoglobin concentration (MCHC)* are ↓ in microcytic anaemias.

*Reticulocytes* are 'young' circulating erythrocytes that normally represent about 1% of RBC. In anaemic patients, reticulocytes may rise to >2%, unless there is a defect in erythropoiesis. Reticulocyte counts are therefore important in the investigation of the aetiology of anaemias.

*White blood cell count (WBC)* In the presence of anaemia:

- ↓ WBC may be due to the same causative factor (e.g. bone marrow disease, cytotoxic drugs)
- ↑ WBC may suggest leukaemia

*Platelets (Plt)* In the presence of anaemia:
- ↓ Plt (thrombocytopenia) may be due to the same causative factor (e.g. aplastic marrow disease, cytotoxic drug therapy)
- ↑ Plt (thrombocytosis) suggest a myeloproliferative disorder or may be part of the acute phase reaction following haemorrhage (so do not be surprised by moderately ↑ Plt following major surgery)

*ESR* is ↑ in anaemia.

## Specific investigations

### Microcytic anaemias

*Iron deficiency* from chronic haemorrhage is the commonest cause of anaemia. Tests that may be needed to confirm diagnosis and establish aetiology include:
- ↓ serum iron, ↑ total iron-binding capacity (TIBC) and ↓ serum ferritin
- Blood film (microcytic and hypochromic cells)
- Gynaecological investigations may be indicated (menorrhagia is the commonest cause in premenopausal women)
- GI investigations (e.g. endoscopy) may be indicated (bleeding from GI pathology is a common cause in the elderly)

*Thalassaemia*—may be confirmed by electrophoresis (↑ Hb F and Hb A2)

### Macrocytic anaemias

$B_{12}$ *deficiency* is confirmed by ↓ serum $B_{12}$. As liver stores last about 3 years, low $B_{12}$ really means a true deficiency. A macrocytic blood film rarely needs to be complemented by a megaloblastic picture in bone marrow aspiration or core biopsy. The commonest cause is pernicious anemia and this can be confirmed by a positive Schilling test (absorption of $B_{12}$ with concurrent administration of intrinsic factor). Other causes may be dietary (vegans), or GI (e.g. Crohn's)—when appropriate investigations may be indicated.

*Folate deficiency* can be confirmed by ↓ serum folate or (much better) ↓ red cell folate. As there are virtually no body stores of folate, serum levels often fluctuate depending upon diet. Folate deficiency is usually dietary in origin, but drugs, alcohol, haemolysis or GI pathology may be implicated.

*Chronic diseases* causing anaemia may have to be diagnosed by exclusion. LFTs, thyroid function tests, ESR and a bone marrow biopsy may be necessary.

### Normocytic anaemias

*Sickle-cell anaemia* is a common haemolytic anaemia in people from a Central African origin. Investigations include:
- Blood film may exhibit sickle cells and target cells
- Sickle solubility tests (e.g. Sickledex) offer rapid screening
- Haemoglobin electrophoresis

*Other causes of haemolytic anaemia* (genetic, autoimmune, malaria etc.) may have to be excluded. Bilirubin and reticulocytes are usually ↑ in haemolytic disorders.

*Some chronic diseases* also cause normocytic anaemias and further investigations may be indicated, if haemolysis or haemorrhage do not appear to be the reason.

# Investigations for bleeding disorders

Most episodes of excessive bleeding have local causes (see page 164). Occasionally though, the history and clinical presentation may raise the suspicion of a systemic cause or the patient may refer to a history of prolonged bleeding.

When a bleeding tendency is suspected, it is important to establish whether there is:

- evidence to suggest a systemic defect
- any family history of bleeding disorders
- a specific pattern, such as:
  - excessive bruising of skin and mucosae and spontaneous prolonged bleeding (vascular or platelet defect)
  - haematomas in muscles and joints and delayed bleeding following trauma (coagulation defect)

Some basic screening investigations are then often warranted, but these only occasionally reveal an abnormality, and then further tests may be necessary to establish the diagnosis.

## Basic screening investigations

### FBC and blood film

*Platelet counts* (Plt) <150 × 10$^9$/L suggest thrombocytopenia.

*Red and white cell counts* may indicate the cause of a thrombocytopenia (e.g. marrow failure if all cells ↓ or marrow infiltration if WBC ↑).

*Morphology* of platelets and other cells on film may be informative.

### Coagulation screen

*Prothrombin time (PT)* tests the extrinsic clotting system and is prolonged in liver disease, vitamin K deficiency and treatment with warfarin. Because PT may vary depending on the laboratory, it is usually expressed as a ratio to an international control sample. This is then called an 'International Normalized Ratio' (INR) and for a healthy patient it should be 1.

*Activated (or Kaolin) partial thromboplastin time (APTT or KPTT)* tests the intrinsic clotting system and is prolonged (>50 s) in haemophilia and in treatment with heparin.

*Thrombin time (TT)* is prolonged (>15 s) in treatment with heparin, and in fibrinogen deficiency (or dysfunction).

## Specific investigations

*Bleeding time (BT)* is an *in vivo* test to assess mainly platelet function. It is pointless to carry out a BT in known ↓ Plt and may even be dangerous. BT >10 min indicates Plt dysfunction, but not the cause.

*Platelet aggregation or adhesion tests* may be useful in identifying the cause of the dysfunction when BT is ↑ with *normal* Plt counts.

*Antiplatelet IgG* may indicate autoimmune (idiopathic) thrombocytopenic purpura (ITP).

*Bone marrow biopsy* allows the study of megakaryocytes and other bone marrow cells.

*Coagulation factor assays* can confirm deficiencies of specific clotting factors (e.g. VIII [haemophilia A or von Willebrand's disease], IX [Haemophilia B] or von Willebrand Factor [vWF in von Willebrand's disease]).

*Other tests*—fibrinogen levels (FL), fibrin-degradation products (FDP), LFTs and GI investigations may be needed to elucidate the cause of a clotting defect.

Table 3.10 summarizes findings in some of the more common causes of a bleeding tendency (see also Chapter 4).

**Table 3.10** Laboratory findings in bleeding disorders

|  | PT (INR) | APTT (KPTT) | TT | Plt | BT | Other |
|---|---|---|---|---|---|---|
| Disseminated intravascular coagulopathy (DIC) | ↑ | ↑ | ↑ | ↓ | ↑ | ↓ FL and ↑ FDP |
| Haemophilia A |  | ↑ |  |  |  | ↓ VIII |
| Haemophilia B |  | ↑ |  |  |  | ↓ IX |
| Heparin | (↑) | ↑ | ↑ |  |  |  |
| Liver disease | ↑ | ↑ | (↑) | (↓) | (↑) | Several factors |
| Thrombasthenia/ aspirin |  |  |  |  | ↑ | Platelet dysfunction |
| Thrombocytopenia |  |  |  | ↓ | ↑ |  |
| Von Willebrand's disease |  | ↑ |  |  | ↑ | platelet dysfunction and ↓ vWF |
| Warfarin/vitamin K deficiency | ↑ | ↑ |  |  |  |  |

Blank spaces mean normal results.

# Investigations for common endocrinopathies

## Diabetes mellitus (DM) (Table 3.11)

*Fasting blood glucose* >7 mmol/L—usually establishes the diagnosis.

*Random blood glucose* >11 mmol/L—diagnostic in the presence of symptoms.

*Glucose tolerance test*—indicated if blood sugar values are borderline. Blood sugar is measured 2 h after an oral administration of 75 g of glucose. Values >11 mmol/L are diagnostic.

*Urinalysis* is a simple screening method for DM but has a low sensitivity (many false negatives), as glucosuria does not occur until blood glucose is very high. The presence of glucose ± ketones in urine is strongly suggestive of DM (high specificity), although rarely this may be caused by a low renal threshold for glucose. Specific tests for glucosuria and ketonuria are simple and may be used at home for monitoring of hyperglycaemic crises.

*Glycosylated haemoglobin (HbA$_{1c}$)* levels are reliable in diagnosing DM, as they accurately reflect blood glucose levels over the past 2 months (levels >7% are strongly suggestive of DM). HbA$_{1c}$ is also an excellent way to assess long-term control, and an indicator of the risk of vascular complications (7–9% suggests good control, >12% shows poor control and suggests a bad prognosis).

*Finger-prick* tests—though not perfectly accurate, are useful for home monitoring. They offer rapid results, useful when hypoglycaemia is suspected.

*Blood insulin* levels may be useful in certain cases where the diagnosis is problematic.

*Other* investigations may be necessary to assess vascular and neurological complications of DM.

**Table 3.11** Investigations in diabetes

| Test | Confirms diabetes | Excludes diabetes |
|---|---|---|
| Fasting plasma glucose (after a person has fasted for 8 h) | >7.0 mmol/L | <6 mmol/L |
| Random blood glucose (taken any time of day) | >11.1 mmol/L | <8 mmol/L |
| Plasma glucose taken 2 h after a person has consumed a drink containing 75 g of glucose in oral glucose tolerance test (OGTT) | >11.1 mmol/L[a] | <11.1 mmol/L[a] |

[a] Persons with equivocal results are usually said to have 'impaired glucose tolerance'. Some may eventually progress to diabetes.

## Adrenocortical function

If history and clinical examination suggest adrenal dysfunction (e.g. low BP in hypoadrenocorticism [Addison's disease] or high BP in hyperadrenocorticism [Cushing's syndrome]), certain investigations may be useful, such as:

*Diurnal rhythm of plasma cortisol* is a sensitive index of adrenal function; plasma cortisol values are normally highest between 6 and 10 am (5–25 microgram/100 mL) and lowest between midnight and 4 am. Samples taken at 8 am should be at least 5 microgram/100 mL higher than at 4 pm. Plasma cortisol at 8 am is often below 6 microgram/100 mL in *hypoadrenocorticism*, and the diurnal variation is lost in *hyperadrenocorticism*.

*ACTH stimulation test (Synacthen test)* measures the rise in cortisol level following stimulation with synthetic ACTH [Synacthen] (normally >18 microgram/100mL). This is ↓ early in hypoadrenocorticism before the low cortisol level is found.

*Dexamethasone suppression test* may reveal hyperadrenocorticism (if cortisol levels fail to decrease following administration of dexamethasone).

*Abdominal radiography* may show calcified adrenals, if tuberculosis is the cause of hypoadrenocorticism.

*Adrenal serum autoantibodies* may be detected in Addison's disease.

*U&Es* will show ↓ Na$^+$ and ↑ K$^+$ in hypoadrenocorticism.

## Thyroid function

*T$_3$, T$_4$ and TSH* values are very informative.

- Hyperthyroidism: ↓ TSH and/or ↑ T$_3$ and/or ↑ T$_4$
- Hypothyroidism: ↑ TSH and/or ↓ T$_4$

*Thyroid autoantibodies* may signify Hashimoto's disease (hypothyroidism).

*Thyroid-stimulating antibodies* may signify Graves' disease (hyperthyroidism).

*Radionuclide scanning* can be very informative in thyroid gland disease.

*US* can differentiate between thyroid cystic and solid nodules.

*FNA cytology* is the most useful test for detecting malignant disorders.

*FBC* may reveal anaemia in hypothyroid patients.

*Ophthalmological investigations* may be necessary in Graves' disease.

## Parathyroid function

*Parathyroid hormone (PTH)* levels are ↑ in hyperparathyroidism and ↓ in hypoparathyroidism.

*Blood calcium* levels should be collected early in the morning without tourniquet (venous stasis and fall in pH alter calcium levels), and from a fasting patient. Albumin levels should also be measured, as they influence calcium levels. Ca$^{2+}$ is ↑ in 1° hyperparathyroidism, and ↓ in 2° hyperparathyroidism and in hypoparathyroidism.

*Blood phosphate* is ↓ when Ca$^{2+}$ is ↑ and vice versa.

*Alkaline phosphatase (ALP)* is ↑ in hyperparathyroidism (↑ bone resorption).

*Radiographs* may show osteolytic lesion in several bones.

# Investigations for sexually transmitted diseases

## Herpes simplex virus
- Detection of viral nucleic acid (with PCR) or antigens (rapid and specific but expensive)
- Culture
- Detection of antibodies

## Human immunodeficiency virus
- Lymphopenia
- Severe T-helper lymphocyte defect (reduced CD4+ cells)
- ↓ Ratio of helper (CD4+) to suppressor (CD8+) lymphocytes
- HIV antibodies (sero-testing), mainly in the asymptomatic phase
- PCR (for nucleic acid detection) and detection of HIV P24 antigen give more rapid results in early disease, and an indication of viral load (important for monitoring disease process at later stages)
- Diagnosis of acute symptomatic HIV infection may be from other causes of glandular fever syndromes such as:
  - Infectious mononucleosis (Epstein–Barr virus antibodies; positive Paul-Bunnell test)
  - Cytomegalovirus infection (CMV antibodies; PCR)
  - Toxoplasmosis (*Toxoplasma gondii* antibodies; Sabin-Feldman dye test)
- Tests for other associated STDs may be indicated
- Counselling is necessary before and after investigations

## Syphilis
- Dark field microscopy of a lesion may demonstrate *Treponema pallidum* (wash oral lesions first with saline to remove oral commensal treponemes)
- Serology
  - VDRL as a screening test (false positives are common)
  - A more specific test, such as the Fluorescent Treponemal Antibody-Absorbed (FTA-Abs) or IgM-FTA-Abs must be used where VDRL proves positive
- Tests for other STDs that may be associated.

## Gonorrhoea
Gonococcal pharyngitis may be seen, particularly in men who have sex with men. Investigations include:
- Direct smear for Gram-staining (Gram-negative diplococci).
- Bacteriological swab for culture and sensitivities.
- Tests for other STDs that may be associated.

## Viral hepatitis (B and C)
- Test for HBV or HCV antigens, antibodies or DNA
- Patients positive for hepatitis B surface antigen ($HB_sAg$) should be screened for $HB_eAg$ (e antigen). About one in five patients with HBV

are $HB_eAg$ positive and at high risk of infectivity. Appearance of anti-$HB_e$ though, relates to ↓ infectivity.
- Those who have $HB_sAg$ should be screened again at 3 months and again if still positive. Those positive at 9 months are 'chronic carriers'.
- Anti-$HB_s$ implies immunity
- Anti-$HB_c$ (antibody to core antigen) indicates past infection
- LFTs are important for monitoring liver damage.

# Investigations for connective tissue diseases

ESR and C reactive protein (CRP) may be raised in connective tissue disease. Serology may be helpful as SS-A (anti-Ro) and SS-B (anti-La) autoantibodies are useful diagnostic indicators of Sjögren's syndrome, RF and ANA may reveal systemic disease (e.g. rheumatoid arthritis or systemic lupus erythematosus) (Table 3.12; Fig. 3.2).

**Table 3.12** Significance of the more common antinuclear antibodies

| Antibodies | Associated with antibodies to | Significance[a] |
|---|---|---|
| Rheumatoid factor[b] (against IgG) | Latex test >1 in 20 SCAT >1 in 32 DAT >1 in 16 | RA (sometimes SLE) |
| Salivary duct antibody | | Sjögren's syndrome, particularly SS-1 |
| Nuclear | | |
| DNA antibodies | ds-DNA (*Crithidia lucillae*) ss-DNA | High titres: SLE Rheumatic diseases and chronic inflammatory disorders (not specific, but sensitive) |
| Extractable nuclear antigens (ENA) | | to Smith (Sm) antigen: very specific for SLE but only seen in minority of cases |
| | | PM-SC1[c]: polydermatomyositis, and scleroderma |
| | | JO-1: polydermatomyositis |
| | | to La soluble substance B antigen (SS-B): SLE and SS-1 and SS-2 |
| | | to Ro soluble substanceA antigen (SS-A): SLE skin disease; some Sjögren's syndrome |
| | | to Ribonuclear protein (nRNP or UIRNP) antigen: mixed connective tissue disorder, scleroderma, SLE |
| | | To Centromere; CREST syndrome |
| Indirect immunofluorescence | | |
| Speckled | | Mixed connective tissue disease |
| Diffuse (homogeneous) | deoxyribonucleoprotein | High titres: SLE Low titres: other connective tissue diseases |
| Rim (peripheral) | double stranded DNA(DS-DNA) | Antibody with the highest specificity for SLE and found in most patients |

**Table 3.12** Contd.

| Antibodies | Associated With antibodies to | Significance[a] |
|---|---|---|
| Centromere | | CREST syndrome |
| Nucleolar | nucleolus-specific RNA | Scleroderma |
| Cytoplasmic | | |
| Anti-neutrophil cytoplasmic antibodies (ANCA) | cytoplasmic proteinase 3 (anti-PR3) | Wegener's granulomatosis |
| Anti-neutrophil cytoplasmic antibodies (ANCA) | perinuclear myeloperoxidase (anti-MPO) | Polyarteritis nodosa |

ss-DNA = single stranded DNA; ds-DNA = double stranded DNA; SLE = systemic lupus erythematosus; CREST = calcinosis, Raynaud's, oesophageal, sclerodactyly and telangiectasia.
[a] The presence of autoantibodies does not always indicate disease.
[b] Agglutination tests, SCAT = sheep cell agglutination test; DAT = direct agglutination test, detect only IgM antibodies.
[c] SC1-70 = anti-topoisomerase 1.

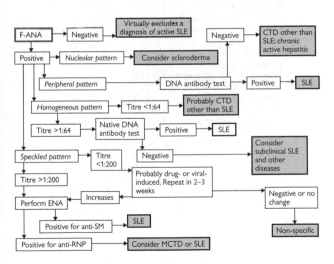

SLE = systemic lupus erythematosus; SM = smooth muscle; RNP = ribonucleoprotein;
ENA = extractable nuclear antigen; CTD = connective tissue disease;
ANA = antinuclear antibody; F = fluoresceinated;

**Fig. 3.2** Distinguishing the connective tissue diseases

# Relevant medicine

*Preventive oral health care and minimization of trauma and stress is crucial in all these groups.*

# Cardiovascular disease

Common features are shown—Appendix 8

## Ischaemic heart disease (IHD)

IHD is when the myocardium is receiving inadequate oxygen to meet its demands, and is the most common single cause of death in the developed world. IHD results mainly from coronary atherosclerosis (atheroma), risk factors for which include diabetes mellitus, hypertension, family history of IHD, male gender, hyperlipidaemia (especially ↑ low-density lipoproteins [LDL]), smoking and lack of exercise.

The atheromatous plaques cause narrowing of the coronary vessels, with resulting ischaemia and sometimes chest pain (*angina*) after exertion or stress. Management involves modification of life-style and risk factors (e.g. statins to reduce hyperlipidaemia), symptom relief with fast-acting vasodilators (e.g. sublingual glyceryl trinitrate [GTN] spray), prophylaxis with long-acting vasodilators (e.g. isosorbide mononitrate, nicorandil and calcium-channel blockers [nifedipine, amlodipine, verapamil, diltiazem, etc.]), reduction of myocardial oxygen demand with beta-blockers (e.g. atenolol), prevention of thrombosis (daily aspirin) and more definitive correction with angioplasty or coronary artery bypass grafting (CABG). Special care is required if angina is unstable (recent onset, increasing frequency or at rest) (Table 4.1).

Rupture of an atheromatous plaque with subsequent thrombus formation can cause coronary vessel occlusion and ischaemic necrosis of part of the myocardium (*MI*). This presents with 'crushing' chest pain (not relieved by rest or fast-acting nitrates), nausea, sweating, anxiety, ↑cardiac enzymes (e.g. Troponin T; Table 4.2) and ECG changes (ST elevation, T inversion, Q waves). MI has a high mortality rate, and survivors may suffer further MI or complications such as arrhythmias and/or heart failure. Acute management of MI is directed towards early pain relief and thrombolysis (page 163) and pain relief; long-term management includes aspirin, beta-blockers (unless heart failure is present), angiotensin-converting enzyme (ACE) inhibitors (e.g. captopril, lisinopril), modification of risk factors and rehabilitation.

## Hypertension

Hypertension is a persistently ↑ BP resulting from ↑ peripheral arteriolar resistance. Hypertension is commonly 1° (essential), the cause of which is unknown (genetics, alcohol, salt and obesity are implicated). Secondary hypertension may be associated with a number of causes (page 28).

Hypertension is usually asymptomatic but may manifest with complications (e.g. cerebrovascular accidents [CVAs; haemorrhagic or thromboembolic], MI and heart failure). Ocular and renal complications as well as encephalopathy may also occur, especially in malignant hypertension (BP >200/130).

Management includes modification of risk factors and a healthier life-style, but drugs are increasingly used, as they appear to improve significantly the outcome, especially if other risk factors for cardiovascular disease (e.g. diabetes) coexist, or complications have occurred. Thiazide diuretics (e.g. bendrofluazide) and beta-blockers (e.g. atenolol) are the usual first line treatments, but there is increasing evidence that ACE-inhibitors considerably improve survival—especially in diabetics (Table 4.3).

# Heart valve disease

The valves of the left side of the heart (aortic and mitral) are the most commonly diseased. Valves may be congenitally defective, but more commonly are damaged by rheumatic fever (changing murmurs and 'flitting' arthritis; due to cross-reaction of tissues with anti-streptococcal antibodies, following a Group A β-haemolytic streptococcal pharyngitis), infective endocarditis (usually of streptococcal [often oral S. viridans such as S. sanguis] or staphylococcal [typically in IV drug users] origin; presents predominantly with fever, malaise and changing murmurs) or senile calcification (stenotic valves).

Although it can be asymptomatic, valve disease often manifests with fatigue, palpitations, or signs and symptoms of cardiac failure. Valvular disease is diagnosed by characteristic heart murmurs. In severe cases, management involves treatment of heart failure, or valve replacement. Prophylaxis of infective endocarditis is necessary (see below).

# Heart failure

Heart failure can result from disorders that strain the heart muscle beyond its capacity to sustain adequate blood circulation.

Left-sided failure is usually due to IHD, hypertension or aortic and mitral valve disease, but anaemia, thyrotoxicosis, cardiomyopathy and arrhythmias are other possible culprits. Left-sided failure manifests mainly with pulmonary oedema and cardiomegaly.

Right-sided heart failure is usually caused by chronic obstructive pulmonary disease (COPD) or other pulmonary disease (cor pulmonale). It manifests with pitting oedema, ascites and ↑ jugular venous pressure (JVP). Failure of one side of the heart usually results in failure of the other.

Acute heart failure management is discussed in Chapter 5 (emergencies). Chronic heart failure management is with a healthier life-style, treatment of the cause and drug therapy. Diuretics are usually the first choice, but ACE-inhibitors and other vasodilators such as alpha-blockers (e.g. prazosin) are also commonly used.

# Arrhythmias

Almost any cardiac pathology may cause abnormal cardiac rhythms—arrhythmias (see also page 27). Arrhythmias may be asymptomatic, or can present with palpitations, dizzy spells, faints, cardiac failure or sudden death. Thromboembolism is a hazard. ECG is used to confirm diagnosis. Management involves treatment of causal or contributing factors, drug therapy (beta-blockers, digoxin, verapamil, adenosine or lidocaine in tachycardias; atropine in bradycardias), cardioversion (with transthoracic electric shock or amiodarone) or pacemakers.

Atrial fibrillation (AF) is a common arrhythmia resulting from cardiac or other conditions (e.g. alcohol or caffeine intoxication). AF presents with an 'irregularly irregular' pulse. Following the standard CVS investigations, expert help is indicated, as the patient may need cardioversion. Any causal factors must be treated, and drug therapy is with digoxin or a beta-blocker (to control the ventricular rate—usually 100–150 bpm). If AF is chronic, patients are usually anticoagulated (with aspirin or warfarin) to prevent thromboembolism.

**Table 4.1** Predictors of high cardiovascular risk

| Very high risk | Medium risk | Lower risk |
|---|---|---|
| MI in previous month | MI >1 month previously | Old age |
| Unstable or severe angina | Mild angina | ECG abnormalities |
| Atrioventricular block | Compensated cardiac failure | Atrial fibrillation |
| Ventricular arrhythmias | | Stroke |
| Severe cardiac valve disease | | Uncontrolled hypertension |
| Advanced cardiac failure | | |

**Table 4.2** Serum enzyme changes after MI

| Enzyme | Abbreviation | Number of days after MI that maximum rise seen |
|---|---|---|
| Troponin T (troponin 1) | TT | 0.5–1.0 |
| Creatine kinase MB | CK-MB | 1.5 |
| Aspartate transaminase | AST | 2.0 |
| Lactic dehydrogenase | LDH | 3.0 |

**Table 4.3** Hypertension; ASA (American Society of Anesthesiologists) grading and management considerations

| BP mmHg (systolic, diastolic) | ASA | Hypertension stage | Key considerations |
|---|---|---|---|
| <140, <90 | I | — | Routine dental care |
| 140–159 and 90–99 | II | 1 | Recheck BP, before starting Routine dental care |
| 160–179 and 95–109 | III | 2 | Recheck BP, before starting<br>Medical advice before routine dental care<br>Restrict use of adrenaline (epinephrine)<br>Conscious sedation may help |
| >180 and >110 | IV | 3 | Recheck BP after 5 min quiet rest<br>Only emergency care until BP controlled<br>Medical advice before routine dental care<br>Avoid vasoconstrictors |

# Peripheral vascular disease

## Peripheral arterial disease

Atherosclerosis is the main cause of peripheral arterial disease, with genetics, obesity, diabetes, smoking, hypercholesterolaemia and hypertension playing a significant role.

Atherosclerosis can manifest as:

*Leg ischaemia* is usually *chronic* (presenting with intermittent claudication [IC; leg pain following exertion and relieved by rest] and occasionally pale and pulseless feet), and rarely *acute* (presenting with cold, pale and pulseless feet, and occasionally neurological manifestations [pain and paralysis] and ulceration).

*Cerebral ischaemia* may manifest with *transient ischaemic attacks* (TIAs), which may precede a *stroke* (CVA). Features depend on the site of the brain affected, last for a few hours in TIAs, but can be permanent following CVA.

*Aortic aneurysms* are localized dilatations (usually of the abdominal aorta), and are life-threatening if they rupture (*aortic dissection*).

*Raynaud's disease* results from spasm of terminal finger or toe arteries (see pages 25 and 231).

Management of peripheral arterial disease involves a healthier life-style with moderate exercise, aspirin and sometimes angioplasty.

## Peripheral venous disease

*Deep-vein thrombosis (DVT)* is usually caused by prolonged venous blood stasis, following:

- a long journey ('economy class syndrome');
- leg trauma and immobilization;
- major operation;
- prolonged bed rest.

Obesity, malignancy, pregnancy, oral contraceptives or a genetic tendency to coagulation also predispose.

DVT may be 'silent' (symptomless) if the thrombus has not caused occlusion of the deep vein. Calf tenderness and a warm, painful and swollen leg may be presenting features. There is a risk of dislodgement of the thrombus and subsequent potentially lethal embolism of a pulmonary artery (*pulmonary embolism [PE]*) especially in silent DVTs. Prophylaxis of DVTs, using leg exercises, elastic stockings, and/or anticoagulants (heparin or warfarin—see page 162) is necessary for patients at risk.

Once DVT has occurred, thrombolysis may be necessary, although anticoagulation (initially with heparin and then warfarin) is needed to prevent PE. Mobilization and pressure stockings should then be started.

*Superficial thrombophlebitis* manifests as inflammation and thrombosis of superficial veins, associated with *varicose veins* (e.g. in pregnancy), malignancy or following intravenous injections. PE may be a complication.

Both superficial and deep vein thrombosis may cause *chronic venous insufficiency* and leg ulceration (usually above the medial maleolus).

# Dental aspects of cardiovascular disease

The severity of cardiac disease may not always be fully appreciated by the patient. Further, some serious cardiovascular defects may lay undiagnosed, particularly in diabetics (who could well be suffering from 'silent' IHD) and children with congenital abnormalities (cardiac defects are associated with many syndromes). If in any doubt, consult the physician.

Of paramount importance in most cardiac patients is stress control—achieved largely by a gentle, reassuring, patient and confident approach by the clinician. Dental appointments should be kept as short as reasonable to achieve some treatment.

There is no evidence that local anaesthetics (LA) containing adrenaline (epinephrine) cannot be used in patients with cardiovascular disease (especially hypertension, IHD, arrhythmias and aortic stenosis). In fact, a profound and long-lasting LA effect as achieved with these is advantageous. The risks of stress-related endogenous adrenal release of adrenaline, which may result from inadequate LA, far outweigh any risks from adrenaline in LA in moderate doses. Nevertheless, care should be taken to avoid high doses of vasoconstrictor entering the circulation, and this is achieved by restricting the volume of LA given at any single time (multiple short appointments are better), using low concentrations of adrenaline ($\leq$1:100 000) and using aspirating syringes (to avoid intravascular injection). Prilocaine with felypressin is an alternate, with no evidence it is safer than either lidocaine or articane with adrenaline.

Conscious sedation can be helpful. Perioperative sedation with oral diazepam or temazepam is useful and safe. Relative analgesia with nitrous oxide is also useful and safe. IV midazolam, as well as postoperative analgesia with opiates can also be useful, but care must be taken, as they can cause respiratory depression or hypotension. GA constitutes a risk for many cardiac patients, and is also generally contraindicated for 3–12 months following an MI.

Many cardiac patients are anticoagulated, and the risk of bleeding should then be assessed. Antihypertensive drugs may cause postural hypotension (raise patient slowly following treatment in the dental chair). Diuretics may affect the length of treatment the patient can tolerate (especially early in the morning) before a visit to the toilet becomes necessary. Calcium channel blockers may cause gingival swelling.

## Specific problems

*MI:* Although there is no evidence to suggest that treatment under LA may be hazardous in the early months following an MI, it is probably wiser to delay elective treatment for ~6 months if possible.

*Cardiac surgery* (e.g. coronary artery bypass graft; CABG), if the operation has been successful, should reduce the risks compared with the preoperative state. Dental treatment should therefore be safe after the immediate postoperative period but it is probably wiser to delay elective treatment for ~6 months if possible.

*Angina:* Unstable angina is a contraindication for elective treatment, as the risk of MI is very high. It is important to liaise with the patient's physician, and any urgent treatment is best performed in hospital. In stable angina, two puffs of sublingual GTN spray before dental treatment may prevent an attack.

*Hypertension*, if poorly controlled, is a risk, as malignant hypertension, MI or CVA may supervene. Dental treatment should only proceed under constant BP monitoring, and is best deferred until BP is under control.

*Cardiac failure* may cause breathlessness if the patient is laid flat (as in the dental chair). Elective treatment is best deferred, until the patient has been treated and is well compensated. In hospitalized patients, monitor fluid balance carefully, and avoid fluid overload. Hypoxia and anaemia will also increase the risk.

*Pacemakers:* as the function of pacemakers can be disturbed by some electronic devices (e.g. MRI, diathermy), and others (e.g. ultrasonic scalers, electric pulp testers) can sometimes interfere, their use should be avoided unless essential (Table 4.4 below).

**Table 4.4** Devices that may have an effect on cardiac pacemakers

- **Diathermy**
- Electronic dental analgesia
- **Electrosurgical units**
- Ferromagnetic (magnetostrictive) scalers
- Lithotripsy
- **Magnetic resonance imaging (MRI)**
- Radiotherapy
- Transcutaneous electric nerve stimulation (TENS)
- Ultrasonography
- Ultrasonic instrument baths

Those in **bold** are the most significant risks.

# Infective endocarditis (IE)

IE is a dangerous, often life-threatening infection of the heart valves. Abnormal heart valves and prosthetic valves are especially at risk from IE.

## Causes

IE is mainly caused by bacteria (*Streptococcus viridans* such as *Strep. sanguis* and *Strep. mutans* [common oral commensals] are the commonest oral culprits). These bacteria can colonize damaged valves following a bacteraemia. Dental operative procedures, particularly those disturbing the periodontium, may be responsible for a significant bacteraemia, and hence antimicrobial prophylaxis may be indicated.

In IV drug users, organisms such as staphylococci may be implicated, but these often originate from the skin and the endocarditis is right-sided.

## Clinical features

Characteristic features include signs of systemic infection (fever, malaise, night sweats and anaemia) and a new or changing cardiac murmur (often resulting in heart failure). Haematuria, and petechial lesions are also common findings, while arthralgia, splinter haemorrhages, clubbing and cerebral emboli are less common.

**Diagnosis** is based primarily on the detection of new valvular damage (usually confirmed by echocardiography) and at least two positive blood cultures.

**Treatment** involves several weeks of antibiotics (usually a penicillin) and occasionally surgical correction of the diseased valves.

# IE Prophylaxis*

If the history or examination suggest a congenital or acquired cardiac valve defect, the dentist must consider whether the patient is at risk of IE. Such patients often carry detailed warning cards, but this is not always the case, so clinicians should be cautious and, if in doubt, obtain expert cardiological advice. The risk of IE may be classified as high (special prophylactic regimens required), moderate, or low (no antibiotic prophylaxis needed). If the patient is at risk of IE (Table 4.5), the next step is to determine whether the procedure you are planning to carry out is likely to cause a significant bacteraemia (Table 4.6). If this is the case, then an appropriate antibiotic prophylaxis regimen should be planned and implemented.

**Table 4.5** Risk of IE

**High-risk patients**

Prosthetic heart valves
Previous IE
Complex cyanotic congenital heart disease (e.g. Fallot's tetralogy)
Mitral valve prolapse with significant regurgitation or thickened leaflets

**Moderate risk patients**

Acquired valve disease (e.g. from rheumatic fever)
Aortic stenosis or regurgitation
Mitral regurgitation
Other non-corrected simple congenital cardiac (e.g. septal) defects

**Low-risk patients (no prophylaxis needed)**

Surgically repaired simple cardiac defects
Mitral valve prolapse without regurgitation
Innocent (functional) murmurs
Previous coronary artery bypass surgery

**Table 4.6** Procedures requiring antibiotic prophylaxis (see also Appendix 12)

- Periodontal probing
- Scaling or polishing of teeth (any method)
- Root planing and any other subgingival procedure (e.g. placement of retraction cords or antibiotic fibres)
- Surgical procedures such as tooth extraction, exposure, reimplantation of avulsed tooth, periodontal and implant surgery and any involving mucoperiosteal flaps (❶ Biopsy, incision and drainage of abscess and suture removal do NOT require antibiotic cover)
- Rubber dam, matrix band and wedge placement
- Root canal instrumentation beyond the apex
- Orthodontic tooth separation
- Sialography
- Intraligamentary local anaesthesia

---

*Based on the recommendations of the British Cardiac Society and Royal College of Physicians (Dental Aspects of Endocarditis Prophylaxis, 2004 [http://www.bcs.com/library])

The antibiotic regimen recommended depends on the risk level, the type of anaesthesia used and the presence of any allergies or recent antibiotic therapy (see 2004 antibiotic advice in Table 4.7). Important changes include:

1. Eight (cardiac) categories of patients now require *IV antibiotics* before invasive dental procedures.
2. All patients with prosthetic heart valves now require IV antibiotic cover.
3. The *first* alternative for patients allergic to penicillin at high risk of IE is now vancomycin and gentamicin. Vancomycin must be given by slow IV infusion over 2 h, and then dental surgery should be done after that. (Total surgery time potentially 3 h)
4. Vancomycin is highly allergenic, hence the 2-h delivery time.

## Some considerations

- The history is often unreliable in determining the need for antibiotic cover. If in doubt, get expert advice but, if treatment is urgent, it is advisable to provide antibiotic cover, and for future reference seek an expert opinion on the level of risk.
- The use of antibiotics carries its own risks and overall patient management may become unnecessarily complicated. Furthermore, antibiotic prophylaxis does not totally eliminate the possibility of IE.
- Bacteraemia is also caused by everyday procedures such as tooth-brushing, but daily antimicrobial prophylaxis would be impractical (and would lead to antibiotic resistance).
- Remember that the cardiac lesion may also make the patient a poor risk for GA.
- Patients with prosthetic valves may be on anticoagulants and have a consequent bleeding tendency.
- Patients at risk from IE should be advised to immediately report any unexplained fever or malaise in the weeks or months following dental procedures.

**Table 4.7** Recommendations on antibiotic prophylaxis of IE for dental procedures

| Risk (see page 142) | Type of anaesthesia | Allergic to penicillin or received >1 dose or course of penicillin in the previous month? | Regimen |
|---|---|---|---|
| Low risk | Any | | No prophylaxis needed |
| Moderate risk | LA or no anaesthesia | No | Oral amoxicillin 3 g (1 h before procedure) |
| | | Yes | Oral clindamycin 600 mg or Oral azithromycin 500 mg suspension (1 h before procedure) |
| | IV sedation or GA | No | IV amoxicillin 2 g (immediately before procedure) |
| | | Yes | IV clindamicin 300 mg (infused over 15 min before procedure) followed by: oral or IV clindamycin 150 mg (6 h later) |
| High risk | Any | No | IV amoxicillin 2 g plus IV gentamicin 1.5 mg/kg (30 min before the procedure) followed by: oral or IV amoxicillin 1 g (6 h after procedure) |
| | | Yes | IV vancomycin 1 g (infused over 2 h before procedure) plus IV gentamicin 1.5 mg/kg (at the same time) |

Notes: 1. Children 5–10 years: give 1/2 adult dose; <5 years give ¼ adult dose. 2. If multiple visits are needed: alternate amoxicillin and clindamicin or leave >1 month between visits.

# Respiratory disease

Common symptoms and signs are listed on Appendix 9.

## Asthma

Asthma is a common obstructive airways disease characterized by reversible airways narrowing due to bronchial mucosal inflammation, ↑ mucus, and smooth muscle contraction, caused by allergy or precipitating factors (e.g. cold, drugs, infection, stress). Asthma presents with episodic dyspnoea, wheezing and cough. Symptoms are worse in the early morning and severe attacks can be life-threatening.

When assessing risk level of an asthmatic patient, previous hospitalizations for attacks are very telling, as is the patient's medication, which may vary from simple 'as required' inhaled bronchodilators (short-acting $\beta_2$-agonists [e.g. salbutamol]) to combinations of long-acting $\beta_2$-agonists (e.g. salmeterol), other bronchodilators (e.g. theophylline, ipratropium) and varying strengths of inhaled or oral corticosteroids. Peak expiratory flow rates (PEFR) are impaired but usually improve with use of bronchodilators, and between exacerbations.

## Chronic obstructive pulmonary disease (COPD)

COPD, encompasses both chronic bronchitis (narrowed airways and chronic productive cough) and emphysema (destruction of alveolar walls with enlarged distal air spaces [↓ surface area for gas exchange]), is a common chronic non-reversible narrowing of the airways presenting with similar symptomatology as asthma, but the cough is characteristically more productive, and PEFR shows little or no improvement between exacerbations. COPD usually results from chronic smoking.

Some patients with COPD compensate by hyperventilating ('pink puffers') keeping blood $CO_2$ levels down within the normal range (type I or no respiratory failure). Other patients with COPD do not appear breathless but present with hypercapnia (chronically ↑ $CO_2$; type II respiratory failure), cyanosis ('blue bloaters') and right heart failure (cor pulmonale).

Although most patients do not fit precisely into either group, those with hypercapnia have lost the normal respiratory drive, rely on hypoxia to stimulate the respiratory centres, and therefore, as some authorities suggest, high $O_2$ concentrations (>30%) must not be given to them. Nevertheless, this risk is mostly theoretical; most patients die from lack of $O_2$ and not excess of it, so do not deny an ill patient much needed $O_2$.

Treatment of COPD involves smoking cessation, bronchodilators (usually nebulized), systemic corticosteroids, chest physiotherapy, antibiotics (exacerbations are usually caused by chest infections) and $O_2$ administration (hypoxia must be corrected but with care [start with low concentrations and monitor arterial blood gasses] to avoid causing ↓ respiration and therefore severe hypercapnia that can lead to unconsciousness).

## Pneumonia

Lower respiratory tract infections (LRTI) are often initially viral (e.g. influenza, but readily become bacterially infected (pneumonia) and may be localized (lobar-) or diffuse (broncho-pneumonia). They present with fever, malaise, dyspnoea, productive cough, chest pain and confusion.

Pneumonia has a high mortality in the elderly and those with underlying disease.

The most common cause of community-acquired pneumonia is *Streptococcus pneumoniae* (pneumococcus), while hospital-acquired pneumonias are usually caused by Gram-negative bacteria (e.g. *Klebsiella*, *Pseudomonas*) or staphylococci.

Inhalation of teeth, tooth fragments or infected material from the mouth may cause pneumonia, lung abscess and some times septicaemia. TB is discussed on page 196.

In an elderly in-patient with a sudden onset pyrexia and confusion, even without chest symptoms, pneumonia should be suspected, the chest carefully examined and a CXR, sputum and blood cultures should be performed. Empirical treatment must be started, if possible after discussion with the microbiologist (penicillins or cephalosporins are commonly used; metronidazole is added if aspiration is suspected). The patient will also need rehydration, $O_2$ and analgesia.

**Cystic fibrosis (CF)** is one of the most common autosomal recessive disorders in Caucasians, caused by a mutation in the CF transmembrane conductance regulator (CFTR) gene, resulting in a defective chloride channel. This leads to ↓ salt and water excretion and therefore secretions thicken. This means ↓ airways clearance and predisposition to infection. Other exocrine glands (e.g. pancreas, salivary glands) are also impaired. Failure to thrive (because of pancreatic insufficiency and malabsorption), diabetes and recurrent chest infections are the important features, and result in a reduced life expectancy of ~30 years.

**Bronchiectasis** is characterized by infected bronchioles and permanently dilated airways caused by severe, chronic or recurrent lung infections (as in CF). Persistent cough and purulent sputum follow.

**Obstructive sleep apnoea (OSA)** is relatively common and characterized by narrowing of the upper airways during sleep → loud snoring and episodes of recurrent apnoea and hypoxia that wake the patient. OSA typically affects middle-aged overweight men who complain of daytime sleepiness. Occasionally, nasal or pharyngeal pathology may be present and is usually surgically correctable. Weight reduction and avoidance of respiratory depressants (e.g. alcohol) are helpful.

**Pulmonary embolism (PE)** usually arises from DVT (see page 136) and presents with acute dyspnoea, pleuritic pain, fever, cyanosis, ↓ BP and ECG changes. Mortality is high. PE is a medical emergency; anticoagulation and 100% $O_2$ should be started immediately.

**Lung cancer** is predominantly caused by smoking and presents with cough, haemoptysis, dyspnoea and cachexia. Patients may have second primary cancers such as in the mouth. The prognosis is very poor.

**Respiratory failure**

*Type I*—hypoxia, resulting from ventilation/perfusion mismatch can be caused by almost any pulmonary disease and is managed by treatment of the primary pathology and by the administration of $O_2$.

*Type II*—hypoxia and hypercapnia, resulting from hypoventilation, may have pulmonary or neurological causes and is managed by treating the cause, careful administration of $O_2$ and, occasionally, artificial ventilation.

# Dental aspects of respiratory disease

Patients with respiratory disease are sensitive to respiratory depressants, e.g. sedatives, hypnotics and opiate analgesics. Physical or emotional stress may lead to respiratory failure.

*Upper respiratory tract infection (URTI)* is a contraindication to non-urgent GA, because the infection may be spread to the lower respiratory tract. URTI may result in sinusitis, usually associated with *Streptococcus pneumoniae* or *Haemophilus influenzae*. Sinusitis is treated, if necessary, with analgesics and decongestants. Amoxicillin or erythromycin may also be needed. In chronic sinusitis, metronidazole can be added against the anaerobes involved.

*LRTI* is an absolute contraindication to GA. Dental treatment should also be deferred until after recovery or limited to pain relief.

*Inhalation* of material from the mouth is more likely if the airways are unprotected, or swallowing is defective, as for instance following major surgery for oral cancer. Aspiration of tooth fragments, instruments and other materials can occur during dental treatment, if rubber dam is not used, or during GA if an inadequate throat pack has been used.

*Legionnaire's disease* can theoretically be caused by Legionellae (usually *L. pneumoniae*) disseminated during aerosolization of water from dental units that have stood idle for long periods. Flushing the system before treating patients may minimize this possibility.

*Asthmatic patients* can experience an attack during dental treatment, precipitated by anxiety. Dental appointments should therefore be kept short and without stress. Ensure that patients have got their inhalers to hand before treatment starts and, if there is reason to believe an attack is likely, consider asking them to take two puffs of salbutamol before starting. GA should be avoided. Sedatives should also be avoided as they may lead to respiratory failure (relative analgesia [RA] is preferable). Drugs such as NSAIDs and beta-blockers may precipitate asthma attacks. Patients who use steroid inhalers may suffer from oropharyngeal thrush, while those on systemic steroids are at risk from an Addisonian crisis (see page 208).

*COPD* sufferers present similar problems to asthmatics and in addition, are prone to chest infections and more likely to exhibit adrenocortical insufficiency. RA can also be problematic due to the relatively high concentrations of $O_2$ used.

*Cystic fibrosis* patients may be compromised by diabetes and lung and liver disease. Major salivary glands may be enlarged, enamel hypoplasia may be seen and dental development and eruption are both delayed. Pancreatin, if held in the mouth, may cause oral ulceration.

*Lung cancer* may be a second 1° neoplasm in patients with oral cancer (tobacco smoking being the common culprit), but lung cancer may also metastasize to the jaws. Some lung tumours can also be caused by chronic inhalation of certain dust particles. Dental technicians appear to be at ↑ risk.

*Granulomatous lung diseases* such as sarcoidosis may appear with orofacial manifestations (e.g. gingival and salivary gland swellings).

*Obstructive sleep apnoea* can occasionally be improved by mouth appliances that displace the mandible anteriorly, or surgery such as uvulopalatopharyngoplasty or advancement osteotomy.

# Gastro-intestinal (GI) disease

*Dysphagia*—difficulty in swallowing, can be caused by oropharyngeal disease (e.g. infection or cancer), infective or reflux oesophagitis (caused by persistent gastro-oesophageal reflux disease [GORD: lower oesophageal sphincter dysfunction]), cancer (usually arising in the lower end of the oesophagus from metaplastic intestinal columnar epithelium [Barrett's oesophagus] resulting from acid reflux), benign stricture (also resulting from acid reflux), webs (e.g. in Plummer–Vinson syndrome [with glossitis and angular cheilitis] resulting from iron deficiency anaemia), rings or pouches, hiatus hernia (herniation of part of the stomach into the chest), oesophageal motility disorders (e.g. achalasia [non-relaxation of the lower sphincter]), systemic sclerosis, diffuse oesophageal spasm (neuromuscular diseases), extrinsic pressure (e.g. neck and intrathoracic tumours), gastric carcinoma and globus hystericus (psychogenic).

Antacids and avoidance of excessive alcohol, smoking and large meals (especially before bed time) as well as weight reduction and propping up the head of the bed at night, should help reduce acid reflux, which seems to be the cause most commonly implicated in dysphagia.

*Dyspepsia (indigestion) and epigastric pain* are also common complaints associated with GORD, gastritis, peptic (duodenal or gastric) ulceration and gastric carcinoma. Peptic ulceration is strongly associated with *Helicobacter pylori* (as are gastritis and gastric carcinoma) and NSAIDs. Gastric ulcers are less common than duodenal, but appear mainly in older people and are likely to be malignant. *H. pylori* may be detected by serology, $^{13}C$ breath test or directly from specimens collected by endoscopic biopsy (necessary in older patients with gastric ulcers). Eradication of *H. pylori* is with 'triple therapy' (for 1 week): a proton pump inhibitor (PPI, e.g. omeprazole or lansoprazole) + clarithromycin + amoxicillin or metronidazole.

*Nausea and vomiting* are common symptoms of GI disease (peptic ulceration, gastroenteritis, GI obstruction, acute pancreatitis and cholecystitis), as well as migraine, ↑ intracranial pressure, MI, blood in the stomach, pregnancy, diabetic ketoacidosis, alcohol and drugs (opiates, GA, cytotoxics and some antibiotics such as erythromycin).

The cause must be investigated and any dehydration corrected. Useful antiemetics include metoclopramide (for nausea of GI origin—may cause dystonic reactions especially in young women), cyclizine (antihistamine; useful postoperatively and when some sedation is advantageous), phenothiazines (centrally acting; may cause dystonic reactions), domperidone (useful in the elderly; especially for cytotoxic-induced nausea), ondansetron ($5HT_3$ antagonist; useful postoperatively).

*Haematemesis and melaena*—i.e. blood in the vomit and dark stools signify upper GI bleeding. Causes include oesophageal, gastric or duodenal inflammation, ulceration or carcinoma, oesophageal varices (a result of portal hypertension caused by liver disease or right heart failure) and drugs (steroids, anticoagulants, aspirin and other NSAIDs). Small amounts of chronic bleeding may cause anaemia and usually remain undetected, but acute presentation with obvious symptomatology is an emergency, usually needing blood transfusion, urgent endoscopy and treatment (e.g. sclerotherapy of varices).

*Diarrhoea* may be a feature of gastroenteritis, inflammatory bowel disease (see next), irritable bowel syndrome (IBS; abdominal pain, bloating and altered bowel habit; stress related), bowel cancer, thyrotoxicosis, alcohol and drugs (e.g. cytotoxics and antibiotics, e.g. pseudomembranous colitis caused by *Clostridium difficile* following antibiotic therapy especially with clindamycin). Rehydration and antimotility drugs such as loperamide (Imodium) or (if analgesia is also required) codeine phosphate, are needed.

*Constipation* is common. In hospital in-patients it is usually due to coexistence of factors such as pain, environment, immobility, low-fibre diet, dehydration and drugs (e.g. codeine, opiates, iron, antimuscarinics). Other causes include intestinal obstruction (bowel cancer or other pathology), anorectal pathology (e.g. fissure), hypothyroidism, or $\downarrow K^+$ and $\uparrow Ca^{2+}$.
The laxatives most commonly used to relieve constipation are senna (stimulant that takes about 10 h to act), lactulose (osmotic laxative; a non-absorbable disaccharide that retains water in the GI tract; takes 1 or 2 days to work) and ispaghula (bulk-forming laxative; long-term management, although natural fibre is preferable).

*Malabsorption* is due to small intestinal or pancreatic disease and may present with diarrhoea, steatorrhoea, weight loss, bleeding tendency and haematinic-deficiency anaemia. Commonest cause in the UK is coeliac disease (gluten-sensitive enteropathy), which may present also with recurrent aphthous ulcers and angular cheilitis. Diagnosis depends on the detection of $\alpha$-gliadin and anti-endomyseal antibodies, but is confirmed by villous atrophy and transglutaminase on jejunal biopsy. Treatment is a gluten-free diet. Other causes of malabsorption include small bowel resection, chronic pancreatitis (e.g. alcohol abuse) and Crohn's disease.

## Inflammatory bowel disease (IBD)
IBD consists of two conditions with fever, malaise, weight loss, abdominal pain and diarrhoea.

*Crohn's disease* is characterized by chronic patchy transmural (full thickness) inflammation of the GI tract (including the mouth) but predominantly the terminal ileum and ascending colon. Granulomas are common.
*Ulcerative colitis* is characterized by chronic diffuse superficial inflammation of the colon. The distal colon is mainly affected and ulcerated, causing diarrhoea with blood and mucus.
Management of IBD is based on corticosteroids and other immunosuppressive agents.

# Dental aspects of GI disease

*Dysphagia* is most often caused by common oropharyngeal disorders such as tonsillitis, pharyngitis, infectious mononucleosis, herpetic stomatitis, herpangina, recurrent aphthous stomatitis, xerostomia, pericoronitis and very occasionally TMJ pain/dysfunction syndrome (difficulty in the initiation of swallowing). Serious infections involving the fascial spaces of the neck (particularly those tracking to the parapharyngeal space, Ludwig's angina and peritonsilar abscesses) can also cause severe dysphagia. Cranial nerve pathology (e.g. from brain-stem lesions) can also present with dysphagia. Carcinoma of the posterior lateral tongue is not an uncommon cause, but can be missed if examination of the mouth is not thorough.

*Chronic acid reflux (GORD)* can cause dental erosion, especially if there is impaired salivation.

*Peptic ulceration* is a contraindication for aspirin and other NSAIDs, especially if given with steroids, because of the risk of bleeding.

*Stomach cancer* may occasionally present with a left lower cervical lymph node enlargement. Metastases to the jaw are uncommon.

*Crohn's disease* may present with facial or labial swelling, mucosal tags or cobblestone proliferations, or oral ulcers. Melkersson–Rosenthal syndrome (facial swelling, facial palsy and fissured tongue) and cheilitis granulomatosa are incomplete manifestations. Biopsy shows granulomas (differentiate from orofacial granulomatosis [OFG]—most likely a reaction to foods or drugs). Look also for signs of steroid and immunosuppressive therapy (e.g. thrush, ulcers), malabsorption and anaemia.

*Malabsorption* may cause vitamin K deficiency and a bleeding tendency, and anaemia ($B_{12}$ deficiency [e.g. pernicious anaemia, gastrectomy, Crohn's, bowel resection] or folate deficiency [e.g. alcohol abuse, coeliac disease]).

*Anaemia* may also be the result of chronic GI bleeding (especially in elderly males). Oral signs of anaemia include recurrent aphthous stomatitis, glossitis, angular cheilitis and oral dysaesthesiae. Anaemia can cause complications with GA, particularly if considerable blood loss is incurred during surgery.

*Nausea and vomiting* are common symptoms in patients with GI disease and may cause difficulty even with simple dental procedures. Gastric disorders may also increase the risk of vomiting after GA.

# Liver disease

*Signs and symptoms* *Acute hepatitis:* Fever, malaise, anorexia, jaundice, pale stools, dark urine, hepatomegaly, or may be subclinical. *Chronic liver disease:* Pain, fatigue, palmar erythema, finger clubbing, leuconychia, liver flap, Dupuytren's contracture, sialosis, spider naevi (telangiectasia) on the chest, gynaecomastia, testicular atrophy, splenomegaly, jaundice, pruritus (due to circulating bile salts; scratch marks may be seen as a result) and purpura (↓ clotting factors). If liver disease is not compensated, additional features may develop such as GI bleeding (from oesophageal varices due to portal hypertension), ascites, ankle oedema (fluid retention from hypoproteinaemia), drowsiness and confusion (encephalopathy). However, liver disease may show few if any signs.

*Jaundice* (yellow discoloration of the skin, conjunctivae and sclerae) is the result of ↑ plasma bilirubin. Bilirubin is the breakdown product of haemoglobin. In hepatocytes, the non-water-soluble (unconjugated) bilrubin is conjugated into a water-soluble form, secreted into the gut with the bile. Gut bacteria convert it to urobilinogen, part of which is excreted in the faeces (as stercobilinogen, which gives faeces their dark colour), while the remainder is absorbed into the blood, from where it either re-enters the liver or is excreted by the kidneys (colouring the urine).

*Pre-hepatic* jaundice is caused mainly by ↑ bilirubin production, as in haemolysis (e.g. Rhesus incompatibility, large transfusion, autoimmune haemolysis, malaria, hypersplenism, sickle cell disease, thalassaemia). Hyperbilirubinaemia then is with unconjugated bilirubin and presents few signs other than jaundice. A similar picture results from Gilbert's syndrome (enzyme deficiency → ↓ conjugation in the liver).

*Intra-hepatic* disease (viral and alcohol hepatitis, cirrhosis, drug-induced damage [e.g. halothane, paracetamol/acetaminophen], primary biliary cirrhosis, 1° or 2° tumours) may cause impaired bilirubin metabolism (and therefore ↑ unconjugated plasma bilirubin as in pre-hepatic disease), but more significantly presents with signs of liver disease (haemorrhages, oedema, encephalopathy, etc.) and some degree of cholestasis (↑ conjugated bilirubin in plasma [→ dark urine] rather than in faeces [→ pale stools] and ↑ bile salts in blood [→ pruritus] rather than in bowel [→ steatorrhoea]).

*Extra-hepatic* jaundice is caused by obstructed bile secretion (mainly due to gallstones, pancreatic carcinoma or drugs [e.g. antibiotics]) and is associated with features of cholestasis (dark urine, pale fatty stools and pruritus).

**Acute hepatitis** (acute inflammatory and degenerative changes in hepatocytes with some degree of necrosis and cholestasis; usually reversible) may be caused by viral (e.g. hepatitis viruses) or other infections, drugs (e.g. paracetamol/acetaminophen), alcohol, toxins, shock and pregnancy.

**Chronic hepatitis** (chronic inflammation of the liver parenchyma with some degree of necrosis and fibrosis) may result from viral hepatitis, drugs (e.g. antiepileptics), autoimmune liver disease, alcohol abuse or hereditary liver disease (e.g. haemochromatosis [disorder of iron metabolism],

Wilson's disease [disorder of copper metabolism], $\alpha_1$-antitrypsin deficiency [deficiency of anti-inflammatory agent → chronic hepatitis and emphysema]).

**Drug-induced liver disease** Hepatotoxic drugs include paracetamol/acetaminophen (overdose → acute hepatitis or fulminant liver failure → encephalopathy) and anti-TB drugs (usually after sustained use). Susceptible individuals may develop acute liver failure following small doses of drugs such as halothane (this should never be given within 3 months of a previous administration, nor to patients with unexplained jaundice or pyrexia after exposure to halothane) and antiepileptics (non-dose related damage). Aspirin given to children <12 years old with a viral infection may lead to Reye's syndrome (liver failure with encephalopathy).

**Alcohol-related liver disease** is the result of toxic ethanol metabolites → fatty changes in the liver as well as hepatitis and cirrhosis.

**Cirrhosis** is the late result of parenchymal liver damage, characterized by irreversible fibrosis, nodular regeneration and vascular derangement. It may be idiopathic or can complicate any chronic liver disease, most commonly alcoholic or viral hepatitis. Cirrhosis may present with features or complications of chronic liver disease, including renal failure and hepatocellular carcinoma. Management involves nutritional supplements, avoidance of alcohol, NSAIDs and excessive salt, as well as prevention and treatment of complications.

**Liver failure** can be the end result of any liver disease. Liver failure can present with any of the signs or symptoms of liver disease, along with severe cerebral oedema (→ ↑ intracranial pressure) and multi-organ failure. The prognosis is poor without a liver transplant.

**Liver tumours** are most often metastases from elsewhere in the body, and indicate a poor prognosis. Hepatocellular carcinoma is the commonest 1° tumour in the liver and is usually either the result of alcoholic cirrhosis or chronic viral hepatitis.

**Gallstones** are common, especially in women and with advancing age. They are usually asymptomatic but, occasionally, passage of stones into the bile ducts may cause obstruction, biliary colic (severe epigastric or right hypochondriac pain) or acute cholecystitis. Cholecystectomy is the treatment of choice.

# Viral hepatitis

## Hepatitis A virus (HAV)

Hepatitis A is the most common cause of childhood jaundice. Endemic throughout the world, HAV is spread via the faecal–oral route and occurs mainly in travellers (ingestion of contaminated food), or in epidemics in institutions and schools. After an incubation period of a few weeks, patients present with non-specific symptoms (fatigue, anorexia, nausea, etc.), and some develop features of cholestasis (jaundice, pale stools and dark urine). The prognosis is excellent, with most patients making a full recovery within a few weeks. A vaccine is available for people travelling in high-risk parts of the world (non-resource-rich areas).

## Hepatitis B virus (HBV)

Hepatitis B is endemic throughout the world, especially in non-resource-rich areas such as parts of South Asia and West Africa. Spread is mainly parenteral (transfusion of blood or blood products, needle-sharing in drug addicts, tattooing), sexually (especially in men who have sex with men), vertical (perinatally) and via close contact with body fluids (e.g. health care workers).

After an incubation period of a few months, two-thirds of patients will have a subclinical infection and recover fully. Another quarter of patients will develop acute hepatitis (seroconversion is often accompanied by non-specific symptoms of fever, malaise, anorexia, arthralgia and rashes, followed by Jaundice and other cholestatic features). The vast majority of these patients will also recover fully within a few months (there is though, ~1% mortality).

Infection persists in <1/10 patients, most of whom are asymptomatic carriers (hepatitis B surface antigen [HB$_s$Ag]-positive [see pages 126–127]), with the remainder suffering features of chronic hepatitis and an ↑ risk of cirrhosis and hepatocellular carcinoma.

Treatment is symptomatic. Those who develop chronic hepatitis may benefit from interferon-$\alpha$ or other antivirals.

Prevention is by active immunization (a recombinant vaccine of HB$_s$Ag given as an IM injection at 0, 1 and 6 months, followed by boosters depending on response; about 90% of healthy adults develop adequate immunity for at least 3 years). In the UK, due to low prevalence, only high-risk groups (e.g. all health care workers) are vaccinated (see page 158). Following a high-risk exposure (e.g. sexual contact or needle-stick injury), non-immune contacts should receive active (vaccine) and passive (specific immunoglobulin) immunization.

## Hepatitis C virus (HCV)

Hepatitis C is transmitted mainly through the IV route (blood transfusion and needle sharing). Prevalence is high among older haemophiliacs (although blood is now routinely tested) and IV drug users. The clinical course is similar to that of hepatitis B, but the majority of patients develop chronic hepatitis and a considerable proportion have long-term complications (cirrhosis ± hepatocellular carcinoma). Early treatment with interferon-$\alpha$ and other antivirals may prevent chronic disease.

## Hepatitis D virus (HDV)

Hepatitis D only exists in the presence of HBV. HDV (delta agent) infection may coincide with HBV infection or superinfect patients with chronic hepatitis B. HDV can cause fulminant hepatitis with a high mortality.

## Hepatitis E virus (HEV)

Hepatitis E has a clinical course similar to that of hepatitis A.

**Non-A-E hepatitis** is the term used when the virus causing hepatitis cannot be typed.

# Dental aspects of liver disease

*Bleeding tendency.* Clotting factors may not be produced by damaged hepatocytes. Bile salt stasis also causes fat malabsorption and impairs absorption of vitamin K. Thrombocytopenia (2° to hypersplenism) and functional abnormalities of platelets are also noted.

Before surgery, parenteral administration of vitamin K (10 mg daily for several days) may improve haemostatic function. If INR (page 162) does not improve, transfusion of blood or fresh frozen plasma (FFP) may be required.

Drugs that may exacerbate the bleeding tendency must be avoided. Anticoagulants (e.g. warfarin) are an obvious hazard. Broad-spectrum antibiotics may destroy part of the gut flora and further reduce the availability of vitamin K. Aspirin and other NSAIDs, as well as corticosteroids may increase the risk of bleeding, especially from the GI tract.

*Impaired drug metabolism.* Both drug detoxification and excretion are compromised and hypoalbuminaemia also reduces protein binding of drugs. Drugs and their metabolites may accumulate. Conversely, some drugs depend on liver metabolism to produce their active form, and their efficacy may be reduced in liver disease.

Drug intolerance is a significant problem in relation to GA. Any CNS depressants, including GA, opioid analgesics, benzodiazepines and other sedatives may be potentiated and can cause respiratory arrest or coma. Relative anaesthesia with $NO/O_2$ is a safer option. Even the maximum safe dose of LA is ↓. The brain is particularly sensitive in hepatic encephalopathy.

Drugs which are directly hepatotoxic and therefore contraindicated include analgesics (e.g. opioids, codeine, aspirin and other NSAIDs), antibiotics (e.g. tetracyclines, erythromycin estolate and ketoconazole), anaesthetics (e.g. halothane and methohexitone), muscle relaxants (suxamethonium), anticonvulsants and oral contraceptives.

Other drugs must be used in considerably lower doses, including metronidazole, clindamycin, temazepam (although probably the safest among CNS depressants) and paracetamol/acetaminophen (although probably still the safest analgesic to be used, if kept to moderate doses).

*Transmission of hepatitis viruses* is a significant risk in dentistry. Blood, plasma and serum of hepatitis patients are highly infectious, with only minute amounts needed to transmit the viruses. Saliva may also be a source of infection, but the risk seems to be very low (except where there is very close contact, or in cases of human bites).

There is clear evidence that unvaccinated dental personnel can be infected. The risk is higher in those performing surgery.

In most countries, it is mandatory for clinical personnel to produce evidence of HBV vaccination and immune status. It is uncertain what should be done about non-responders.

Patients have also been infected with hepatitis following dental treatment, although if adequate care is taken with infection control routines and procedures, this should no longer be occurring. Practitioners ill with hepatitis or $HB_eAg$-positive or HCV-positive should cease practice until fully recovered.

Dental staff must avoid penalizing virus-positive patients. Refusal to treat known carriers is a dangerous practice, because it may lead patients to conceal their disease. Furthermore, most carriers are unidentified, and dentist should now be following standard precautions as if everyone is potentially a source of infection transmission. Standard cleaning, sterilizing and protective (shielding) measures used routinely in dental and hospital practice should prevent the transmission of most serious transmissible diseases including viral hepatitis.

Clinical staff should be particularly careful when collecting specimens from known carriers. Although standard precautions are taken inside laboratories, clinicians should securely seal and label all infective material as 'biohazard', to warn anyone involved in its transport and handling.

*Other considerations*

- Sialosis and dental erosion may be seen in hepatic disease, particularly in alcohol-associated liver damage.
- Poor wound healing may be a feature.
- Treatment of patients awaiting liver transplantation is problematic, as careful attention to oral and dental disease is required before immuno-suppression is started, but the active liver disease may be restrictive. Following transplantation, elective treatment is best deffered for 3 months. Antibiotic and/or steroid cover may be needed. Gingival swelling may be seen in patients receiving ciclosporin.
- Renal failure 2° hepatic failure (hepatorenal syndrome) may also occur, especially following major surgery. This should be avoided by aggressive IV hydration and diuresis with mannitol, in jaundiced patients undergoing major surgery.
- Postoperative jaundice is not uncommon, and may be caused by haemolysis (incompatible blood transfusion or resorption of large haematoma), drug-induced hepatitis (e.g. halothane), aggravation of pre-existing liver disease (e.g. viral or alcoholic hepatitis), Gilbert's syndrome (jaundice can occur if these patients are starved or given a GA), or hepatic necrosis 2° to circulatory failure.
- Disturbed glucose metabolism may cause diabetes.
- Iron deficiency anaemia may be a feature of hepatocellular or cholestatic liver disease, because of chronic GI bleeding. Furthermore, the main cause of prehepatic jaundice is haemolytic anaemia.

# Bleeding disorders

A bleeding tendency can be due to inherited or acquired problems with vessel integrity, platelet numbers or function or coagulation defects. Investigations are discussed in Chapter 3.

## Vascular disorders

Vascular disorders present with easy bruising, and bleeding into the skin and mucous membranes.

### Congenital
- Hereditary haemorrhagic telangiectasia (Osler–Weber–Rendu syndrome)
- Congenital connective tissue disorders (e.g. osteogenesis imperfecta, Ehlers–Danlos syndrome, Marfan's syndrome)

### Acquired
- Easy bruising syndrome (benign and relatively common in women)
- Senile purpura (perivascular atrophy)
- Corticosteroid therapy (due to perivascular atrophy)
- Autoimmune disorders (e.g. SLE, rheumatoid arthritis)
- Vasculitis (e.g. post-infection type III hypersensitivity reactions)
- Severe infections (e.g. meningococcal meningitis, septicaemia)
- Scurvy (vitamin C deficiency)

## Platelet disorders

Platelet disorders present with excessive bruising of skin and mucosae and spontaneous (e.g. epistaxis, gingival bleeding) or prolonged (e.g. during surgery) bleeding. Aspirin is a common cause of platelet dysfunction.

### Thrombocytopenia ($\downarrow$ platelets)
$\downarrow$ *Production (bone marrow failure)*
- Megaloblastic anaemia
- Aplastic anaemia (due to drugs [e.g. cytotoxics, chloramphenicol], viruses, chemicals or irradiation)
- Tumours infiltrating the bone marrow (including leukaemias and multiple myeloma)

$\uparrow$ *Destruction*
- Autoimmune ('idiopathic') thrombocytopenia
- Other immune-mediated thrombocytopenias, caused by:
  - drugs (e.g. heparin may cause a type III hypersensitivity reaction)
  - viruses (e.g. HIV)
  - Systemic lupus erythematosus (SLE)
  - post-transfusion purpura
- Splenomegaly (2° to liver failure and portal hypertension)

*Other causes*
- Large transfusion of stored blood (dilution of platelets)
- Disseminated intravascular coagulation (DIC: consumption of platelets)

### Thrombasthenia (platelet dysfunction)
- Drugs (e.g. β-lactam antibiotics, cytotoxics, NSAIDs [aspirin →↓ thromboxane A →↓ platelet activation and aggregation])
- Inherited thrombasthenias (e.g. Glanzmann's syndrome)
- Myeloproliferative or myelodysplastic disorders
- Liver disease
- Chronic renal failure (uraemia →↓ platelet adhesion)

Management depends on the cause, and may involve corticosteroids, splenectomy, IV immunoglobulins or platelets.

## Coagulation disorders

### Inherited

*Haemophilia A* is an X-linked recessive disorder (it affects males) characterized by deficiency of clotting factor VIII. It usually manifests in childhood with bleeding into muscles and joints (haemarthroses). Internal haematomas may cause serious damage to adjacent tissues or organs, while any laceration or surgery results in delayed bleeding (~1 h later, following initial apparent haemostasis from platelet plug) that persists despite all local measures. A severe and often fatal complication is cerebral haemorrhage.
The disease usually manifests if factor VIII is <25% (mild), is moderate when factor VIII is <5% and is severe when factor VIII is <1%. Management involves factor VIII replacement prophylactically or (plus desmopressin and tranexamic acid) to control haemorrhage.

*Haemophilia B (Christmas disease)* is caused by deficiency of clotting factor IX, is clinically similar to haemophilia A, but 10-fold less frequent.

*von Willebrand's disease (vWD)* is caused by deficiency of von Willebrand factor (vWF), which plays a role in platelet function and as a carrier for factor VIII and is the most common coagulation disorder. Bleeding is due to low factor VIII, and a platelet defect. There are several subtypes of vWD, and the clinical features are variable. vWF or factor VIII replacement may be necessary.

### Acquired

*Anticoagulant treatment* (with warfarin or heparin) is the most common cause (discussed below).

*Vitamin K deficiency* (due to malabsorption [e.g. cholestasis], treatment with antibiotics or inadequate stores [e.g. newborns]) leads to ↓ factors II, VII, IX and X.

*Liver disease* causes a combination of defects (see page 158).

*Alcohol abuse* may damage the liver, and therefore produce a coagulopathy, and may also cause hypersplenism, folate deficiency and bone marrow damage, all of which can impair platelet formation.

*Disseminated intravascular coagulation (DIC)* is a complex condition, where a serious underlying pathology (e.g. severe sepsis, malignancy, incompatible transfusion, extensive trauma or surgery) → extensive thrombotic phenomena → consumption of platelets and clotting factors, and activation of the fibrinolytic system → widespread haemorrhage.

# Anticoagulants

Anticoagulants are used in the treatment of acute thrombotic episodes, and as prophylaxis against thromboses in patients at risk.

---

### Anticoagulant indications

- DVT, PE, unstable angina, MI, cerebral and peripheral arterial thrombosis; prevention and treatment
- AF, rheumatic heart disease and prosthetic heart valves; prevention of embolization
- Peri and postoperative prophylaxis of DVT in high-risk patients (see page 136)

---

### Warfarin

Warfarin is an anticoagulant given orally as a single daily dose of 1–10 mg (usually at night). It is a vitamin K antagonist, reducing the liver production of clotting factors II, VII, IX and X. Warfarin needs at least 48 h to reach its maximum effect. It is important to regularly monitor its effects using the International Normalised Ratio (INR) (monthly checks are usually adequate).

Warfarin is used in outpatients for long-term prophylaxis against thromboembolism. It has a narrow therapeutic range, with target INR being 2–2.5 for DVT, 2.5–3 for AF, and 3–4 for recurrent DVT/PE and for mechanical prosthetic heart valves. Patients with erratic INRs may occasionally need to go on a sliding scale (dose adjusted daily depending on INR), to achieve maintenance at or near target values.

The risk of haemorrhage becomes serious when INR >8. In such cases, warfarin should be stopped and restarted when INR <5. If there is another risk or evidence of bleeding, give vitamin K 5 mg orally or IV. Fresh frozen plasma may also be needed if major bleeding occurs. (See below for management of oral surgery).

### Heparin

Heparin is an anticoagulant given by injection, which acts rapidly, but has a short-lived effect and is limited to short-term management of inpatients. It inhibits thrombin formation. It is used in the acute treatment of thromboses, during the initiation of prophylactic treatment (until warfarin comes into effect) and for DVT prophylaxis following surgery. Heparin effect is monitored by activated partial thromboplastin time (APTT). Heparin can be reversed by stopping the drug or, in an emergency, by giving protamine sulphate.

*Standard (unfractionated) heparin* has a particularly short-lived effect. For the prophylaxis of at risk patients from DVT during major surgery, give 5000 units SC 2 h before surgery, then every 12 h for a week (or until patient is mobile). If DVT occurs, contact the medical team (need for higher doses and daily monitoring of APTT).

*Low molecular weight heparins* have a longer duration of action and can be administered as a single daily dose, but the anticoagulation effect is not easily reversed. For DVT prophylaxis use enoxaparin (clexane) 2000 units SC 2 h before surgery, then every 24 h for a week.

**Other drugs** used in thromboembolic diseases include:
- Antiplatelet drugs (primarily for the prevention of arterial thrombosis [angina/MI, TIA/stroke, intermittent claudication])
  - Aspirin (cyclo-oxygenase inhibitor)
  - Clopidogrel (inhibitor of ADP-mediated platelet aggregation)
- Thrombolytics (used after MI or severe DVT/PE to degrade clot)
  - Streptokinase (derived from haemolytic streptococci)
  - t-PA (recombinant tissue plasminogen activator)

# Dental aspects of bleeding disorders: general considerations

*Local causes* are responsible for most bleeding following tooth extraction, and include:
- Excessive trauma (to soft tissue in particular)
- Inflamed mucosa at the extraction/operation site
- Poor compliance with postoperative instructions
- Post-extraction interference with the socket (e.g. mouth rinsing, sucking and tongue pushing)
- Reactive hyperaemia

*Blood blisters or petechiae* in the mouth may occasionally cause concern regarding a possible bleeding disorder, but are usually due to:
- Trauma
- Vesiculobullous disorders (e.g. mucous membrane pemphigoid)
- Viral infection causing thrombocytopenia (e.g. Coxsackie A [herpangina], EBV [infectious mononucleosis], HIV, rubella virus)
- Angina bullosa haemorrhagica (benign idiopathic condition; diagnosed after exclusion of all other possible causes)

*Significant histories* suggesting a bleeding tendency include:
- Previous diagnosis of a bleeding tendency
- Previous bleeding for more than 36 h, or bleeding restarting more than 36 h after operation, particularly if on more than one occasion
- Previous admission to hospital to arrest bleeding
- Previous blood transfusions for bleeding
- Spontaneous bleeding (e.g. haemarthrosis, deep bruising or menorrhagia) from little obvious cause
- A convincing family history of one of the above, combined with a degree of personal history
- Recent therapy by significant drugs (anticoagulants or, occasionally, aspirin)

The situation should be considered as *urgent*, if the patient is:
- losing large quantities of blood
- hypotensive
- bleeding internally

The **general approach**, when faced with a patient who seems to be bleeding excessively, is discussed in Chapter 6.

*Things to restrict or avoid* in anyone with a bleeding tendency:
- Trauma (operate with extreme care)
- Surgery (use preventive and conservative methods, if possible)
- Regional or floor of mouth LA injections (may bleed into fascial spaces of the neck and obstruct the airways)
- IM injections
- Drugs causing ↑ bleeding tendency (e.g. aspirin or other NSAIDs)
- Drugs causing gastric bleeding (e.g. aspirin, other NSAIDs and steroids)

# Dental aspects of bleeding disorders: specific conditions

## Vascular disorders

Echymoses into skin and mucous membranes are common, serious bleeding is rarely caused but vessel fragility may lead to chronic small bleeds and subsequent iron deficiency.

*Hereditary haemorrhagic telangiectasia* may need cryosurgery to treat telangiectasias. Nasal bleeding is an ever-present danger, and nasal intubation is best avoided.

## Platelet disorders

*Thrombocytopenia* assessment depends on platelet counts (Table 4.8).

**Table 4.8** Thrombocytopenia: manifestations and management

| Platelets (× 10⁹/L) | Purpura | Postoperative bleeding | Platelet transfusion needed |
|---|---|---|---|
| 100–150 | Mild | ↑ | for major surgery |
| 50–100 | Moderate | ↑ | even for minor surgery |
| 25–50 | Severe | ↑ even from venepuncture | even for regional anaesthetic blocks |
| <25 | Spontaneous | ↑ may be life threatening | usually, and avoid surgery if possible |

Contact the haematologist well in advance when platelets are necessary for a planned operation, and give immediately preoperatively, repeating if necessary, as sequestration is rapid. The need for platelet transfusions may be reduced by local haemostatic measures (e.g. absorbable oxidized regenerated cellulose [Surgicel], desmopressin or antifibrinolytics (tranexamic acid or epsilon amino caproic acid).

Antiplatelet drugs (e.g. aspirin, β-lactam antibiotics, cytotoxics, furosemide, diazepam and some antihistamines) should be avoided.

Patients on long-term corticosteroids (autoimmune thrombocytopenia) may need corticosteroid cover and are prone to develop infections.

Splenectomized patients do not usually need antimicrobial prophylaxis before dental procedures.

## Coagulation disorders

*Haemophiliac* patients present a special difficulty in dental management. Prevention of dental and periodontal disease is imperative, and all necessary treatment (including conservation and surgical procedures) should be co-ordinated in specialized centres.

Regional block anaesthesia should be avoided, as must injections in the floor of the mouth (danger of bleeding into fascial spaces → airways compromise). Infiltration anaesthesia can be performed with caution (avoid lingual infiltrations), but intraligamentary anaesthesia is safe.

Matrix bands and rubber dam are protective for the gingivae, but must be applied with care. Saliva ejectors must also be used with caution. Endodontic treatment is usually safe if not going beyond the apex. Periodontal scaling can be carried out under antifibrinolytic cover.

When surgical procedures are planned, the haematology unit should be contacted and collaboration ensured (Table 4.9). Patients require:
- Factor VIII (for haemophilia A)
  - dentoalveolar surgery:    >50% of normal, given preoperatively
  - major surgery:    100%, repeated twice daily for 7–10 days
  - head and neck trauma:    100%, repeated for ~3 days
- Desmopressin (twice daily IV infusion, for up to 4 days)
- Tranexamic acid (1 g orally × qds × 7–10 days)
- Local haemostatic measures (Surgicel, good suturing, etc.)
- Antibiotics (e.g. oral penicillin V 250 mg × qds × 7 days) to reduce the risk of 2° haemorrhage from wound infection
- Careful postoperative care (soft diet, etc.) and in-hospital stay (for up to 10 days)

If GA is required (especially for major surgery), assess by full haemostatic screening, LFTs and viral assays (possibility of hepatitis or HIV infection in older haemophiliacs). Any pre-existing anaemia should be assessed, and blood should be grouped and cross-matched. An oral laryngeal mask is recommended to minimize trauma to the nasal and tracheal lining. Aspirin and NSAIDs must be avoided.

*von Willebrand's disease:* The commonest type of the disease (type I) can be managed with desmopressin, tranexamic acid and local measures. Types II and III require clotting factor replacement (vWF ± factor VIII) and can be difficult to manage. Aspirin and NSAIDs must be avoided.

*Other coagulopathies* are usually due to defects in the synthesis, absorption or utilization of *vitamin K*.
- Synthesis may be impaired by destruction of the gut flora by prolonged antibiotic therapy or parenteral feeding; such patients will benefit from parenteral vitamin K (prior to surgery or if bleeding occurs).
- Malabsorption may be due to various gut disorders causing steatorrhoea (e.g. biliary obstruction). Parenteral 10 mg of vitamin K (a water soluble form for oral administration is also available) is necessary to allow control of bleeding (response though, is not rapid).
- Utilization may be ↓ due to:
  - hepatocyte damage (vitamin K will have no effect)
  - oral anticoagulant therapy (see below)

**Table 4.9** Management of patients with haemophilia A requiring oral surgery

| Surgery schedule | Factor VIII level required | Preoperatively give | Postoperative |
|---|---|---|---|
| Dentoalveolar | Minimum of 50% at operation | Factor VIII IV[a] Tranexamic acid 1 g qds (starting 24 h preop.) | Rest for 3 days Soft diet. For 10 days give tranexamic acid 1 g qds and penicillin V 250 mg qds. If there is bleeding during this period give repeat dose of Factor VIII[a] |
| Maxillofacial | 100% at operation 50% for 7 days | Factor VIII IV | Rest inpatient for 10 days. Soft diet. Factor VIII[b] twice daily IV for 7–10 days postop |

[a] Factor VIII dose in units = weight in kg × 25 given 1 h preoperatively.
[b] Factor VIII dose in units = weight in kg × 50 given 1 h preoperatively.

# Dental aspects of bleeding disorders: antithrombotic drugs

## Aspirin

Aspirin may cause prolonged peri- and postoperative bleeding, despite the low doses (75 mg daily) used for protection from arterial thombosis. One aspirin can impair platelets for 1 week. Although bleeding is not usually problematic, consider stopping the drug (patients on aspirin are not usually at high risk from thrombosis) 1 week prior to a major operation. If in doubt, discuss with the patient's physician.

## Warfarin

Patients on warfarin should carry a diary, where their INR results are recorded after every review at the anticoagulation clinic. Patients who need checking more than monthly are usually those with erratic INRs, who need warfarin frequently adjusted. If an operation is needed, check the diary, to get an indication of problems you may face.

Do not interfere with the warfarin prior to surgery unless so directed by the physician: the benefits of a reduced risk of bleeding by reducing the warfarin (which can usually be controlled easily using local measures), must be weighed against the risk of thrombosis, which is usually high and has potentially lethal consequences. If in any doubt, discuss with the patient's physician.

Simple extraction of 1–3 teeth is usually safe if INR <3.5, even in general practice, so long as a recent INR (<24 h preoperatively) can be obtained (Table 4.10). A useful approach for the general practitioner is to book the extraction appointment on the afternoon of the day that the patient will have their routine INR check, or, at the latest, the next morning (INR can fluctuate considerably from day to day). Special attention should be given to minimizing trauma, and using local haemostatic measures (Surgicel and sutures). If INR >3.5, reschedule around next blood test or ask the coagulation clinic for an earlier review if necessary.

If management becomes difficult, or if the INR is very erratic and there are other reasons to suspect potentially serious bleeding, consider referring the patient to the local Oral and Maxillofacial Surgery Unit. Unless target INR ~4, discontinuation of the drug for 48 h will be considered (after communication with the clinician treating the condition that necessitates coagulation), followed by a re-check of the INR the morning before the operation. Warfarin should be restarted the same evening after the operation. INR will need at least 48 h to rise back to therapeutic levels, and therefore an INR is arranged 2–4 days postoperatively.

If a more major operation is needed, this must be performed in hospital, where a variety of approaches may be employed. The surgeon may be happy to perform the procedure if INR <2.5, possibly with some extra precautions such as tranexamic acid. If a GA is required or there are added risks of thrombosis, it may be decided to stop the warfarin, admit the patient and start them on heparin, which allows a much better control over a bleeding episode, not usually necessitating monitoring by APTT. Warfarin is re-started postoperatively, but heparin is only discontinued after the INR has reached its therapeutic range. This usually takes 2–3 days; the patient can then be discharged from hospital, if appropriate.

If postoperative bleeding occurs, local haemostatic measures should be reviewed and tranexamic acid should be considered. If the INR is also found to be very high (e.g. >8), as can occur several days postoperatively (bleeding due to infection, or ↑ INR due to prolonged antibiotic therapy) or when the patient presents unexpectedly (e.g. trauma), consider giving 5 mg of vitamin K (but discuss with medical team as vitamin K may cause rebound hypercoagulability and complicate subsequent anticoagulation).

Bear in mind that other factors, such as irregular tablet-taking, obstructive jaundice, alcohol abuse, malabsorption and NSAIDs may exacerbate the bleeding tendency.

Also remember that the condition for which anticoagulant therapy is being given, may affect dental management (e.g. prosthetic valves are a high risk for IE).

## Heparin

Heparin produces a very controlled bleeding tendency, which is easily reversed by discontinuing the drug or giving protamine sulphate. Low molecular weight heparins are slightly more difficult to reverse. Patients undergoing renal dialysis are heparinized for the procedure. Surgical treatment is best performed the day after the dialysis, when the effect of heparin has ceased (and there is maximum benefit from dialysis; see page 214).

**Table 4.10** Oral anticoagulant therapy and oral surgery

|  | Prothrombin time | Thrombo test | INR |
|---|---|---|---|
| Normal level | <1.3 | >70% | 1 |
| Therapeutic range | 2–4.5 | 5–20% | 2–5 |
| Levels at which dentoalveolar surgery can be carried out[a] | <2.5 | >15% | <3.5 |

INR= international normalized ratio.
[a] e.g. the uncomplicated forceps extraction of 1–3 teeth.

# Anaemia

Anaemia is a ↓ haemoglobin (Hb) level for the patient's age and gender. The causes include:

- loss of blood from haemorrhage;
- ↓ production of Hb (due to deficiency of haematinics);
- ↑ destruction of erythrocytes (haemolytic anaemia).

Patients with anaemia may complain of fatigue, shortness of breath, headaches, dizziness or palpitations. Although there might be no clinical signs, inspect the conjunctivae and palms for pallor, and check for tachycardia or a systolic flow murmur (↑ cardiac output). Classification of anaemias depends mainly on mean cell volume (MCV) and blood picture (see Chapter 3).

## Deficiency anaemias

*Iron deficiency* is a common cause of anaemia, usually due to chronic blood loss (e.g. menorrhagia in premenopausal women; GI bleeding in older people). Poor iron intake and iron malabsorption are infrequent causes. Special features of this anaemia include brittle nails and hair, koilonychia, atrophic glossitis, mouth ulcers and angular cheilitis. A severe form of the disease, Plummer–Vinson syndrome, presents with glossitis and post-cricoid web (causing dysphagia and ↑ risk of oesophageal cancer).

Management depends largely on identification and treatment of the cause. Iron deficiency is corrected by giving enough iron to correct the anaemia (usually improvement of 1 gm/dL per week of treatment) and replenish stores (~3 months treatment). Blood transfusion is rarely needed (see Chapter 10).

---

*Iron preparations*
- Ferrous sulphate 200 mg × tds (GI side-effects)
- Ferrous gluconate 600 mg × bd (↓ side-effects, but ↓ iron per tablet)
- Ferrous fumarate 15 mL (420 mg) × bd (syrup for nasogastric [NG] or percutaneous endoscopic gastrostomy [PEG] feed)
- Iron sucrose IV infusion—according to body weight (for malabsorption)

---

*Vitamin B$_{12}$ deficiency* is mainly caused by ↓ absorption due to lack of intrinsic factor (pernicious anaemia or gastrectomy), and less frequently by dietary deficiency (vegans) or malabsorption in the terminal ileum (e.g. Crohn's disease). Chronic exposure to $NO_2$ may impair vitamin B$_{12}$ metabolism. Neurological complications such as paraesthesiae of extremities may occur if untreated. Treatment is with vitamin B$_{12}$ (hydroxocobalamin) 1 mg IM every 3 months.

*Folate deficiency* is usually caused by ↓ intake (poor diet ± alcohol abuse). Other causes include ↑ demand (e.g. pregnancy, malignant disease, haemolysis), malabsorption, and folate antagonist drugs (e.g. methotrexate, trimethoprim). Treatment is folic acid 5 mg daily for 4 months.

## Haemolytic anaemias

*Sickle cell anaemia* is hereditary, found mainly in patients originating from Africa, Mediterranean countries and Asia. It is characterized by abnormal haemoglobin, HbS. GA may be dangerous, particularly in the *homozygous form (sickle cell disease)*, because at low oxygen tensions (about 45 mmHg), the red cells become inelastic, sickle-shaped and then either 'sludge', blocking capillaries and causing infarcts (e.g. in bone marrow and brain), or rupture, causing haemolysis. A thrombotic sickle crisis (typically presenting with bone and abdominal pain) may be precipitated by hypoxia, infection, cold or dehydration. A crisis is usually managed with strong analgesics, $O_2$, IV fluids and antibiotics. Haemolysis presents with anaemia, jaundice and splenomegaly. Blood transfusions are occasionally needed.

In the *heterozygous form (sickle cell 'trait')*, where there is HbS along with normal Hb (HbA), sickling occurs only at much lower $O_2$ tensions (<20 mmHg), uncommon in normal clinical practice.

*Thalassaemia* is a hereditary condition affecting mainly people from the Mediterranean and South Asia (*thalassa*: Greek for sea). Patients with *homozygous thalassaemia* present with severe anaemia from infancy, failure to thrive and expanded haemopoietic tissues (hepatomegaly, facial and skull bone enlargement). Management involves frequent transfusions, iron-chelators (e.g. desferrioxamine mesilate or deferiprone, to delay damage from iron deposition [transfusion haemosiderosis]), and splenectomy.

*Other haemolytic anaemias* include malaria, glucose-6-phosphate dehydrogenase (G6PD) deficiency, hereditary spherocytosis, haemolytic anaemia of the newborn (maternal–fetal blood group ABO or Rhesus incompatibility) and autoimmune haemolytic anaemia.

## Aplastic anaemia

Aplastic anaemia is due to bone marrow failure, with ↓ RBC, WBC and Plt. It is usually idiopathic, but can be congenital, or 2° to drugs (NSAIDs, chloramphenicol, cytotoxics and other immunosuppressants), chemicals, viruses or radiation. Pancytopenia may also be the feature of bone marrow infiltration (e.g. by leukaemia or myeloma). Anaemia, susceptibility to infections and bleeding tendency may manifest.

Management involves removal of any possible causes, protection from or treatment of bleeding or infection, and bone marrow transplantation (haematopoietic stem cell transplantation; HSCT).

## Anaemia of systemic disease

Anaemia may be a feature of systemic diseases, such as malignancy, connective tissue diseases, chronic inflammatory diseases, liver disease, renal disease (↓ erythropoietin, ↑ urea), hypothyroidism, hypopituitarism and hypoadrenocorticism.

# Dental aspects of anaemia

When assessing a patient's fitness for GA and major surgery, always enquire, examine and, if appropriate, investigate for anaemia. A significantly ↓ Hb is an absolute contraindication for elective surgery, and every effort should be made to correct this prior to operation. GA can be a hazard for anaemic patients, as an already strained myocardium may be unable to respond to the increasing demands of anaesthesia. Bleeding during the operation will further compromise the patient's haemodynamic status. An Hb <10 g/dL for a male or <9 g/dL for a female should cause serious concern.

The priority is to identify and treat the cause of anaemia and, if possible, define its course. If for instance, you can confirm that the patient's Hb has been low for some time, they are asymptomatic and the cause is known and predictable, it may be appropriate to proceed with the operation, if this is urgent. However, always liaise with the anaesthetist; it is they who are responsible for the decision-making.

Even in patients with a normal Hb, you should bear in mind that some degree of anaemia may develop following any major operation. Anaesthetists always record intra-operative blood loss and can usually provide a good estimate of the problem. Always ask and look for symptoms and signs of anaemia postoperatively, and remember that it may sometimes present as a deterioration of a pre-existing problem such as angina or pulmonary disease. Anaemia often presents with a simple systolic flow murmur, but may potentially precipitate heart failure.

Remember also that, following acute blood loss (e.g. trauma or surgery), declining Hb levels will not become evident until the blood fluid volume is replaced, and this can take days.

❶ Therefore, never be reassured by a normal Hb following acute blood loss; treat if necessary, relying on history and clinical picture, and repeat the Hb test the following day.

Iron therapy may be adequate for treating mild anaemia caused by an operation or injury, and may also be preferable for correcting anaemia prior to elective surgery. However, urgent or severe cases usually necessitate blood transfusion. Whole blood transfusion is appropriate for young fit patients but, as this may cause significant fluid overload in an older patient, especially if there is a pre-existing heart condition, packed red cells given with diuretics are preferable. Rising Hb estimations are just as unreliable as falling, and are useless for at least 12 h post-transfusion. Blood transfusion is discussed in Chapter 10.

*Deficiency anaemias* often present with oral mucosal lesions, such as:
- Sore or burning tongue (no depapillation; often normal Hb)
- Moeller's glossitis (a pattern of red lines; may resemble erythroplakia)
- Atrophic glossitis (red, glossy, smooth and sore; severe anaemia)
- Plummer–Vinson syndrome (glossitis and dysphagia; ↑ risk of oral and post-cricoid cancer; mainly seen in northern European women)
- Candidosis (especially chronic mucocutaneous; iron deficiency)
- Angular cheilitis (*Candida albicans* usually associated)
- Ulcers (especially late onset; folate deficiency)

### Haemolytic anaemias

*Sickle cell anaemia (HbSS)* must be investigated for in all patients of African origins, before GA is given. In all sufferers, anaemia must be corrected preoperatively. Folic acid may be valuable while, in some cases, exchange blood transfusion is required. It is always better to treat the patient under LA, avoiding vasoconstrictors (risk of infarction) and prilocaine (risk of methaemoglobinaemia).

If GA is necessary, special precautions must be taken to avoid hypoxia (↑ $O_2$ and avoid respiratory depressants), acidosis, hypotension, dehydration, hypothermia, trauma or infection (prophylactic antimicrobials; aggressive treatment if infection occurs). Blood should be available for transfusion.

Some patients have such severe pain during crises that they over-use analgesics and may have become drug addicts. As a consequence of this or of multiple transfusions they may also be infected with blood-borne viruses.

Infarcts may occur in the mandible, or cause pulpal symptoms or cranial neuropathies. Radiographic findings may include bone marrow hyperplasia in the jaws or skull (with apparent osteoporosis), delayed skeletal maturation, hypercementosis and a dense lamina dura.

*Sickle cell trait (HbSA):* Provided the Hb level is normal, patients may be safely treated as outpatients, using either GA or LA. Avoid hypoxia, but only extreme anoxia is likely to produce sickling and its consequences. Consult a physician first.

*Thalassaemia:* patients with homozygous β-thalassaemia have a characteristically enlarged maxilla (↑ haemopoiesis) with spacing of the teeth. Consider the possibility of blood-borne viruses and of multi-organ damage (iron deposition) following multiple transfusions. Iron deposition may also cause parotid swelling and xerostomia, while folate deficiency may manifest with glossodynia or oral ulceration.

**Aplastic anaemia** presents with the problems of anaemia, but also with:
- Susceptibility to infection
- Bleeding tendency
- Effects of corticosteroid therapy
- Hepatitis B and other viral infections
- Problems associated with bone marrow transplantation
  - Painful mucositis, parotitis or sinusitis (complications of immunosuppression, cytotoxic treatment and radiotherapy)
  - Lichenoid reactions or xerostomia (if graft-versus-host disease)
  - Gingival swelling (from ciclosporin)

# Haematological malignancy I

## Leukaemias

Leukaemias are neoplastic proliferations of white blood cells released into the blood. In acute leukaemias, the malignant cells are primitive blast leucocytes whereas, in chronic leukaemias, the malignant cells retain most of the morphological features of their normal counterparts. Treatment of acute leukaemias is with cytotoxic drugs singly or in combination (see page 186). Treatment of chronic leukaemias may be with α-interferons and corticosteroids. Supportive care against the complications of leukaemia or its treatment is necessary.

### Acute leukaemias

Acute leukaemias account for ~50% of malignant disease in children, and are the most common cause of non-accidental death. Clinically they present with weight loss, fatigue and anorexia, as well as features due to leukaemic infiltration of:

- bone marrow
  - anaemia (weakness, tiredness, breathlessness, pallor)
  - ineffective leucocytes (infections, recurrent fever)
  - thrombocytopenia (bruising, and bleeding from mucosae)
- lymphoreticular system (enlargement of lymph nodes, spleen and liver)

Diagnosis is confirmed by blood count (↓ RBC and usually ↑ WBC and ↓ Plt), film (blast cells), bone marrow biopsy and immunophenotyping (categorization of blast cells).

Acute lymphoblastic leukaemia (ALL) is the most common leukaemia of childhood: most patients respond to chemotherapy and 2/3 are cured.

Acute myeloid leukaemia (AML) is the most common acute leukaemia of adults. Remission is increasingly achieved with combination chemotherapy, but recurrences are common, especially in older patients.

### Chronic leukaemias

Chronic lymphocytic leukaemia (CLL) is the most common leukaemia overall. Many patients remain asymptomatic for years, often being discovered coincidentally and life expectancy may be unaffected. Conversely, CLL may present with any of the features of the acute leukaemias, and then often requires treatment (usually with chlorambucil and/or steroids).

Chronic myeloid leukaemia (CML) is seen almost exclusively in adults. In most cases, the leukaemic cells are characterized by the Philadelphia chromosome, an abnormal chromosome 22 resulting from a translocation. CML is progressive, and sooner or later develops an acute phase that is usually refractory to treatment. Interferon is the treatment of choice, with good results if given early. Bone marrow transplantation is also helpful.

## Myeloproliferative disorders

The term 'myeloproliferative disorders' refers to proliferation of the bone marrow cells other than leucocyte stem cells, i.e. erythrocytes and thrombocytes.

*Polycythaemia* is an expansion of the erythrocyte (RBC) population, which may be primary (polycythaemia rubra vera), secondary (e.g. altitude, chronic lung disease) or relative (↓ plasma volume due to severe dehydration).

*Polycythaemia rubra vera* is a rare erythrocyte neoplasia characterized not only by ↑ RBC, but also ↑ WBC, ↑ Plt and platelet dysfunction (thromboses/haemorrhages). Patients usually succumb to hyperviscosity syndrome (↑ thrombosis) or myelofibrosis (→ bone marrow failure → myeloid metaplasia of spleen and liver). Treatment is by repeated venesection.

*Thrombocythaemia* is an expansion of the thrombocyte population with ↑ Plt, which may be primary (essential thrombocythaemia) or secondary to bleeding (e.g. acute phase reaction following major surgery), splenectomy or connective tissue disease.

*Essential thrombocythaemia* is characterized by gross thrombocytosis with functionally abnormal platelets resulting in thrombosis or haemorrhage. Treatment is with hydroxyurea (hydroxycarbamide), or radioactive phosphorus. Aspirin may help prevent thrombosis.

# Haematological malignancy II

## Plasma cell diseases (monoclonal gammopathies)

Plasma cell diseases are B-lymphocyte disorders characterized by over-production of a paraprotein detectable on electrophoresis (specific monoclonal immunoglobulin). This may arise from any class of immunoglobulin (usually IgG) and the production is defective with an overproduction of light chains (Bence-Jones protein) or heavy chains (Table 4.11).

**Table 4.11** Paraproteins found in the serum and urine in different monoclonal gammopathies

| Monoclonal gammopathy | Serum paraproteins | Bence-Jones proteinuria |
|---|---|---|
| Heavy chain disease | Usually alpha chain | — |
| Idiopathic monoclonal gammopathy | Usually IgG | — |
| Multiple myeloma | IgG or IgA or IgD | + |
| Waldenström's macroglobulinaemia | IgM | Rarely |

*Multiple myeloma* is a disseminated plasma cell neoplasm characterized by:
- extensive bone infiltration and destruction (→ bone pain, ↑ serum calcium, pathological fractures, neurological lesions, anaemia, leucopenia and thrombocytopenia)
- ↑ paraprotein in the blood (→ hyperviscosity syndrome and renal failure)

There is no curative treatment, but temporary remission may be achieved with cytotoxic drugs, immunosuppressants, radiotherapy or bone marrow transplantation.

*Solitary plasmacytoma* is a localized plasma cell neoplasm, usually with no immunoglobulin production. Occasionally seen in the jaws, it may respond to local radiotherapy. Multiple myeloma may eventually develop.

*Waldenström's macroglobulinaemia* is a plasma cell malignancy with overproduction of IgM → hyperviscosity syndrome. It shares some of the features of lymphomas including lymph node enlargement. Despite temporary responses to chemotherapy, patients usually succumb to the effects of hyperviscosity and bone marrow infiltration.

*Heavy chain disease* may present with palato-pharyngeal lymphoid swelling (involvement of Waldeyer's ring).

*Benign monoclonal gammopathy* is a benign overproduction of monoclonal immunoglobulin seen in older patients and requiring no treatment, though some patients may develop multiple myeloma or amyloid disease.

## Amyloid disease

Amyloid disease (amyloidosis) is the result of the deposition in tissues and organs of an eosinophilic hyaline material (amyloid), which may be:

- primary—with amyloid derived from immunoglobulin light chains (AL amyloid), as a complication of plasma cell diseases;
- secondary—with an acute phase protein amyloid produced by the liver (AA amyloid) in chronic infections, inflammation or neoplasms;
- familial—various types.

Amyloidosis may affect any tissue or organ (especially liver, spleen, kidneys, adrenal and heart) causing enlargement and compromising function. Oral tissues and other organs may be affected. Diagnosis can be made from biopsy of the gingivae or rectum. Management may involve immunosuppression (1° amyloidosis) or treatment of the cause (2° amyloidosis).

# Haematological malignancy III

## Lymphomas

Lymphomas are solid neoplasms arising from lymphocytes. The main difference from lymphocytic leukaemias is that lymphomas affect *mainly* the lymphoreticular system (lymph nodes and extranodal lymphoid tissue) while leukaemias affect primarily the bone marrow and blood. Unfortunately, this is only an oversimplification if one considers the various histological types of lymphomas.

Lymphomas are classified into Hodgkin's (HL) and non-Hodgkin's lymphomas (NHL), based on histology; the clinical course is also different. Further sub-classification is complex and even confusing; do not worry—even histopathologists despair with this!

*HL* affects mainly males, with a peak incidence in the fourth decade. The aetiology is unclear. HL is characterized by binucleate cells on histology (Reed–Sternberg cells). Prognosis depends on

- histological grading (with the 'lymphocyte depleted' type being the only one associated with poor prognosis), and
- clinical staging, as follows:
  - I: Involvement of a single group of lymph nodes
  - II: Involvement of two or more groups of lymph nodes on the same side of the diaphragm
  - III: Involvement of lymph nodes on both sides of the diaphragm
  - IV: Involvement of extralymphatic organs (liver, bones, etc.)

HL typically presents with progressive lymph node enlargement (often beginning in the neck). Some patients also complain of remittent fever, night sweats, weight loss, malaise, pain and pruritus. HL responds well to radiotherapy (for localized disease) and combination chemotherapy (for more advanced disease). Haematopoietic stem cell transplant (HSCT) further increases cure rates.

*NHL* is a diverse group of neoplasms with variable but generally poor prognosis. NHL may be caused by Epstein–Barr virus (EBV) and the incidence is rising, mainly because of the HIV epidemic. NHL usually begins in lymph nodes, with enlargement of cervical lymph nodes being the commonest presenting complaint. Involvement of Waldeyer's ring and mucosa-associated lymphoid tissue (MALT) in the mouth is common. NHL may also present in salivary glands, particularly in ~6% of patients with Sjögren's syndrome. Extranodal spread is usually early and therefore disseminated disease should always be suspected. Clinical staging is important, but histological grading plays a greater role in prognostication and treatment planning.

*Low-grade* NHLs have a chronic course, which may be so slow that treatment is not then required. Others progress to cause disseminated disease with bone marrow involvement and systemic symptoms. Chemotherapy, radiotherapy or occasionally splenectomy may then help, but cure rates are generally low.

*High-grade* NHLs are generally aggressive, often seen in younger age and mostly respond better to combination chemotherapy than do low-grade lymphomas. Burkitt's lymphoma is a high-grade lymphoma, often EBV-related, seen particularly in African children, which often presents with fast-growing jaw swellings, but responds very well to chemotherapy.

Midline granuloma, a destructive maxillary lesion, is usually a T-cell lymphoma.

## Langerhans cell histiocytosis (formerly histiocytosis X)

Langerhans cell histiocytosis is a group of tumours characterized by Langerhans cells (antigen-presenting cells). There are 3 main types:

*Solitary eosinophilic granuloma:* a relatively benign osteolytic bone lesion with a predilection for the mandible. It usually affects adults and responds well to curettage, radiotherapy or chemotherapy.

*Multifocal eosinophilic granuloma:* seen in children, with multiple osteolytic skull lesions, exophthalmos and diabetes insipidus (Hand–Schüller–Christian syndrome). Lymphadenopathy, hepatomegaly and splenomegaly are also common. Although some lesions may resolve spontaneously, chemotherapy is often necessary.

*Letterer–Siwe disease:* typically affects children <5 years, with enlarged lymph nodes, liver and spleen, and bone and skin lesions. Treatment is rarely successful and death occurs rapidly soon after diagnosis.

# Dental aspects of haematological malignancies

*Acute leukaemias* predispose to *infections*. Antimicrobial cover is needed for any surgery. If patients have received multiple transfusions of blood products or bone marrow transplants, they may be carriers of blood-borne viruses. Patients with ↓ Plt have a *bleeding tendency*. Regional LA injections are best avoided and any surgical interventions are best deferred until a remission phase. If oral surgery is necessary, local haemostasis should be used, and antibiotics should be taken for a week to prevent delayed bleeding from 2° infection. *Anaemia* may be a contra-indication to GA.

*Oral manifestations,* which may be the presenting features include purpura, gingival bleeding, and opportunistic infections. Gingival swelling from leukaemic infiltration is usually a sign of myeloblastic leukaemia. Lymph node enlargement is common in lymphoblastic leukaemia.

Prophylactic antimicrobial therapy is useful, as candidosis and herpetic infections are common. Established infections must be treated vigorously. Cytotoxic or steroid drugs used in the treatment of leukaemias may present with oral side-effects and can cause other management problems (see pages 186 and 208).

*Chronic leukaemias* present similar management problems as the acute leukaemias. The dentist is likely to encounter these diseases, as they have a more indolent course.

*Myeloproliferative disorders* may present problems similar to those of the acute leukaemias, particularly if myelofibrosis has occurred.

*Plasma cell diseases* are often complicated by anaemia, infections and haemorrhages. Renal failure may arise because of the paraproteinaemia. Radiation, steroid and cytotoxic treatment further complicate management of these patients. Skull lesions are present in ~70% of patients with multiple myeloma, while osteolytic lesions may also appear in the jaws.

*Amyloidosis* may complicate management because of the underlying disorder (e.g. multiple myeloma, chronic infection, inflammatory disease), or through renal involvement, or disease affecting the adrenal glands, heart, salivary glands or other organs. Amyloid deposition, particularly in primary amyloidosis may cause macroglossia and gingival swelling.

*Lymphomas* may cause management difficulties similar to those in leukaemias (anaemia, infections, bleeding, complications of treatment). Involvement of the cervical lymph nodes is common. Extranodal disease in the gingivae or fauces is also common, especially in NHL.

*Eosinophilic granuloma* has a predilection for the mandible, presenting as a radiolucent bone lesion or a painful tumour-like swelling. It must be differentiated histologically from a traumatic eosinophilic granuloma, which needs no treatment. Bone scans are necessary to exclude multifocal disease. Whether treatment is with curettage, radiation or cytotoxic drugs, the oral side-effects may be significant.

# Other malignant disease

**Oral cancer** is usually squamous cell carcinoma (see Chapter 12). Salivary gland tumours are usually benign (mostly pleomorphic adenomas affecting the parotid). Lymphomas and Kaposi's sarcoma in the mouth are increasing due to the HIV/AIDS epidemic.

**Antral carcinoma** is rare, but appears to be ↑ among woodworkers. It is usually diagnosed late, when the tumour has expanded into neighbouring structures, then presenting with pain, unilateral nasal obstruction or epistaxis, swelling or ulcer in the palate or vestibule, epiphora (from nasolacrimal duct obstruction), infraorbital anaesthesia, ophthalmoplegia or proptosis. Treatment is usually by maxillectomy, often with orbital exenteration.

**Nasopharyngeal carcinoma** is associated with EBV and common in southern Chinese, Tunisian and Inuit populations. It usually remains undetected, until local advancement of the disease causes unilateral conductive deafness (obstruction of Eustachian tube), elevation of the soft palate or neurological symptoms (invasion of mandibular nerve), or until metastasis in the neck nodes. Treatment is usually by radiotherapy.

**Other tumours** may affect management or have oral manifestations. The commonest type of cancer is lung cancer, which has a predilection for males. Smoking is the main cause, although inhalation of dust plays a role in some occupation-associated lung cancers.

Bladder cancer is also commoner in males and is associated with smoking and some industrial chemicals.

The commonest cancer in females is breast cancer. Treatment approach tends to be less radical these days and 5-year survival rate is >50%.

Stomach and colon cancers are common in both sexes.

Prostate cancer in males and cervical cancer in females round off the commonest types of cancer in humans.

Cancer survival rates vary, and life expectancy must be a factor when dental treatment is planned. It is important to have good communication with the patient, partner or family, and anyone involved in their treatment, so that all are aware of the prognosis, the patient's state of mind and insight of their disease and its prognosis, and any treatment plans for the future. The dentist may need to modify care plans accordingly, but should always keep in mind that quality of life is more important than life expectancy. Pancreatic cancer has a particularly grave prognosis, with >90% of patients dying within a year of diagnosis. Lung, eosophageal and stomach cancers also have very poor survival rates, as do myeloid leukaemias.

Dental management may be complicated by the cancer treatment. Extensive surgery may leave the patient with some form of disability. The effects of cytotoxic and radiation therapy are discussed below.

Anaemia complicates many cancers by several mechanisms, such as folic acid consumption, bone marrow invasion or chronic bleeding from GI tumours.

Oral manifestations of internal tumours are rare but may represent metastases (particularly from lung, breast and prostate cancer), organ dysfunction (e.g. bleeding tendency in liver cancer) or tumour metabolites effects (e.g. pigmentation in ACTH-secreting tumours).

Some inherited neoplastic disorders may also initially present with oral lesions (e.g. neuromas in multiple endocrine neoplasia syndromes, osteomas in Gardner's syndrome, neurofibromas in neurofibromatosis, basal cell carcinomas and keratocysts in Gorlin–Goltz syndrome).

**Childhood neoplasms** are most commonly leukaemias. Brain tumours are the most frequent solid tumours, and are most commonly astrocytomas. Wilm's tumour of the kidneys, neuroblastomas and retinoblastomas are also characteristic tumours of childhood. Treatment is usually associated with significant disabilities and prognosis is overall poor.

# Cytotoxic chemotherapy

Chemotherapy is used as the $1°$ treatment in some malignancies, especially haematological ones. Cytotoxic drugs may be given with an intention to treat or occasionally as a palliative measure. The doses vary accordingly. They are often administered in combinations of cytotoxic drugs or with other types of treatment.

Cytotoxic drugs may be divided in the following 5 classes:
• Alkylating agents (e.g. chlorambucil, busulphan, cyclophosphamide)
• Antimetabolites (e.g. methotrexate, fluorouracil, cytarabine)
• Cytotoxic antibiotics (e.g. bleomycin, dactinomycin, doxorubicin)
• Antimicrotubular agents (e.g. vinblastine, vincristine, etoposide)
• Others (e.g. cisplatin, interferon alpha, hydroxycarbamide)

## Adverse effects of chemotherapy

Most cytotoxic agents target rapidly dividing cells, aiming to kill cancer cells, but the process is not selective, so there is a degree of damage to all tissues with a high cell turnover. Thus bone marrow, GI tract, skin, hair, oral mucosa and gonads are commonly damaged.

Bone marrow suppression is the most significant consequence, and causes anaemia, susceptibility to infection and a bleeding tendency. GI tract damage causes mucositis, nausea and vomiting. Skin toxicity presents as hair loss or rashes. Other organs such as the liver, kidneys, lungs or heart may also be damaged, but these effects are unpredictable. Doxorubicin may be cardiotoxic. Cisplatin in particular may damage the kidneys or VIIIth cranial nerve.

Oral mucositis and ulceration causes painful ulcers at any site in the mouth, especially the buccal mucosae and fauces (Table 4.12). Ulcers heal within 2–3 weeks of discontinuation of chemotherapy, although they are often so severe, that an 'antidote' may be needed to reverse the effects of the cytotoxic drug (e.g. 'leucovorin rescue' for methotrexate toxicity). Aspirin and other NSAIDs should be avoided in patients on metho-trexate because they may increase toxicity.

Infections, particularly with candida species, herpesviruses and Gram-negative bacteria are also more common in the mouth. Oral purpura and gingival bleeding may result from thrombocytopenia. Xerostomia may also be caused by some agents, especially doxorubicin.

## Dental management considerations

Prior to chemotherapy, patients should be carefully assessed. All dental treatment, and surgical procedures in particular, must be completed before cytotoxic treatment starts. Intensive preventive measures must be taken. Any potential causes of irritation (e.g. sharp teeth, fillings or appliances) must be removed. Similarly any potential sources of infection (e.g. teeth with deep periodontal pockets or partially erupted third molars) must be eliminated.

Oral mucositis may be relieved by benzydamine or lidocaine rinses. Chlorhexidine mouth rinses may also help by preventing $2°$ infection. Prophylactic nystatin suspension and occasionally aciclovir are used in some centres. Any infections that develop must be treated aggressively.

Anaemia, bleeding tendency, nausea and the effects of cytotoxic drugs on other organs may also complicate dental management (Table 4.13).

**Table 4.12** WHO mucositis scale

| Grade | Clinical features |
|-------|-------------------|
| 0 | — |
| 1 | Soreness/erythema |
| 2 | Erythema, ulcers but able to eat solids |
| 3 | Ulcers but requires liquid diet |
| 4 | Oral alimentation not possible |

**Table 4.13** Dental treatment for patients on cytotoxic chemotherapy

| Blood cell type | Peripheral blood count | Precautions |
|-----------------|------------------------|-------------|
| Platelets | $>50 \times 10^9$/L | Routine management, though desmopressin or platelets are needed to cover surgery |
| | $<50 \times 10^9$/L | Platelets needed before any invasive procedure where bleeding is possible |
| Granulocytes | $>2 \times 10^9$/L | Routine management |
| | $<2 \times 10^9$/L | Prophylactic antimicrobials for surgery |
| Erythrocytes | $>5 \times 10^{12}$/L | Routine management |
| | $<5 \times 10^{12}$/L | Special care with GA |

# Radiotherapy

Radiotherapy (DXR) is commonly used to destroy proliferating malignant cells in treatment of solid malignant neoplasms (see also Chapter 12). However, it also damages any healthy tissues in the line of the beam and produces subsequent endarteritis and fibrosis. Treatment can lead to serious complications such as mucositis, xerostomia and osteoradionecrosis (ORN). The most common complication is mucositis—inevitable but transient. Xerostomia may also be inevitable but can be permanent. ORN is disabling, but should be avoidable. Complications are mostly related to DXR type, dose, and duration (Table 4.14). Pre-radiotherapy planning of oral care, and radiation dose and portal can minimize complications. With improved radiation techniques, application of lower radiation doses, shielding of susceptible tissues, and other measures, some complications are preventable. Planning of dental interventions, with treatment designed to avoid postoperative infections, as well as close monitoring of the oral cavity with strict application of preventive measures (dental care protocol) can reduce odontogenic complications.

## Oral complications of radiotherapy

*Mucositis* severity is determined by the radiation dose, field size and fractionation schedules, and appears modified by saliva volume, total epidermal growth factor (EGF) level, and the concentration of EGF in the oral environment. Radiation-induced mucositis is a function of cumulative tissue dose and typically begins at doses of about 15–20 Gy of standard fractionated radiation therapy. Profound ulcerative mucositis is usually noted at doses of 30 Gy.

Mucositis can be reduced by:
• modifying the radiation treatment,
• protecting the mucosa with midline mucosa-sparing blocks, or
• other methods, including the use of amifostine or various mouthwashes.

*ORN* is the most serious complication, and seen particularly in the mandible. Such infection often results from dental extractions carried out after DXR because of reduced bone vascularity following irradiation endarteritis. Oral infections involving bone, e.g. periodontal, and any additional immune or nutritional defect may also predispose to ORN. ORN appears to develop mainly in patients receiving more than 60 Gy, particularly to the floor of the mouth and mandible, may follow months or years after radiotherapy but about 30% of cases develop within 6 months. ORN is, however, a less frequent problem now, as megavoltage has less effect on bone than did orthovoltage DXR.

ORN is characterized by throbbing pain, swelling, cellulitis, suppuration, halitosis and cutaneous fistulae. As ORN progresses, exposed bone, haemorrhage and pathological bone fractures are seen. The area of bone affected is often small (<2 cm) and, with antibiotics, the signs and symptoms of inflammation may clear within a few weeks. Complete resolution can, however, take 2 or more years despite intensive antimicrobial treatment. Hyperbaric oxygen (HBO) may be required (20–50 sessions).

*Xerostomia:* Radiotherapy to tumours of the mouth and oropharynx may damage salivary glands, depress secretion and result in saliva of increased viscosity. Salivary secretion diminishes within a week of DXR in most patients and saliva becomes thick, tenacious and of lower pH.

Sparing at least one parotid gland during irradiation of patients with head and neck cancer will preserve parotid function and substantially reduce xerostomia. Amifostine is cytoprotective of parotid acinar cells exposed to DXR and, given intravenously can reduce both acute and long-term xerostomia.

Some salivary function may return after many months but, meantime there may be discomfort and taste disturbances, and the patient is liable to infections. Hyposalivation increases oral pathogens, particularly *Streptococcus* and *Candida* spp. Caries, oral candidosis and acute ascending sialadenitis may result.

*Radiation caries and dental hypersensitivity:* The dryness and soreness of the mouth, hypersensitive teeth and loss of taste may make oral hygiene difficult and encourage the patients to take a softer, more cariogenic diet, which can cause rampant caries, starting from any time between 2 and 10 months after DXR.

*Loss of taste (hypoguesia)* follows radiation damage to the taste buds, but xerostomia alone can also disturb taste.

Taste may begin to recover within 2–4 months but, if more than 60 Gy have been given, taste loss is usually permanent. Zinc has been administered, but with unreliable results.

*Trismus* may result from replacement fibrosis of masticatory muscles following progressive endarteritis. It becomes apparent 3–6 months after radiotherapy and can be permanent. It must be differentiated from recurrence of the tumour, and from ORN.

### Other problems

Craniofacial defects, tooth hypoplasia, dental agenesis, short roots, premature apical closure, enamel and dentinal alterations, microdontia and retarded eruption can follow DXR. Children treated for neuroblastoma are at particular risk for abnormal dental development.

**Table 4.14** Oral complications of radiotherapy involving the mouth and salivary glands

| Week 1 | Week 2+ | Week 3+ | Later |
|---|---|---|---|
| Nausea<br>Vomiting | Mucositis<br>Taste changes<br>Glossodynia | Dry mouth | Infections<br>Caries<br>Pulp pain and necrosis<br>Tooth hypersensitivity<br>Trismus<br>Osteoradionecrosis<br>Craniofacial defects<br>Tooth development<br>  alterations |

# Immunodeficiencies

## Congenital immunodeficiencies

These rare genetic immune defects (IDs) are due to 1° abnormalities of specific immune components and include:

- B-cell defects (antibody deficiencies)
  - Selective IgA deficiency (with a prevalence of ~1 in 600, this is the most common congenital ID)
  - Other hypogammaglobulinaemias (low immunoglobulins [Ig])
- T-cell defects (defects of cell-mediated immunity)
  - Di George syndrome (thymic aplasia)
- Combined B- and T-cell defects
  - Severe combined immunodeficiency (several variants)
  - Wiskott–Aldrich syndrome (thrombocytopenia plus eczema and ID)
- Phagocyte deficiencies
  - Cyclic neutropenia (↓ neutrophils every 3–4 weeks)
  - Benign chronic neutropenia
  - Phagocyte functional defects (↓ chemotaxis, adhesion, phagocytosis or microorganism killing)
    —Chronic granulomatous disease
    —Chediak–Higashi disease
    —Early onset periodontitis
    —Papillon–Lefevre syndrome
    —Down syndrome
    —Shwachmann syndrome
    —Leucocyte adhesion defects
- Complement deficiencies

## Acquired immunodeficiencies

Acquired immunodeficiency is increasingly common, usually characterized by leucocyte defects as a result of a variety of systemic disorders or as a complication of medical interventions (e.g. immunosuppressive drugs):

- Deficiency states
  - Malnutrition (the most common cause in the developing world)
  - Iron deficiency
  - Protein loss (↓ immunoglobulins)
- Malignant disease
  - Haematological malignancy (e.g. acute leukaemias, lymphomas)
  - Other malignancies (through marrow invasion or folate consumption)
- Bone marrow disease (other than malignant disease)
  - Aplastic anaemia (marrow failure)
  - Myelofibrosis
- Infections
  - HIV/AIDS (discussed below)
  - Other severe viral infections (e.g. influenza, measles, EBV)
  - Tuberculosis
- Autoimmune disorders
  - SLE
  - Rheumatoid arthritis

- Drugs
  - Immunosuppressive drugs (e.g. corticosterids, ciclosporin)
  - Cytotoxic agents (including those used in low doses for rheumatic disorders [e.g. azathioprine, cyclophosphamide and methotrexate])
  - Others (e.g. co-trimoxazole, chloramphenicol, phenothiazines)
- Splenectomy (↓ phagocytosis and ↓ Ig production)
- Diabetes mellitus (phagocytic defects)
- Chronic renal failure
- Tobacco smoking (phagocytic defects; mucociliary damage)
- Severe burns (destruction of skin as a mechanical barrier)

## Dental aspects of immunodeficiencies

All IDs result in defective protection against microorganisms. In general, neutrophil (phagocytic), B-cell (antibody) and complement defects manifest with a liability to bacterial infections, while T-cell defects result in susceptibility to intracellular pathogens (viruses, fungi, protozoa, mycobacteria) neoplasms (e.g. lymphoma, Kaposi's sarcoma, ano-genital carcinoma—which are virally related) and autoimmune disease.

Neutrophil defects, whether congenital (e.g. Down syndrome) or acquired (e.g. diabetes mellitus, tobacco smoking), often cause oral ulceration, gingival inflammation and accelerated periodontal disease.

Bone marrow disease and cytotoxic drugs may cause reduction of any type of leucocyte, and present with fever, malaise, lymphadenopathy as well as oral ulceration and periodontal disease. Septicaemia may be caused by oral viridans streptococci and therefore, antibiotic prophylaxis is indicated for dental surgical procedures.

Patients with selective IgA deficiency and those with congenital or acquired mucociliary defects are prone to recurrent respiratory infections including sinusitis.

Most acquired immunodeficiencies cause mainly T-cell defects and are characterized by opportunistic infections such as oral candidosis and viral diseases. Oral NHL, hairy leucoplakia (caused by EBV) and Kaposi's sarcoma (caused by human herpesvirus 8) can present.

Chronic mucocutaneous candidosis syndromes, a group of cell-mediated immunity disorders present with persistent candidosis.

Immunocompromised patients may also be carrying transmissible diseases or suffering from chronic infections or treatment complications, which may affect their dental management. They may also be at risk from infections caused by dental surgical treatment, and then prophylactic antibiotics as well as chlorhexidine mouthwashes may be indicated.

# HIV infection and AIDS

Infection with HIV (an RNA virus containing reverse transcriptase [retrovirus]), of which there are at least two types (HIV-1 [worldwide] and HIV-2 [mainly in West Africa]) as well as several subtypes, is endemic worldwide. Heterosexual spread is the main route of transmission worldwide. In the developing world, where the infection is widespread, vertical transmission (mother to child) is also a major problem. In the developed world, heterosexuals, men who have sex with men (MSM), IV drug abusers, and, to a much lesser extent, haemophiliacs and children are at risk.

After primary infection, viraemia results in widespread dissemination of HIV, which is trapped in lymphoid dendritic cells. From there, infection is propagated to cells with CD4 receptors (helper T lymphocytes, macrophages and brain glial cells). Acute infection is usually asymptomatic, but seroconversion (development of antibodies 3–6 months later) may present with fever, malaise, lymphadenopathy, pharyngitis, mouth ulcers, a rash and rarely encephalitis.

Infection may remain asymptomatic for ~10 years, although generalized lymphadenopathy may persist. However, CD4 cells are damaged and, as CD4 blood counts start to fall, minor opportunistic infections, such as oral candidosis, hairy leucoplakia and herpetic infections, may develop (AIDS-related complex).

Inevitably, AIDS ensues, characterized (and defined) by CD4 counts <200/μL and clinical features resulting from the defective cell-mediated immunity. Fungal (mycotic), viral, parasitic and mycobacterial infections predominate. Tumours and neurological involvement are also common. Clinical presentations include:

- Pulmonary infections
  - *Pneumocystis carinii* pneumonia (a mycosis)
  - Tuberculosis
- Mucocutaneous infections
  - Disseminated cytomegalovirus (CMV) infection
  - Disseminated herpes simplex infection
  - Herpes zoster infection
- Eye infections (mainly CMV retinitis)
- GI involvement
  - Oral and oesophageal candidosis
  - Anorexia and weight loss
  - Diarrhoea (mainly due to cryptosporidiosis)
- Neurological involvement
  - Meningoencephalitis (associated with CMV, *Toxoplasma gondii* [a parasite] or *Cryptococcus neoformans*)
  - Progressive multifocal leucoencephalopathy
  - AIDS-related dementia
- Neoplasms
  - Kaposi's sarcoma (vascular tumour)
  - Lymphomas (mainly central nervous system), associated with EBV
  - Cervical and anal carcinomas, associated with human papillomaviruses (HPV)

- Autoimmune disorders (e.g. thrombocytopenic purpura)
- Oral manifestations
  - Candidosis
  - Hairy leucoplakia (EBV-associated)
  - Kaposi's sarcoma (HHV-8 associated; presenting as a purple macule or nodule)
  - Cervical lymphadenopathy
  - Herpetic infections
  - Herpes simplex- or CMV-associated ulcers
  - Aphthous-like ulcers
  - Severe gingivitis or periodontitis
  - HIV-salivary gland disease (parotitis and xerostomia)
  - Non-Hodgkin's lymphomas
  - Many other lesions

Diagnosis is based on clinical features and laboratory-based tests usually for HIV antibodies (page 126). Management includes prophylaxis and treatment of the above conditions. Nucleoside analogues such as zidovudine (Retrovir), dideoxyinosine (Didanosine), dideoxycytidine (Zalcitabine), Stavudine and Lamivudine have been the main anti-retroviral drugs used but protease inhibitors such as Saquinavir, Ritonavir, Indinavir, and Nelfinavir are now also used. Highly active anti-retroviral therapy (HAART) involves combinations of these drugs, and can suppress disease for some time.

Attempts to produce a vaccine have been compromised by the intracellular location of the virus and its continuous mutations.

Therefore, the most important method of HIV prevention is by safe sexual practices using barrier precautions and monogamy.

## Dental aspects of HIV infection

Oral manifestations are seen in most patients with HIV disease at some time. Enlargement of cervical lymph nodes is a common early sign. Oral candidosis is seen in at least half of the patients and is often the initial manifestation. Hairy leucoplakia usually affects the lateral borders of the tongue. The common sites of Kaposi's sarcoma are the palate, gingivae and the skin of the nose and face.

The long latent period, when the disease is not yet diagnosed but the patient is infective, stresses the importance of standard cross-infection control measures. The chief occupational risk is injury by contaminated sharp instruments, but the risk of HIV transmission is ~100 times less than that of viral hepatitis transmission, and prophylactic treatment must be decided upon the particular circumstances.

Dental unit water systems must be decontaminated before treatment. Use chlorhexidine mouthwash pre- and postoperatively. If possible, avoid surgical extractions or any bone exposure. Minimize stripping of mucoperiosteum. In patients who are severely immunocompromised, antimicrobial prophylaxis should be considered. Bleeding tendency may further complicate management.

# Infectious disease

The widespread use of vaccines, better understanding of modes of transmission of infectious agents and the effectiveness of antibiotic therapy have controlled diseases such as diphtheria, poliomyelitis, pertussis (whooping cough) and tetanus, and eradicated others, notably smallpox. Certain diseases that were fatal in the past are now easily curable. Surgery has also become much safer following the appreciation of aseptic techniques and the use of antibiotic prophylaxis in certain cases.

Nevertheless, travel, sexual liberation and iatrogenic immune compromise and global warming are resulting in resurgence of some diseases, appearance of new ones and ↑ virulence or treatment resistance of others. The incidence of sexually transmitted diseases (STDs) is increasing exponentially and with the ↓ uptake of certain vaccines, the incidence of some diseases is likely to ↑ again (e.g. measles, mumps and rubella, due to ↓ MMR vaccination rates resulting from recent controversy suggesting an unproved link with autism). Outbreaks of diphtheria, poliomyelitis and other infections appear where vaccination has lapsed.

*Commensal organisms* are the host's normal flora. *Pathogens* may be endogenous (arising from commensals) or exogenous (acquired from other humans, animals or the environment). *Transmission* may be via airborne droplets (e.g. TB), direct contact (e.g. STDs), indirect contact (e.g. faecal–oral route or hands of clinical staff), food, water, blood (transfusion of blood or blood products, needle sharing, needle-stick injury, etc. → hepatitis or HIV) or insects (e.g. malaria). Vertical transmission (from mother to fetus) can also occur with some pathogens (e.g. rubella, hepatitis B, HSV, HIV).

*Nosocomial (hospital-acquired) infections* are increasingly serious, with nearly 1 in 10 people infected with microorganisms while in UK hospitals. This is due to inadequate hygiene and an ↑ pool of vulnerable patients, because of disease (e.g. cancer) or medical intervention (e.g. corticosteroids, surgery, prostheses and catheters). The use of common facilities by patients and staff acting as vectors further promote spread.

*Resistance* to antimicrobial agents is one of the most significant problems in medicine today and has arisen primarily because of inappropriate antibiotic use. Meticillin-resistant *Staphylococcus aureus* (MRSA: see below) is most important, but vancomycin-resistant enterococci, multi-resistant *Pseudomonas aeruginosa* and *Clostridium difficile* are becoming a problem. Prudent antibiotic use involves serious consideration before treatment is instigated, use of specific and narrow-spectrum agents based on culture and sensitivity results, constant review of treatment in the light of laboratory or clinical developments, shortening of unnecessarily long courses and switching from IV to oral regimens when appropriate. Communication with the microbiologist is always advantageous.

*MRSA* is a problem endemic in most UK hospitals. MRSA compromises treatment, lengthens in-patient stay, causes fatalities and is difficult to treat. Nasal carriage in patients or staff is treated with chlorhexidine and neomycin cream (Naseptin) or mupirocin ointment (Bactroban nasal).

Wound colonization may be treated with topical mupirocin or povidone iodine. Chlorhexidine baths are also useful.

MRSA does not respond to traditional antibiotics (e.g. flucloxacillin or erythromycin). Clinically significant infections must be treated with oral fucidin combined with doxycycline, vancomycin or teicoplanin. Both topical and systemic treatments must be guided by culture and sensitivity results, and clearance monitored by further samples. Standard isolation procedures must remain active until clearance is achieved.

# Some important infections

Some of the most important and relevant infectious diseases are summarized on Appendix 10. Notifiable diseases are listed on Appendix 11.

## Tuberculosis (TB)

TB is one of the most prevalent infections, affecting one third of the world's population. In the UK, it is an increasing problem affecting primarily immigrants and the immunocompromised (e.g. HIV-infected patients). In the latter it may be multiple drug resistant.

TB is caused by *Mycobacterium tuberculosis*. Initial infection affects primarily the lungs and may be asymptomatic or present with fever, sweats and productive cough. Immune response rapidly contains the disease, but the bacilli survive intracellularly and may be reactivated if the patient becomes immunocompromised → disseminated (miliary) TB, which can affect the GI tract, genito-urinary tract, bones (especially the spine), lymph nodes, etc.

*Diagnosis* is aided by: sputum microscopy (acid-fast bacilli on Ziehl–Nielsen stain) or culture (on Lowenstein–Jensen medium); histology (caseating granulomata); CXR (consolidation, calcifications and cavitating lesions); and immunology (tuberculin skin test).

*Treatment* is with at least three different antibiotics in the initial phase (2 months) and two drugs in the continuation phase (further 4 months). Resistance is common and requires additional drugs. Compliance is often problematic and the adverse effects of treatment may be serious, dictating different regimens depending on the patient's expected reliability with treatment (supervised [3-weekly doses] or unsupervised treatment).

## Prions

Transmissible spongiform encephalopathies (TSEs) are a group of lethal degenerative brain diseases (encephalopathies) characterized by microscopic vacuoles in the brain grey matter, giving a sponge-like (spongiform) appearance. TSEs are associated with an abnormal form of a host-encoded protein termed a prion (proteinaceous infectious particle) composed of a cell surface glycoprotein called PrP. Prion diseases appear to be associated with the accumulation of an isoform ($PrP^{sc}$) in the brain, resistant to inactivation by conventional sterilization.

All TSEs have prolonged incubation periods leading to death over months or years. There are several animal TSEs, including bovine spongiform encephalopathy (BSE; 'mad cow disease') in cattle, and scrapie in sheep. The human TSEs exist in several forms (Table 4.15), and are frequently referred to collectively as Creutzfeldt–Jakob disease or CJD.

## Skin infections

Common infections that affect the face and, although usually treated by other specialists, often require dental input are discussed here.

*Impetigo* is a highly contagious superficial skin infection that affects mainly children and young adults. Caused by *Staphylococcus aureus* ± group A streptococcus, lesions often start on the face, as blisters that soon rupture leaving a characteristically weeping area covered by yellow to brown crust. Take swabs and give advice to prevent further spread to other sites or to other people. Topical fucidic acid or mupirocin ± povidone iodine are usually adequate therapy for localized lesions. Widespread lesions require treatment with oral flucloxacillin or erythromycin.

*Boil (furuncle)* is a skin abscess caused by *Staphylococcus aureus*. Treatment is with incision and drainage, and systemic antibiotics.

*Erysipelas* is a superficial well-defined erythematous area of skin representing localized streptococcal infection. Antibiotics are indicated.

*Cellulitis* is a more widespread streptococcal skin and subcutaneous infection, often causing the patient to be systemically unwell. Treatment of choice is oral or IV penicillin.

*Herpes zoster (shingles)* usually affects older or immunocompromised people. It is due to reactivation of varicella-zoster virus (VZV), which has remained latent in sensory nerve ganglia following 1° VZV infection (chickenpox). Branches of the trigeminal nerve are commonly involved → prodromal symptoms of tingling or pain followed by a unilateral cropping vesicular eruption within the relevant dermatome. Involvement of cranial nerve VII leads to Ramsay–Hunt syndrome, which includes facial paralysis and vesicles around the ear. Complications include ocular involvement and post-herpetic neuralgia. These may be ameliorated or avoided by early antiviral treatment (e.g. with high doses of aciclovir).

**Table 4.15** Types of CJD

| Causes | Type | Abbreviation | Comments |
|---|---|---|---|
| Genetic | Familial | fCJD | Autosomal dominant |
| Uncertain | Sporadic | sCJD | Most common form |
| Acquired | Iatrogenic | iCJD | Contaminated surgical instruments, or human dura mater grafts or pituitary hormones |
| | Variant | vCJD Sometimes termed nvCJD | Consumption of BSE infected material |
| | Kuru | — | Ritualistic cannibalism (Fore tribe Papua New Guinea) |

# Infection control

## Sterilization of instruments (Appendix 5)

All instruments should be sterile. Use disposable equipment and materials wherever possible. For others, autoclaving at 134°C for 3 min, in a vaccum sterilser, chemiclave (formaldehyde vapour) or gamma radiation are adequate. Boiling in water is inadequate.

If sterilization is impossible because the instrument will be damaged by heat, and for surfaces, effective disinfectants include:

• Sodium hypochlorite 10% (at least 30 min exposure required; corrosive; unstable in presence of cationic detergents)
• Povidone-iodine (at least 15 min exposure required)
• Glutaraldehyde 2% (at least 30 min exposure to fresh alkaline glutaraldehyde required; solutions are toxic [take care not to carry glutaraldehyde over on to tissues or to expose staff to the vapour]).

▶ None of the above destroy prions.

## Control of cross-infection

All members of the dental team have a duty to ensure that all necessary steps are taken to prevent cross-infection, in order to protect their patients, colleagues, themselves and their families. All tissues/body fluids are potentially infected. Most of the carriers of blood-borne viruses are not identified and they are unaware of their condition. It follows, therefore, that the routine practice adopted for all dental patients must be adequate enough to prevent cross-infection—*standard precautions*.

Where the history or clinical condition of a patient warrant HBV (or HCV or HIV) testing, the information obtained will not alter the control of infection measures routinely adopted, except when a patient is immunocompromised. HIV testing, if indicated, should first be discussed with a senior member of staff, before suggesting the necessity to a patient. Specialist counselling is mandatory, prior to HIV testing.

▶ The local Health Authorities should always be notified if certain infectious diseases are suspected (Appendix 11).

### Routine clinical practice

The following recommendations are made in the light of current knowledge and may be subject to alteration and updating as further information becomes available.

• All health-care workers should be immunized against HBV. They should also consider protection against other infectious diseases, such as diphtheria, poliomyelitis, tetanus, tuberculosis, and rubella (in the case of females). No special measures are required by those who have not seroconverted after HBV immunization, as the routine measures should afford all necessary protection.
• Gloves should be worn routinely by all dental staff, clinical professionals complementary to dentistry, students, and close support dental staff. Wash hands before gloving, and after gloves are removed. Cuts and abrasions should be protected with waterproof dressings and/or double gloving as appropriate. Gloves must be changed if punctured and after treatment.

- Masks and eye protection should be worn when aerosols or tooth fragments are generated. High volume aspiration must be used and waste should go into a central drain or sanitary suction unit. The patient's eyes must also be adequately protected.
- Clean white coats, or clean surgical gowns in surgical areas, must be worn. These must be changed if contaminated. Surgical gowns must not be taken into any food/drink area. Similarly, food/drink must not be consumed in clinical areas.
- All 3-in-1 syringe tips, handpieces and ultrasonic scaler tips should be changed after use, and cleaned and autoclaved before re-use.
- Ultrasound scaler handpiece ends, which cannot be sterilized, must be thoroughly cleaned and disinfected before re-use.
- Cling-film or other protectives can be placed across the dental chair control buttons, operating light handles, ultrasonic scaler handpieces and 3-in-1 syringe bodies. The film must be changed or decontaminated with chemical solution after every patient.
- Restorative care must be performed under rubber dam, with high volume suction.
- Work surfaces in the operating area should be protected with disposable material and changed after every patient or the surface should be sanitized.
- The operator should avoid touching unprotected surfaces, the patient's notes, etc. Should extra instruments or other items be required, a non-operating assistant should perform these tasks.
- All 'sharps' must be disposed of in rigid-sided containers. This must include any steel burs, polishing cups or brushes, local anaesthetic cartridges, orthodontic wire, syringe needles, matrix bands and suture needles. 'Sharps' bins must be replaced when not more than 2/3 full.
- Disposable polythene sleeving must be used routinely in oral surgery, for the tubing leading to the handpiece motor.
- Benches and other work surfaces must not be used as seats.
- Resheathing of needles should be avoided wherever possible. Where resheathing is necessary, this must be done using two instruments, or special resheathing devices.
- When cleaning an operation area or instruments, heavy-duty gloves should be worn.
- Before despatch to a laboratory, all impressions and other items, which have intra-oral contamination, should be thoroughly rinsed in running tap water, sprayed with disinfectant and placed in a polythene bag.
- Items received from a laboratory must be thoroughly washed in running tap water before further handling.

### In the event of accidental injury to operator:
- Ensure that the accident is not repeated.
- Wash the wound under running water with soap.
- Consult the occupational health authority immediately.
- The patient's serum must be tested for hepatitis B antigens, and the possibility of HIV positivity must be enquired.
- Discuss with the local occupational health department whether any further action or treatment is necessary.

# Diabetes mellitus

Diabetes mellitus (DM) is a common endocrine disorder. It affects >2% of the population, many patients are undiagnosed and the incidence is constantly rising. DM is caused by deficiency of, or resistance to, insulin → persistently ↑ blood glucose (hyperglycaemia).

**Classification** of DM is as:
- Primary
  - Type I: insulin-dependent; juvenile onset; usually immune-mediated; ↓ insulin production; patients are usually thin; prone to ketoacidosis and needing insulin treatment.
  - Type II: non-insulin-dependent (although insulin often needed); maturity onset; strong genetic component; ↓ sensitivity of insulin receptors; patients are usually obese; no ketoacidosis and usually controlled by diet ± drugs.
- Secondary to
  - pancreatic damage (e.g. pancreatitis, pancreatectomy, haemochromatosis, cystic fibrosis);
  - other endocrine abnormalities (e.g. Cushing's syndrome, corticosteroid therapy, phaeochromocytoma, acromegaly, glucagonoma).

**Presentations** *Type I DM* typically has an acute onset, in a child, who complains of tiredness, weight loss, polyuria and polydipsia. Ketoacidosis (↓ insulin → ↓ glucose usability → ↑ fat metabolism → accumulation of ketone bodies → metabolic acidosis) with hyperventilation (compensates for the acidosis) and a characteristic acetone breath may also be features. *Type II DM* typically has a more insidious onset, in a middle-aged obese patient complaining of fatigue, polyuria and polydipsia. However, many diabetic patients are asymptomatic and detected only through routine blood or urine tests, or present with complications, e.g. infections.

**Diagnosis** of DM is based on two positive laboratory tests (mainly, fasting blood glucose >7 mmol/L) or one positive test in the presence of symptoms (see Table 3.11).

**Acute complications** of DM include:
*Hypoglycaemia* (blood glucose <2.5 mmol/L): a dangerous complication of insulin therapy, usually resulting from ↓ food intake, or overdosage of insulin. It manifests with signs of adrenaline release (anxiety, tremor, rapid pulse, warm and sweaty skin, and dilated pupils) and cerebral hypoglycaemia (neuroglycopenia; confusion, agitation and finally unconsciousness). Hypoglycaemia is at the top of the differential diagnostic list of a collapse of unknown cause, and its management involves the urgent administration of glucose (see Chapter 6).
*Diabetic ketoacidosis:* a feature of poorly controlled type I DM. It presents with signs of metabolic acidosis (hyperventilation, vomiting, ↓ blood bicarbonate, ketonuria and acetone breath) and osmotic diuresis (polyuria, dehydration, hypotension, tachycardia, dry mouth and abdominal pain). The patient may be confused or in coma. Management includes rehydration and administration of insulin and potassium.

**Chronic complications** of DM include:
- Macrovascular disease (atherosclerosis)
  - Ischaemic heart disease (angina, MI)
  - Cerebrovascular disease (TIA, CVA)
  - Peripheral vascular disease (may lead to gangrene)
- Microvascular disease
  - Diabetic nephropathy (→ renal failure)
  - Diabetic retinopathy (→ blindness)
- Diabetic neuropathy
  - Autonomic neuropathy (e.g. postural hypotension)
  - Symmetrical sensory polyneuropathy (starting distally [feet])
- Infections (↑ glucose → abnormal neutrophil function → staphylococcal abscesses, candidosis, accelerated periodontal disease, etc.)
- Diabetic foot (neuropathy [→ calluses]; ischaemia [→ ulcers]; susceptibility to infection [→ spreading foot infection → amputation])

**Management** of DM is aimed at a tight control of blood glucose (<10 mmol/L), which reduces both short and long-term complications, avoiding hypoglycaemia or medicalizing the patient's life.
- *Close monitoring* of blood glucose by home use of a glucometer (recording these in a diary guides adjustments of therapy) and 3-monthly lab. measurements of glycosylated haemoglobin [HbA$_{1c}$] (long-term control).
- *Diet* based on ↑ complex carbohydrates (starch) and ↓ sugar and fats usually helps and may suffice in some patients with type II DM.
- *Healthier life-style* (exercise, avoidance of smoking, etc.) may help the control of diabetes and ↓ cardiovascular complications.
- *Oral hypoglycaemic drugs* are used in type II DM and include:
  - Sulphonylureas (e.g. chlorpropamide, tolbutamide, gliclazide), which stimulate insulin release
  - Biguanides (metformin), which ↑ glucose utilization and ↓ liver gluconeogenesis
  - Thiazolidinediones (e.g. pioglitazone), which ↓ insulin resistance
  - Other drugs (e.g. acarbose)
- *Insulin* is needed in all patients with type I DM as well as some with type II DM. It can only be given parenterally (mainly SC, using a syringe, a 'pen' injection device or an insulin pump). Finding the right regimen for each patient is a challenging task, often involving a combination of short-acting insulin before main meals and intermediate-acting insulin once or twice daily.
  - *Short-acting* insulins: Insulin lispro (Humalog), insulin aspart (Novorapid) and soluble insulin (Actrapid, Humulin S, etc.). Soluble insulin can also be given IV (useful for emergencies and perioperatively).
  - *Intermediate- and long-acting* insulins: Isophane insulin (Insulatard, Humulin I, etc.), insulin zinc suspension (Humulin lente, Monotard, etc.), insulin glargine (Lantus).
  - *Mixtures* of different insulins are available, for example soluble and isophane insulin (e.g. Mixtard).

# Dental aspects of diabetes mellitus

## Oral manifestations

- Periodontal disease is more common and aggressive in poorly controlled diabetics.
- Dry mouth from dehydration.
- Oral candidosis from the immune defect and dryness.
- Salivary gland enlargement (sialosis) from autonomic neuropathy.
- Lichenoid reactions from oral hypoglycaemic drugs.
- Dentoalveolar abscesses may be more common and severe.
- Dry socket may also be more common following dental extractions.

### Infections

Although there is evidence that poorly controlled diabetics have phago-cytic dysfunction, evidence this causes a significantly ↑ susceptibility to infections is not convincing. Equally, the evidence that control of perio-dontitis significantly aids diabetic control is equivocal.

Antimicrobial prophylaxis therefore, should not be used routinely for diabetic patients. It is certainly true nevertheless, that diabetic patients do not tolerate infections well. Insulin requirements ↑ in time of infection → hyperglycaemia and ↑ risk of ketoacidosis. Oral infections also disrupt normal diet → ↑ risk of hypoglycaemic episodes. A prophylactic course of antibiotics may therefore be indicated for some high-risk procedures, especially in patients whose diabetic control is less than satisfactory. When acute infections do occur, they should be treated vigorously.

## General management considerations

Hypoglycaemia may occur during dental treatment, especially if the patient misses their meals. It is best to give diabetic patients early morn-ing appointments (↓ risk of delays and therefore ↓ risk of hypoglycaemia) and advise them not to miss their breakfast or lunch.

►In the short-term, it is always preferable to err on the side of short-term hyperglycaemia; so always have a glucose drink available and use if necessary, or if you are concerned.

Diabetic patients have ↑ risk of conditions such as ischaemic heart dis-ease or renal failure, which may be undiagnosed.

Care must be taken when patients rise from the dental chair, as they may have postural hypotension (due to autonomic neuropathy).

All the above health problems become more relevant if the patient needs GA. Liaise with the anaesthetist. Assess other risk factors for cardio-vascular disease and discuss with the patient's physician.

When treating a diabetic patient who has been severely traumatized, remember that insulin requirements are likely to increase and there is ↑ risk of ketoacidosis. Finally, delayed wound healing should be anticipated.

## Surgery in diabetics

*Patients controlled with diet alone* do not require any special precautions apart from monitoring finger-prick blood glucose before and after sur-gery. If major surgery is planned, blood glucose should be monitored 2-hourly.

*Patients on oral hypoglycaemics*, *if well controlled and only requiring a short GA*, can be managed by stopping their hypoglycaemics for 24 h and monitoring blood glucose levels pre- and postoperatively, 2-hourly until eating again, when medication can be restarted. *If diabetic control is poor or if major surgery is planned*, perioperative insulin infusion is needed as described below.

*Patients on insulin*, *if well controlled and only requiring a short GA*, may be managed safely by operating early in the morning and withholding food and insulin until after the operation. *Longer procedures* are best carried out taking the following measures:
- Patient can have their normal insulin the day before operation.
- Admit early on the morning of operation (or the night before) and take blood 1 h preoperatively for glucose estimation.
- Start IV infusion of:
  - 10% glucose, at a rate of 100–140 mL/h
  - $K^+$ 10 mmol/L added in the infusion fluid
  - 1 unit/mL soluble insulin must be infused constantly, at a rate of 2 units/h (2 mL/h) using a syringe pump
- Blood glucose must be measured hourly throughout the operation (and 2-hourly after), and the rate of insulin infusion adjusted accordingly (↓ if glucose <4 mmol/L and ↑ if glucose >15 mmol/L).
- Once patient is eating again, start normal SC insulin regimen and, when that takes effect (usually 30 min after injection), discontinue the IV soluble insulin (effects of the latter last only for a few minutes).

▶Following most oral and maxillofacial operations, food intake may be ↓ for a period of time, and patients need to adjust their insulin regimen accordingly. Most diabetics are capable of estimating their own insulin requirements according to food intake. Nevertheless, insulin requirement may be ↑ by about 10–20% after surgery, so regular blood glucose monitoring is advisable for a few days postoperatively (patients may prefer to use their glucometer for this).

# Adrenocortical disease

## Adrenocortical hyperfunction

*Glucocorticoid excess (Cushing's syndrome) Causes*—most cases (excluding steroid pharmacotherapy, which is discussed below) are due to adrenal hyperplasia 2° to ACTH excess from a pituitary tumour (Cushing's disease). Less commonly, the cause may be ectopic ACTH production from a small cell lung carcinoma, or excess cortisol production from an adrenal adenoma or carcinoma. *Features* of Cushing's syndrome include fat redistribution (particularly affecting the face [moon face], interscapular region [buffalo hump] and trunk, but with relative sparing of the limbs [central obesity]), hyperglycaemia (2° DM), hypertension, osteoporosis, muscle weakness, thinning of the skin, purpura, skin striae, acne and hirsutism. *Treatment* involves excision or radiotherapy of the responsible gland (pituitary or adrenal). Medical treatment is possible, but only provides temporary effect. *Dental aspects* Once treated, patients are maintained on corticosteroid replacement therapy and then are at risk from an adrenal crisis (see page 208).

*Mineralocorticoid excess (hyperaldosteronism) Causes*—usually 1° due to an adrenocortical adenoma (Conn's syndrome), but occasionally 2° to ↑ renin from renal artery stenosis, severe cardiac failure or liver cirrhosis. *Features* include hypertension (from sodium retention), as well as muscle weakness, polyuria, polydipsia and tetany (from loss of potassium). *Treatment* Spironolactone is given until the affected glands can be excised. *Dental aspects* Risk of adrenal crisis in those who have had the adrenals removed.

*Androgen excess* is usually due to congenital adrenal hyperplasia, and results in hirsutism and virilism (amenorrhoea, deepening of voice and male hair pattern in females).

## Adrenocortical hypofunction

*Primary adrenal insufficiency (Addison's disease) Causes*—usually autoimmune (circulating autoantibodies detected in most cases). Adrenal tuberculosis, sarcoidosis, amyloidosis, malignancy or haemorrhage are rare causes. *Features* Both cortisol and aldosterone are ↓ → hypoglycaemia, hyponatraemia, hyperkalaemia, hypotension, weakness, dizziness, anorexia, weight loss, nausea and vomiting. Skin and mucosal pigmentation are common due to pro-opiomelanocortin excess (an ACTH precursor). Patients are vulnerable to any stress (infection, injury, surgery or GA) → an acute adrenal crisis (Addisonian crisis), which manifests with hypotension, bradycardia, hypoglycaemia, vomiting, dehydration and collapse. *Treatment* is replacement of corticosteroids ± mineralocorticoids. *Dental aspects* Oral hyperpigmentation and risk of adrenal crisis (steroid cover required for dental treatment—see page 208).

*Secondary adrenal insufficiency* may be due to ↓ ACTH (pituitary disease) or, more commonly, corticosteroid therapy.

# Corticosteroid therapy

Corticosteroids (steroids) are commonly used as immunosuppressives in allergic and autoimmune diseases, or to prevent graft rejection. They are also used as a replacement in Addison's disease or after adrenalectomy.

## Adverse effects of steroids

A single high dose of steroids, or short courses (<5 days), are safe. Long-term treatment may be associated with potentially serious complications, including adrenal suppression, hypertension, 2° DM, osteoporosis, growth retardation, peptic ulceration, ↑ susceptibility to infection, delayed healing, proximal myopathy, mood changes or psychosis, fat redistribution (as in Cushing's syndrome), skin striae, bruising and acne. Topical steroids also cause skin thinning.

Pre-existing hypertension or DM are contraindications to systemic steroids. Complications may be reduced if the smallest effective doses of steroids are used, and if they are given on alternate days instead of daily.

### Adrenal suppression

The most significant effect is suppression of ACTH secretion → adrenal atrophy → failure to respond to stress. The length of treatment or doses required for ↓ adrenal function, and the time required for recovery are unpredictable. However, adrenocortical function is likely to be suppressed if the patient is on systemic steroids or has taken daily steroids in excess of 10 mg prednisolone, or equivalent, within the last 3 months.

Patients on steroids should carry a warning card, and all clinicians must be aware that the dose should be ↑ if there is systemic illness, infection, trauma or operation.

Systemic steroids should never be withdrawn abruptly.

## Dental aspects of corticosteroid therapy

Patients in whom adrenocortical function is likely to be suppressed (see above) are at risk of an adrenal crisis if stressed, and are best given steroid cover for dental treatment (despite controversy). If there is doubt as to the need for steroid supplementation, it is possible to examine adrenocortical function with an ACTH stimulation test. Unless you are certain that adrenal function is normal, it is best to provide steroid cover.

- *For minor operations (including conservative dentistry) under LA,* oral steroid supplements (50 mg hydrocortisone or 20 mg prednisolone) 2–4 h preoperatively should suffice, although IV hydrocortisone immediately before operation is preferable.
- *For longer operations (e.g. multiple extractions) under LA or GA,* give hydrocortisone 100 mg IV preoperatively and then 50 mg 6-hourly for a further 24 h. BP should be monitored regularly, and further supplementation given if indicated (↓ BP).
- *For major maxillofacial surgery or trauma* give hydrocortisone 100 mg IV preoperatively and then 50 mg 6-hourly for a further 72 h.

In all the above, normal steroid medication should be continued throughout. Avoid hypoxia, hypotension or severe haemorrhage. Wound healing can be impaired, and antimicrobial prophylaxis should therefore be considered (susceptibility to infection). Other problems such as hypertension, DM, or psychosis may complicate management.

*Oral manifestations*

Long-term and profound systemic immunosuppression may predispose to oral Kaposi's sarcoma, hairy leucoplakia, lymphomas or lip cancer. Topical steroids for use in the mouth rarely produce significant systemic effects, but predispose to oral candidosis.

# Other endocrinopathies

**Hyperthyroidism** *Cause*—mainly Graves' disease (autoimmune disorder with thyroid-stimulating autoantibodies). *Symptoms* Heat intolerance, sweating, ↓ weight, tremor, irritability, ↑ activity, diarrhoea, psychosis, infertility. *Signs* Tachycardia, arrhythmias, warm hands, hair thinning, goitre (thyroid gland enlargement), exophthalmos. *Treatment* Drugs (e.g. carbimazole, propranolol), radioactive iodine, thyroidectomy. *Dental aspects* Anxiety, pain, trauma or GA may precipitate thyroid crisis with tremor, dyspnoea and arrhythmias (e.g. AF). Relative analgesia sedation may be advantageous. Oropharyngeal ulceration (if carbimazole → agranulocytosis).

**Hypothyroidism** *Causes*—Hashimoto's thyroiditis (autoimmune), or anti-thyroid treatment (carbimazole, radioiodine, thyroidectomy). *Symptoms* Cold intolerance, lassitude, ↑ weight, hoarseness, constipation, depression, dementia. May be asymptomatic. *Signs* Bradycardia, dry skin, hair loss, anaemia, myxoedema. Macroglossia and learning disability are features of congenital hypothyroidism. *Treatment* Thyroxine. *Dental aspects* Anaemia and IHD are common complications of hypothyroidism. Sedatives, opioids or GA may precipitate myxoedema coma.

**Hyperparathyroidism** *Causes*—primary (hyperparathyroid adenoma), secondary (caused by ↓ $Ca^{2+}$ due to vitamin D deficiency or renal disease), or tertiary (follows prolonged 2° hyperparathyroidism, which has become autonomous). *Features* Hypercalcaemia (↑ $Ca^{2+}$). Often asymptomatic, but may present with arrhythmias, renal stones, hypertension, peptic ulceration, abdominal pain, ↑ bone resorption (punched-out lesions, pathological fractures and bone pain), psychiatric disorders, weakness, constipation, pancreatitis. *Treatment* Parathyroidectomy. *Dental aspects* Loss of lamina dura, brown tumours (osteolytic giant cell lesions). Management may be complicated by renal disease and arrhythmias.

**Hypoparathyroidism** *Cause*—surgical removal of the parathyroid. *Features* of hypocalcaemia (↓ $Ca^{2+}$) include tetany, epilepsy, psychiatric disorders, perioral and limb paraesthesiae, Chvostek's sign (twitching of facial muscles upon tapping over the facial nerve). *Treatment* Calcium. *Dental aspects* Dental hypoplasia and chronic mucocutaneous candidosis in congenital hypoparathyroidism (candida-endocrinopathy syndrome).

**Phaeochromocytoma** is a catecholamine (adrenaline and nor-adrenaline)-producing tumour of the adrenal medulla. *Features*—of sympathetic over-stimulation, including episodes of anxiety, sweating, flushing, tachycardia, palpitations, hypertension, pyrexia, headache, epigastric pain or 2° DM. *Treatment* Alpha- (e.g. prazosin) and then beta- (e.g. propranolol) blockers, before surgical excision of the adrenal. *Dental aspects* Dental treatment is best avoided in untreated patients. Potent analgesia and sedation are necessary, while adrenaline-containing LA is best avoided (although evidence is weak). Phaeochromocytoma is occasionally associated with oral mucosal neuromas and medullary carcinoma of the thyroid (multiple endocrine neoplasia IIb [Sipple] syndrome).

**Pituitary gland:** pituitary tumours may produce excess pituitary hormones and/or deficiency, visual defects (e.g. bitemporal hemianopia), headaches and other neurological signs. *Treatment* Dopamine agonists may help in some cases (e.g. prolactin-secreting tumours) but transsphenoidal gland excision or radiotherapy are often needed.

Deficiency of pituitary hormones may also results from hypophysectomy or cranial lesions pressing on the hypophysis; hormone replacement is usually necessary.

**Prolactin excess** *Causes* Physiological (breast feeding), pituitary tumour or ↓ dopamine (e.g. antidopaminergic drugs [antipsychotics]). *Features* Galactorrhoea, ↓ libido, infertility and vaginal dryness in women. Galactorrhoea and impotence in men.

**Growth hormone excess** causes gigantism before the epiphyses have fused, and acromegaly thereafter. In gigantism, the skeleton, soft tissues and all organs are enlarged. Features of acromegaly include enlargement of mandible, hands and feet, supraorbital ridges, and soft tissues, plus coarse oily skin, deepening of the voice, macroglossia and tooth spacing. Cardiovascular complications may occur, due to DM, ↑ BP or cardiomyopathy. Kyphosis and other deformities affecting respiration may make GA hazardous.

**Growth hormone deficiency** results in short stature (in children), obesity and weakness.

**Syndrome of inappropriate antidiuretic hormone secretion (SIADH)** may occur after intracranial lesions, head or maxillofacial trauma or surgery. It is characterized by water retention and overhydration causing confusion, ataxia and behavioural disturbances. Fluid restriction and corticosteroids are needed.

**Antidiuretic hormone deficiency (diabetes insipidus)** may be caused by trauma or other intracranial lesions, and results in the production of an excessive volume of dilute urine and thirst.

**Gonadotrophin deficiency** may result in amenorrhoea, infertility, ↓ libido or osteoporosis.

# Renal disorders

Investigations relevant to the kidneys and the urinary tract have been discussed in Chapter 3 (U&Es, urinalysis and abdominal investigations).

**Urinary tract infections (UTIs)** are common in normal sexually active women arising from transfer of bacteria up the short urethra during intercourse. They are also common in patients with urinary catheters. In other men and children, however, UTIs often indicate renal or urinary tract abnormalities or impaired host defences. The commonest culprit is *E. coli*. *Lower UTIs (cystitis)* present with urinary frequency, urgency, dysuria and haematuria, and are treated with trimethoprim, unless culture and sensitivity indicate otherwise. *Upper UTIs (pyelonephritis)* present with fever, vomiting and loin pain, and are treated with cefuroxime IV. ↑ Fluid intake helps treatment and prevention. Some patients suffering with recurrent UTIs need to be on long-term antibiotic prophylaxis.

**Renal stones (calculi)** may be found anywhere from the renal pelvis to the urethra, and are usually calcified. They are more prevalent following dehydration or ↑ $Ca^{2+}$. Stones may be asymptomatic or present with pain (renal colic) and symptoms of UTI. They may pass spontaneously with ↑ fluid intake, or may be removed by lithotripsy or open operation.

**Urinary retention** is usually due to benign prostatic hyperplasia in men, but may also be caused by pain, GA, anticholinergic drugs, neurological disorders, renal failure, bladder or other pelvic tumours. Catheterization is usually required until the cause is treated.
▶Dehydration is the most common cause of not passing urine.

**Tumours** of the kidney are usually renal cell carcinoma in adults and Wilm's tumour in children. Bladder tumours are usually transitional cell carcinoma and are more prevalent in smokers, and workers in the rubber industry. Prostatic adenocarcinomas are common in older men and may only need monitoring with prostatic specific antigen (PSA) assays. When necessary, treatment is with transurethral resection, radiotherapy or radical prostatectomy ± medical therapy with goserelin.

**Glomerulonephritis** is usually immunological in origin, but the exact cause is established from histology and associated clinical features. It may present with haematuria (macroscopic or microscopic), proteinuria, nephritic syndrome (haematuria with proteinuria), nephrotic syndrome (proteinuria, hypoalbuminaemia and oedema) or renal failure. *Nephrotic syndrome* is treated with ↑ protein intake, fluid and salt restriction, and diuretics for associated hypertension.

## Renal failure

Loss of renal function may be caused by pre-renal disorders (e.g. renal hypoperfusion in severe haemorrhage or shock), renal disease (different causes for acute or chronic failure—see below) or post-renal conditions (e.g. urinary obstruction).

*Acute renal failure (ARF)* usually follows circulatory compromise (e.g. from severe infection, trauma or surgery), but may also be caused by urinary obstruction or nephrotoxic drugs including antibiotics (e.g. tetracyclines, gentamycin, vancomycin), NSAIDs (e.g. aspirin), immunosuppressants/cytotoxics (e.g. methotrexate, ciclosporin) and GA (e.g. with enflurane). ARF manifests with rapid deterioration of renal function with ↓ urine output, ↑ urea and creatinine, and electrolyte abnormalities. ARF is managed with full assessment of cardiovascular status, careful fluid balance, and treatment or withdrawal of the cause.

*Chronic renal failure (CRF)* is progressive and irreversible renal damage as shown by ↓ glomerular filtration rate (see page 65). It may be caused by chronic glomerulonephritis, pyelonephritis, hypertension, urinary obstruction, diabetes, SLE, myeloma or congenital renal anomalies. CRF may be asymptomatic or patients may complain of anorexia and nocturia. Features of advanced CRF may include:
- Polyuria and thirst
- Hypertension (vicious cycle between hypertension and CRF)
- IHD and congestive cardiac failure with peripheral and pulmonary oedema (due to hypertension and hyperlipidaemia)
- GI features (anorexia; nausea; vomiting; peptic ulcer; GI bleeding)
- Dermatological features (bruising, pruritus, yellow pigmentation)
- Neurological disturbances (weakness, visual or peripheral sensory disturbances, headaches, seizures, drowsiness or coma)
- ↑ Serum urea, creatine and lipids, and electrolyte disturbances
- Renal osteodystrophy (↓ vitamin $D_3$ production and phosphate retention → ↓ plasma calcium → 2° or tertiary hyperparathyroidism → bone resorption)
- Bleeding tendency (impaired platelet aggregation and ↑ prostacyclin)
- Anaemia (blood loss in the gut and ↓ erythropoietin production)
- Susceptibility to infections (immunoglobulins may be lost; patients may be immunosuppressed; signs of inflammation are masked; infections are poorly controlled and rapidly spread → clinical deterioration)
- Impaired drug excretion (→ ↑ toxicity of drugs excreted by the kidney)

Management of CRF may include:
- Control of fluid balance and restriction of salt and protein intake
- Treatment of symptoms and complications such as:
  - Hypertension (which may cause further renal damage)
  - Oedema (with diuretics)
  - Anaemia (with iron or erythropoietin)
  - Renal osteodystrophy (with calcium and vitamin D supplements)
  - Hyperlipidaemia (which may worsen renal and cardiac function)
  - Infections (with aggressive antimicrobial therapy)
- Advanced CRF needs dialysis. Peritoneal dialysis is simplest and may be carried out at home. Haemodialysis is usually carried out as an outpatient (three 6-hourly sessions each week), via an arteriovenous (A-V) fistula created surgically at the wrist to facilitate the introduction of infusion lines. Heparinization is necessary during haemodialysis.
- End-stage CRF treatment of choice is renal transplantation.

# Dental aspects of renal disorders

This discussion mainly refers to patients with chronic renal failure (CRF).

*Bleeding tendency* is due to vasodilatation and impaired platelet function. Patients on haemodialysis are also heparinized but, although the effect of heparin is brief, dental treatment is best carried out on the day after dialysis, when there has been maximal benefit from the dialysis (including improvement of platelet function) and the effect of heparin has abated. Local haemostatic measures must be taken. If postoperative bleeding is prolonged, or if more extensive surgery is planned, desmopressin or other measures may be necessary (consult haematologist).

*Infections* are poorly controlled, especially in immunosuppressed patients. Odontogenic infections should be treated vigorously, as they may spread rapidly, accelerating tissue catabolism → clinical deterioration. Consult the nephrologist and consider antimicrobial prophylaxis prior to surgery (IV teicoplanin during dialysis provides cover for at least 24 h). Haemodialysis predisposes to blood-borne infections (e.g. viral hepatitis). Patients with indwelling peritoneal catheters are not at higher risk from infection during dental treatment.

*Impaired drug excretion* can result in undesirably enhanced or prolonged drug activity, unless doses are reduced. In addition nephrotoxic, drugs must be avoided.
*Safe drugs* include phenoxymethyl penicillin, flucloxacillin, erythromycin, ketoconazole, lidocaine, codeine and diazepam.
*Avoid* tetracyclines (except doxycycline and minocycline), some cephalosporins (cephalothin and cephaloridine) and NSAIDs (e.g. aspirin).
*Reduce doses* of amoxicillin, ampicillin, benzylpenicillin, metronidazole, clindamycin, vancomycin, fluconazole, aciclovir, paracetamol/acetaminophen, opioids, antihistamines and barbiturates.

*Veins* of the forearms and saphenous veins are lifelines for patients on haemodialysis, as they are used for A-V fistulas, and the latter are prone to infection and thrombosis, and should never be used for injections, venesection or cannulation. Use veins of the antecubital fossa or above.

*Anaemia* may be a contraindication to GA. If Hb <10 g/dL, consult anaesthetist and haematologist regarding further action needed.

*Postoperative complications* may include hyperkalaemia ($K^+$ is primarily intracellular and is released during tissue damage or haemolysis) → arrhythmias. Other complications may be acidaemia or prolonged bleeding necessitating blood transfusion (further increasing serum potassium).

*Underlying diseases and complications* of CRF e.g. hypertension, diabetes, SLE, IHD, cardiac failure or peptic ulceration may affect dental management.

*Oral manifestations* may include oral ulceration, dry mouth, metallic taste, calculus accumulation, halitosis and sialosis. Enamel hypoplasia and delayed tooth eruption may be seen in children with CRF. Renal osteodystrophy may manifest with loss of the lamina dura, osteoporosis, osteolytic areas (brown tumours) and abnormal bone repair after extractions.

**Patients with renal transplants** may still suffer some of the problems of CRF. The immunosuppression may predispose to oral candidosis or herpetic infections and there is also ↑ incidence of lymphoma, Kaposi's sarcoma and lip cancer. Odontogenic infections may spread rapidly in an immunosuppressed person, and antibiotic prophylaxis is therefore advocated for at least 2 years post-transplantation. Steroid supplementation may also be necessary. Carriage of hepatitis viruses is common. Ciclosporin may cause gingival swelling as may calcium-channel blockers. Erythromycin may ↑ ciclosporin toxicity and is therefore contraindicated.

**Patients with nephritic syndrome** are prone to infections because of loss of immunoglobulins and immunosuppressive therapy. Cardiovascular disease is also more prevalent due to hyperlipidaemia and predisposition to thromboses (↑ clotting factors and loss of antithrombin III).

# Genetic skeletal disorders

**Osteogenesis imperfecta** (OI) is a group of inherited disorders that result from a defect in type I collagen → bone fragility. Multiple fractures follow minimal trauma, and, despite rapid healing, lead to bone distortion and severe skeletal deformity. However, the jaws do not appear to be particularly brittle, and tooth extractions can usually be carried out safely. Some types of OI are associated with blue sclerae, and others (mainly type IV) with dentinogenesis imperfecta, which consists of thicker dentine (→ brown opalescent tooth discolouration) that adheres poorly to enamel (→ rapid tooth wear). Easy bruising, laxity of tendons and ligaments and mitral valve prolapse may be seen. Mitral valve prolapse with regurgitation necessitates antibiotic prophylaxis against infective endocarditis. Cardiovascular disease or chest deformities may complicate management, particularly if GA is required.

**Osteopetrosis** is due to a defective osteoclastic activity → ↑ bone density. In severe forms, bone marrow space is ↓ → anaemia, thrombocytopenia and, occasionally, leucopenia. Blood supply is also ↓ → susceptibility to osteomyelitis. Bones, although denser, are also prone to fracture. Cranial nerve compression may cause pain or other neurological impairments such as blindness, deafness or facial paralysis. Tooth eruption is usually retarded. Patients are often treated with systemic steroids.

**Cleidocranial dysplasia** is an autosomal dominant disorder of membranous bone formation → skeletal defects involving mainly the clavicles and skull. Complete or partial absence of clavicles causes hypermobility of the shoulders. The head is large and brachycephalic with frontal, parietal and occipital bossing, hypertelorism and persisting fontanelles. The middle third of face is hypoplastic and the palate is high-arched. Malformed teeth, retained deciduous teeth, multiple unerupted permanent teeth, supernumeraries and dentigerous cysts may be seen.

**Achondroplasia** is an autosomal dominant disorder of cartilaginous bone formation → short limbs with a relatively large head ('circus dwarf').

**Crouzon's syndrome** is due to premature fusion of the cranial sutures → learning disability and neurological disorders. Patients have a characteristic 'frog-like' facies with hypertelorism, exophthalmos and a hypoplastic middle third. Anterior open bite and high-arched palate are common. Craniofacial surgery may be needed to correct the craniosynostosis and facial deformities.

**Treacher–Collins syndrome** is characterized by mandibular and zygomatic hypoplasia, malformed ears, high-arched or cleft palate and dental malocclusion and downward-slanting palpebral fissures.

**Marfan's syndrome** is an autosomal dominant connective tissue disorder. Patients are tall with particularly long arms and fingers (arachnodactyly). Ligament laxity predisposes to subluxation or dislocation of joints, including the TMJ. Subluxation or dislocation of the lens is common → visual impairment. Aortic dissection is common and may be fatal.

Mitral valve prolapse predisposes to infective endocarditis. Regular medical examinations are necessary and physical activity must be restricted.

**Ehlers–Danlos syndrome** is a group of collagen disorders presenting with hyperextensible and fragile skin (skin and oral mucosa may split following minor trauma; wounds gape; healing is slow), hypermobile joints (e.g. recurrent dislocation of the TMJ) and fragile vessels (rupture of major arteries; widespread purpura; bleeding tendency). In type VIII Ehlers-Danlos syndrome there is early onset periodontal disease. Oral operations should be avoided if at all possible, because of the bleeding diathesis and poor wound healing. Antimicrobial prophylaxis is necessary in those with mitral valve prolapse.

**Cherubism** is an inherited condition, which is similar to fibrous dysplasia (see page 219), but affects the jaws bilaterally, causing facial fullness, upward gazing eyes, malocclusion and abnormalities of teeth.

# Disorders of bone metabolism

**Rickets and osteomalacia** are defective mineralization of bone in children and adults respectively. Causes include

- vitamin D lack (from nutritional deficiency, malabsorption or impaired metabolism due to renal or liver disease, lack of sunlight or prolonged use of certain drugs [e.g. phenytoin, rifampicin, isoniazid]).
- loss of calcium and phosphate (due to renal disease, impaired renal reabsorption of phosphate in familial hypophosphataemia) or
- excessive calcium demands during pregnancy.

In the UK, it is more prevalent among populations of Indian Sub-Continent origin, probably due to lack of sunshine and eating of chapattis, which impair calcium absorption. The bones are soft, weak and readily deformed (a feature more prominent in weight-bearing bones). Green-stick fractures of bones are also common. Bone pain and muscle weakness are prominent features. Teeth seem to be spared from the effects of rickets, although, in familial hypophosphataemia, pulp chambers are larger and prone to pulpitis and subsequent dental abscesses.

**Osteoporosis** is a deficiency of both bone matrix and calcium salts (osteopenia). Post-menopausal women are mainly affected, but other causes include old age, poor diet, hypogonadism, Cushing's syndrome, corticosteroid therapy, hyperthyroidism, alcoholism, smoking, immobilization and family history of osteoporosis. Accurate assessment of diminishing bone mass is now possible with dual X-ray absorptiometers.

Common complications of osteoporosis are vertebral body fractures → gradual spinal collapse and chest deformities, and hip (neck of femur) fractures—which are associated with significant morbidity and mortality in the elderly. Hormone replacement therapy (HRT) is effective for the prevention of osteoporosis in women with an early menopause. The bisphosphonates (e.g. etidronate, alendronate) are also effective for prophylaxis and treatment of osteoporosis. These occasionally cause mouth ulcers, or jaw necrosis, when given parenterally. Calcitonin is a useful alternative. ↑ Dietary intake of calcium and vitamin D are helpful.

**Paget's disease** is a common disorder of bone metabolism with slowly progressing bone enlargement and deformity. It affects mainly older men and the aetiology is unknown. In the early phase, bone resorption predominates but later there is ↑ bone vascularity and apposition. Finally, bones expand and sclerose with ↓ blood supply. Skull radiographs may initially reveal radiolucencies, which are later replaced by a characteristic dense 'cotton-wool' appearance. Laboratory evidence includes ↑ serum alkaline phosphatase and ↑ urine calcium and hydroxyproline.

The hands and feet are usually spared, but the jaws (especially the maxilla) may be affected → ↑ tooth spacing, occlusal abnormalities and root hypercementosis or resorption. Bones may become painful, cranial nerves may be compressed (→ neurological complaints) and pathological fractures may occur. Malignant transformation into osteosarcoma has been reported.

Treatment is with analgesics and bisphosphonates or calcitonin, both of which suppress bone turnover.

At the later stages of Paget's disease, tooth extraction may be problematic, as bone is inelastic and roots hypercementosed. Alveolar bone fractures are likely, so a surgical approach with adequate exposure must be performed. Prophylactic antibiotics should be considered to prevent postoperative infection, which is likely because of ↓ bone vascularity.

**Fibrous dysplasia** is a disease of unknown aetiology, usually presenting in childhood and characterized by replacement of an area of bone by fibrous tissue. A localized swelling appears and gradually ossifies (giving a characteristic 'ground-glass' radiographic appearance) and becomes stabilized. Fibrous dysplasia usually involves only one bone (*monostotic fibrous dysplasia*), this often being the maxilla. When several bones are affected (*polyostotic fibrous dysplasia*), there is also occasionally cutaneous hyperpigmentation (*Jaffe's syndrome*), often with precocious puberty in females (*Albright's syndrome*).

Fibrous dysplasia does not usually require treatment. Radiotherapy must be avoided, as it has been associated with malignant transformation. Surgery is often employed after puberty to correct cosmetic defects.

**Hormonal abnormalities** such as hyperparathyroidism and acromegaly also affect bone metabolism (see pages 210–211).

# Joint disorders

**Back pain** is the most common musculoskeletal complaint. It is usually due to muscle strain, or a prolapsed intervertebral disc irritating a nerve root, a pain then radiates to the relevant dermatome (usually the ipsilateral buttock and thigh). Less frequently, the cause may be trauma or ankylosing spondylitis.

With advanced age, osteoporosis, degenerative joint disease and malignant disease should also be included in the differential diagnosis.

**Osteoarthritis (OA)** is the commonest type of arthritis. It affects many of the elderly, and is particularly symptomatic in women. Weight-bearing or traumatized joints are mainly involved. There is cartilage degeneration (↓ joint space), and underlying bone becomes exposed and proliferates, producing osteophytes and joint deformity. OA cannot be explained simply by a natural wear-and-tear phenomenon.

Clinically, there is joint pain and stiffness, which are worse towards the end of the day and lead to ↓ function. Swellings at distal interphalangeal joints (Heberden's nodes) are characteristic. Crepitus may be palpable in the TMJ.

Treatment is by weight reduction, analgesics and physiotherapy. Arthroplasty (joint replacement) is necessary for severe cases. The patient should not reduce activity; this leads to earlier disability.

**Rheumatoid arthritis (RA)** is an immune-mediated multi-system disease affecting 2% of the population, women in particular. An inflammatory process produced by prostaglandins and cytokines leads to symmetrical deforming polyarthritis, presents with swollen, stiff and painful joints, particularly in the morning. The hands are typically affected with joint swelling, muscle wasting, tenderness and ulnar deviation at the metacarpophalangeal joints. Other features include subcutaneous nodules, lymphadenopathy and anaemia. Radiographically, there is widening of the joint space and adjacent osteoporosis. Rheumatoid factor is typically positive and antinuclear antibodies may also be detected.

*Treatment* consists primarily of encouraging exercise, and NSAIDs. Immunosuppressive therapy early in the disease may significantly slow the disease process and reduce morbidity and disability. Corticosteroids (e.g. prednisolone) have been used with relative success, but disease-modifying antirheumatoid drugs (DMARDs) are now used increasingly. DMARDs include methotrexate (which in low doses [e.g. 5–20 mg weekly] is probably the safest and most effective), sulphasalazine, gold, ciclosporin, penicillamine, hydroxychloroquine and azathioprine. Tumour necrosis factor-α inhibitors (etanercept and infliximab), are gaining ground. Household adjustments and psychological support are valuable aids. Joint replacement may sometimes be necessary.

*Dental management* may be affected by the disease process or treatment. RA commonly affects the TMJ but symptoms are usually slight. Dislocation of the atlanto-axial joint or fracture of the odontoid peg may occur during the induction of GA.

RA is associated with mild immunosuppression, made worse by immuno-suppressive therapy. Oral hygiene can be problematic due to ↓ manual dexterity. Sjögren's syndrome is strongly associated with RA.

Aspirin may cause GI bleeding and worsen anaemia. Steroids may cause oral candidosis. DMARDs may produce mouth ulceration (methotrexate, sulphasalazine, penicillamine), lichenoid reactions (gold, penicillamine, hydroxychloroquine) and severe systemic adverse effects including mar-row depression and hepatic or renal failure.

*Juvenile RA* is a severe form of RA affecting young children. Cases of ankylosis of the TMJ and micrognathia have been reported.

*Felty's syndrome* comprises of RA, splenomegaly, lymphadenopathy, anaemia and leucopenia (predisposing to oral infection and ulceration).

**Psoriatic arthritis** resembles mild RA, but affects primarily the lower spine and sacro-iliac joints, and is associated with psoriasis (see page 225).

**Ankylosing spondylitis** is an HLA B27 +ve chronic inflammatory arthritis, mainly affecting young males. The spine is predominantly affected, with inflammation of the joints and ligament and tendon inser-tions. Subsequent ossification causes fusion of adjacent vertebral bodies, with progressive back pain and stiffness → a fixed flexed spine, and ↓ chest expansion. The TMJ may be affected → ↓ mouth opening, which, together with chest deformity and frequently associated cardiac lesions, makes GA hazardous. Treatment is with NSAIDs and physiotherapy.

**Gout** is an arthropathy resulting from joint deposition of urate crystals, predominantly affecting adult men. Gout may be due to an inborn error of metabolism resulting in ↑ serum uric acid, or 2° to cytotoxic therapy or radiotherapy of myeloproliferative disorders. Excessive alcohol intake may precipitate an acute attack but is not the cause of gout. Deposition of urate crystals and subsequent phagocytosis result in acute inflamma-tion and severe pain of the affected joints, the metatarsophalangeal joint of the big toe in particular. Masses of urate crystals (tophi) may form in joints (causing deformity) or in extra-articular sites (e.g. pinna of ear). Treatment is with NSAIDs (NOT aspirin, which is contraindicated) to relieve attacks, and allopurinol (→ ↓ urate production) between attacks. Allopurinol can cause oral ulceration. Gout is often associated with IHD, DM, hypertension and renal disease—which may affect management.

**Seronegative spondyloarthropathy (Reiter's disease)** is an immunologically mediated disorder affecting young males following a gut or genito-urinary infection. It presents with chronic or relapsing and migratory arthritis, conjunctivitis, urethritis (sterile pyuria), circinate penile lesions, sterile abscesses of the palms and soles (keratoderma blenorrhagica), and oral lesions resembling migratory glossitis, but affecting any part of the mouth. The disease is usually self-limiting, espe-cially if the underlying cause can be treated, but NSAIDs may be used.

# Muscle disorders

**Muscular dystrophies** are genetic disorders characterized by progressive muscle weakness.

*Duchenne muscular dystrophy* is the most common form, affects males (X-linked recessive inheritance) and is due to lack of dystrophin (a muscle protein). Proximal muscles are primarily affected, and the child has difficulty standing and walking, and typically has to climb up his legs in order to stand (Gower's sign). Paradoxically, the affected muscles are enlarged. The hands, head and neck are usually spared. Finally, patients are crippled, and cardiomyopathy and respiratory insufficiency lead to death in early adulthood.

**Myotonic disorders** are genetic conditions characterized by abnormally slow muscle relaxation following contraction. Muscle weakness is a feature of some types. Common complications include cardiac conduction defects, respiratory impairment, behavioural problems and suxamethonium sensitivity (→ malignant hyperthermia).

**Myasthenia gravis** is an autoimmune disorder with circulating autoantibodies against acetylcholine receptors affecting the neuromuscular junction → severe muscle weakness and fatiguability. It mainly affects young adult women, and is associated with thymic hyperplasia or thymoma. All muscles are affected, worse as the day goes on → an expressionless face, hanging jaw, squinting, difficulty speaking and swallowing, and respiratory impairment. *Treatment* is with an anticholinesterase (e.g. pyridostigmine) and a corticosteroid ± other immunosuppressive drugs. Thymectomy is occasionally curative.

*Dental treatment* is best carried out early in the morning: then routine medication has its maximal effect and the patient is not tired. Fatigue or emotional stress may precipitate a myasthenic crisis. GA and IV sedation should be avoided as they may further impair respiration. Myasthenia gravis may be associated with Sjögren's syndrome. Thymoma is associated with chronic candidosis. Corticosteroids may also cause candidosis, as well as pose other management problems. Anticholinesterases cause ↑ salivation.

**Polymyositis and dermatomyositis** are immune-mediated inflammatory myopathies → muscle weakness and pain. Proximal leg muscles are predominantly affected, but patients may also have difficulty speaking and swallowing. The condition is termed dermatomyositis when there is skin involvement, typically with a violaceous rash across the nasal bridge. Other autoimmune disorders may be associated and, in ~10% of patients, there is an underlying malignancy.

**Giant cell arteritis** is an immune-mediated vasculitis, with inflammation affecting medium-sized arteries → luminal obliteration → ischaemic muscle pain. It may affect primarily the temporal region (cranial or temporal arteritis), or be more widespread, affecting several muscles (polymyalgia rheumatica).

*Cranial or temporal arteritis* presents as a severe unilateral throbbing temporal headache. The temporal artery is prominent and tender, and

ESR is ↑, but diagnosis is only confirmed by biopsy of the artery. Treatment is with high dose systemic corticosteroids to avoid complications such as optic nerve ischaemia → blindness. Ischaemia may also affect muscles of mastication or the tongue. Temporal arteritis must be differentiated from other causes of headaches, as well as from TMJ pain-dysfunction syndrome, atypical facial pain and trigeminal neuralgia. It is a medical emergency, requiring systemic steroids.

*Polymyalgia rheumatica* may coexist with cranial arteritis, and typically presents with pain, stiffness and weakness of the shoulders, upper arms, buttocks and thighs (proximal distribution). Small doses of corticosteroids may help, although the disease is usually self-limiting.

# Skin disorders

**Eczema** is another term used for dermatitis, and may result from acute or chronic irritation of the skin. Itchy erythematous dry skin is a consistent feature. Classification can be confusing, but the main types include:

*Atopic eczema (atopic dermatitis)*—very common in childhood and considered to be due to hypersensitivity (e.g. to house dust mite [↑ in warm, carpeted and poorly ventilated homes], animal fur, foods, etc.) and damaged skin barrier (primarily due to detergents, like soap), in susceptible individuals (strong hereditary component). Treatment is by avoidance of irritants and allergens (e.g. home modifications), topical steroids used during exacerbations and frequent use of emollients (to rehydrate and strengthen the skin barrier → ↓ need for steroids).

*Contact eczema (contact dermatitis)*—a localized form of eczema caused by irritation by damaging chemicals (e.g. detergents) or chronic topical exposure to allergens (e.g. nickel, latex).

*Seborrhoeic eczema (seborrhoeic dermatitis)*—an inflammatory disorder associated with overgrowth of the fungus, *Malassezia furfur*. It mainly affects young men and is characterized by a pruritic erythematous rash and scaling of the face (often including the eyebrows) and scalp (severe dandruff). Treatment of facial lesions is with combined steroid and azole antifungal creams (e.g. Daktafort), while scalp involvement usually responds to ketoconazole shampoo. Emollients are helpful.

An *infantile form* of seborrhoeic dermatitis affects most neonates, especially in the scalp ('cradle cap') where a yellowish crust is seen. Treatment is not usually required.

**Acne** is a common chronic facial rash of adolescence with a complex aetiology. Some individuals are predisposed to hyperkeratosis of the pilosebaceous ducts → follicular plugging → formation of open or closed comedones (blackheads or whiteheads, respectively) presenting as red papules. In addition, there may be ↑ androgens and/or progesterone → ↑ sebum production → overgrowth of *Propionibacterium acnes* → formation of inflammatory pustules. The skin is usually greasy and lesions may enlarge considerably, leaving scars after resolution.

Treatment usually consists of regular washing of the face with soap and water in combination with benzoyl peroxide cream, topical antibacterial agents (clindamycin or tetracycline), or topical retinoids (tretinoin or isotretinoin). Long-term oral antibiotic therapy (e.g. oxytetracycline) or co-cyprindiol (oral contraceptive with an anti-androgenic effect) may be used, if topical regimens fail. Oral isotretinoin (Roaccutane) is reserved for severe scarring acne un-responsive to other methods. It reduces sebum, but is toxic and teratogenic.

**Rosacea** is a chronic inflammatory condition that affects middle-aged individuals. Vasomotor instability and the skin mite, *Demodex folliculorum* have been implicated. Alcohol, hot beverages, extremes of temperature and topical steroids may worsen the condition. Rosacea presents with diffuse facial erythema and a papulo-pustular eruption affecting the forehead, cheeks and nose. Treatment is with topical or systemic antibiotics (tetracycline or metronidazole). Topical or systemic retinoids may also be used.

*Rhinophyma* is a form of rosacea affecting the nose, particularly in men. Hypertrophy of the sebaceous glands results in a thickened and greasy nose. Rhinophyma is usually treated with laser surgery.

**Perioral dermatitis** is an inflammatory condition affecting young women and associated with the use of topical steroids or cosmetics. Clinically, it presents as an erythematous papulo-pustular perioral rash. Treatment involves withdrawal of causal agents, and administration of long-term oral oxytetracycline.

**Psoriasis** is a proliferative inflammatory disorder presenting with well-defined red plaques covered by silvery scales, typically on the knees, elbows, ears and scalp. The nails are commonly affected with pitting ('ice-pick pits') and onycholysis. Psoriatic arthritis is a less common feature. Aetiology is unknown; there seems to be a strong genetic influence as well as influence from infections, drugs, trauma, sunlight or stress. Treatment may include emollients, topical agents (keratinolytics [e.g. salicylic acid or coal tar], steroids, dithranol, or retinoids). Phototherapy and low-dose oral methotrexate are considered in unresponsive patients.

**Blistering autoimmune disorders** are rare. *Pemphigus:* Autoantibodies against the desmosomal protein, desmoglein → intraepithelial blisters that rupture easily → widespread severe erosions, potentially lethal. Oral lesions are invariable and >50% of cases present with these. Treatment is with high-dose systemic steroids or other immunosuppressants. *Cicatricial (or mucous membrane) pemphigoid:* Autoantibodies against epithelial basement membrane proteins → subepithelial vesicles or bullae, particularly affecting mucous membranes (mouth, eyes, etc.) → scarring after healing (rare in the mouth, but in the eyes or larynx it is a serious complication). Treatment is usually topical steroids.

Mouth lesions are rare in: *bullous pemphigoid* which is histologically similar to cicatricial pemphigoid, but affects mainly the skin; *dermatitis herpetiformis* which produces an itchy vesicular rash on extensor surfaces, associated with coeliac disease; and *linear IgA disease,* which may produce a similar clinical presentation.

**Cutaneous lichen planus** may be seen in ~10% of patients presenting with oral lesions and occasionally it may be seen as an independent condition. Aetiology is unknown, although a complex immunopathogenesis is suspected. Skin lesions are usually small polygonal red to violaceous itchy papules with a fine network of white striae on the surface (Wickham's striae) and affect particularly the flexor surfaces of the wrists. Treatment is usually topical steroids or tacrolimus.

**Erythema multiforme** is an immune-mediated disorder in response to infections (e.g. HSV, mycoplasma) or drugs (e.g. hydantoin). Target lesions of the skin (red rings with a pale centre) are typical, although any type of rash can develop in any site (mouth, eyes, hands, feet, genitals, etc.). Stevens–Johnson syndrome is a severe form of the disease.

**Infections** affecting the face are discussed on pages 196–197.

# Surgical dermatology of the face

## Benign skin lesions

*Ephelides (freckles)* are small pigmented macules resulting from ↑ melanin production. They affect young people and fade with ↓ sun exposure.

*Lentigos* are similar to freckles, but result from melanocytic hyperplasia. They affect older individuals and are usually permanent.

*Naevi (moles)* are benign neoplasms of naevus cells (almost identical to melanocytes). They affect most people from an early age. They may be macular or papular and are usually pigmented.

*Seborrhoeic warts* are flat, usually pigmented nodules or plaques, with a rough, warty surface. They become common with ↑ age and are completely benign, but may be removed with cryotherapy, curettage, or shave biopsy for cosmetic reasons.

*Viral warts* are caused by human papillomaviruses (HPV). They are typically exophytic with a 'warty' cauliflower-like surface. They are common on the hands, particularly in children and young adults and transmitted by direct contact. Those on the plantar surface of the feet (verrucae) may be flat and inward-growing. Genital warts are usually sexually transmitted and may be oncogenic. Most viral warts will resolve spontaneously, although this may take years. Treatment is usually by cryotherapy; surgical excision is rarely required. Topical keratinolytics (e.g. salicylic acid or podophyllin) or the immunostimulator imiquimod may be helpful.

*Keratoacanthoma* is a rapidly-growing nodule with a central keratin plug. It usually resolves over a few months but is best excised to exclude squamous cell carcinoma (SCC).

*Epidermoid cysts* (previously thought to be sebaceous cysts) appear as cutaneous nodules with a punctum on the surface. They are filled with keratin, which can spill, causing inflammation (although inflammation is often due to 2° infection). Problematic lesions may be excised.

## Premalignant skin lesions

*Actinic keratosis* is relatively common in sun-exposed sites of fair-skinned older persons. Lesions present as red plaques up to 1 cm in diameter with a rough surface occasionally scaly or hyperkeratotic. There is epithelial dysplasia and actinic damage of the underlying connective tissue. Cryotherapy is usually effective, as is topical cytotoxic therapy with fluorouracil cream (Efudix). Excision may be needed to exclude SCC.

*Bowen's disease (carcinoma-in-situ)* is basically an SCC confined to the epidermis (not yet invaded beyond the basement membrane). Clinical presentation and treatment are similar to actinic keratosis.

*Lentigo maligna* is an irregular pigmented macule affecting sun-exposed skin of elderly people. It is basically a 'melanoma-in-situ', which may take decades to enter an invasive phase. Excision is the treatment of choice.

## Malignant skin tumours

*Basal cell carcinoma (BCC; rodent ulcer)* is the most common form of skin cancer and affects sun-exposed sites, the midface in particular. Elderly patients with fair skin and a history of excessive sun exposure are typically affected. BCC usually (nodular) presents as a slow-growing nodule with an ulcerated/crusted centre, raised pearly margins and telangiectatic surface vessels. The morphoeic type presents as an indurated yellow plaque, resembling a scar. Sebaceous adenomas may have a similar appearance.

BCCs rarely metastasize but are locally destructive; therefore, surgical excision (>3 mm margin) is the standard treatment, with recurrence rate ~5%. Mohs' microscopically guided surgery provides the highest clearance rates. If surgery is contraindicated, radiotherapy may be equally effective and is more practical for wide superficial lesions (morphoeic and superficial types), which tend to recur more commonly following surgery. Nevertheless, it requires several visits, and aesthetic results are usually sub-optimal. Curettage and cryotherapy are occasionally used, but recurrence rates are higher.

*Gorlin's syndrome* is an autosomal dominant condition consisting of multiple basal cell naevoid carcinomas, odontogenic keratocysts and skeletal abnormalities.

*SCC* of the skin is more aggressive than BCC, and can metastasize, but is more indolent than mouth SCC. Sun exposure is the main aetiological factor. Clinically it appears as an ill-defined keratotic lesion with an ulcerated/crusted surface and slightly raised indurated margins. The ears and lower lip are predominantly affected. Treatment is with excision (>5 mm margin) or radiotherapy.

*Malignant melanoma* is the most aggressive form of skin cancer, with early metastases. Sunburns at an early age seem to be implicated. There are two major types, including a superficially-spreading type (irregular pigmented macule) and a nodular type (rapidly-growing pigmented nodule that may ulcerate—the most aggressive). Melanoma may be difficult to differentiate from a mole and, in some cases, it arises from a pre-existing mole. Suspect features are mainly changes in size, shape or colour. Treatment is with wide surgical excision (>10 mm margin) but, occasionally, lymph node dissection, radiotherapy and/or chemotherapy may also be employed. Microscopical measurement of tumour thickness (Breslow's thickness) is the major determinant of prognosis, with survival rates rapidly declining in thicknesses >1 mm.

*Kaposi's sarcoma* is a tumour caused by human herpesvirus 8 (HHV-8), arising from endothelium, and presenting as a purple plaque or nodule. The face and mouth are mainly involved in the immunodeficiency-related type of Kaposi's sarcoma, which primarily affects persons sexually infected with HIV, and may be multifocal. Treatment is usually with radiotherapy, but immunotherapy or chemotherapy for multifocal disease.

# Hypersensitivity

### Type I: acute (atopy and anaphylaxis)

*Pathogenesis:* Within minutes of exposure, antigens (allergens) combine with antibodies (IgE) on the surface of mast cells or basophils (in a patient previously sensitized to the antigen). Degranulation of the mast cells, found mainly beneath the skin and mucous membranes of the eyes, nose and throat, releases inflammatory mediators, which may be early (histamine, adenosine, neutrophil chemotactic factor, proteases, heparin) or late (leukotrienes, prostaglandin, platelet activating factor, cytokines), causing vasodilatation, ↑ vascular permeability, chemotaxis and contraction of smooth muscle (bronchoconstriction).

*Allergens:* Pollen, dust, foods (peanuts), insect stings (bees and wasps) drugs (penicillin, codeine, aspirin), latex, physical stimuli (hot and cold).

*Clinical manifestations:* Urticaria, allergic rhinitis and conjunctivitis, angio-oedema, asthma, anaphylaxis.

### Type II: cytotoxic (antibody mediated)

*Pathogenesis:* Antibodies (IgG or IgM) are directed against intrinsic (auto-immune diseases) or exogenous (e.g. transfusion reaction) antigens. Destruction of cells carrying the antigens may occur through phagocytosis (antibody acting as an opsonin), complement-dependent lysis (as in transfusion reactions, fetal erythroblastosis and autoimmune haemolytic anaemia) or by killer cells. In some cases, the antibodies cause cellular dysfunction (as in Graves' disease).

### Type III: immune-complex (IC) disease (complex mediated)

*Pathogenesis:* Antigen–antibody (immune) complexes are commonly formed and usually eliminated by phagocytes. Some ICs are deposited in tissues → complement activation and attraction of polymorphs (i.e. inflammation). The antigens may be:

- Exogenous (e.g. micro-organisms [streptococci, HBV] or drugs [heroin]), as in:
  - Rheumatic fever (following streptococcal infection)
  - Polyarteritis nodosa (hepatitis B antigen carriage)
  - Serum sickness (from repeated injections of drugs)
- Endogenous (antigens of collagen diseases or tumours may form persistent ICs, which are then deposited on vessels, joints, kidneys or skin)

### Type IV: delayed type hypersensitivity (cell mediated)

These reactions occur a few days after exposure to the antigen. A central role is played by antigen-presenting cells and T lymphocytes.

*Contact hypersensitivity* Low molecular weight antigens (haptens) bind to host proteins before being taken up by Langerhans' cells in the epidermis and presented to T cells in the lymph nodes. Subsequent exposure to the antigen will elicit large numbers of cytokines from T cells → further recruitment of lymphocytes and macrophages. Contact dermatitis (nickel allergy) is a good example.

*Graft-versus-host-disease* follows bone marrow transplantation (haemo-poeitic stem cell transplantation). Donated T cells attack the recipient, mainly mucocutaneous and liver tissues. Orofacial lesions may be liche-noid or sclerodermatous.

*Granulomatous diseases* (tuberculosis, sarcoidosis, Crohn's disease, orofacial granulomatosis, foreign body reactions, leprosy, leishmaniasis) result from the inability of macrophages to destroy certain pathogens or foreign bodies → granulomas (central zone of macrophages, epithelioid cells and giant cells surrounded by lymphocytes and fibrous tissue).

# Immunologically mediated disorders

## Allergies

Allergies are exacerbated responses of the immune system to an exoge-nous substance, including hay fever, extrinsic asthma (see page 146), food allergy, allergic angioedema, urticaria, and systemic anaphylaxis. These may present singly or, not infrequently, in combinations.

*Laboratory tests* for allergies include:
• Total serum IgE levels (paper radioimmunosorbent test [PRIST])
• IgE to specific antigens (radioallergosorbent test [RAST])
*Clinical (skin) tests* need controls, and for identification of allergens include:
• Prick test (intradermal injection of allergen), for type I hypersensitivity
• Patch test (application of allergen on a disk, which is then taped on to the skin), for type IV hypersensitivity

It must be emphasized that no tests can reliably predict the possibility of an allergic or anaphylactic reaction; diagnosis may need to be based largely on the patient's history regarding previous reactions.
Furthermore, there is risk of anaphylaxis following prick tests.

**Food allergy** is common but also commonly overdiagnosed. Furthermore, it is not the same as food intolerance, which is far more common (e.g. dose-related reactions to food toxins, preservatives, etc.). *Oral allergy syndrome* is an acute allergic reaction (precipitated usually by fruits or vegetables) → pruritus, irritation and swelling of the lips, tongue and throat. *Orofacial granulomatosis (OFG)* may be a delayed type of food hypersensitivity → granulomas in the face and mouth.

**Allergic angioedema** is characterized by rapid development of oedematous swelling, typically of lips, eyelids, and/or larynx. In severe cases, the airways may be threatened, constituting an emergency. Acute cases are treated as for anaphylaxis (see Chapter 6). Uncomplicated cases are treated with antihistamines (adverse effects include sedation and dry mouth).
*Hereditary angioedema* is not an allergy but a familial deficiency of C1 esterase inhibitor. The precipitant is usually blunt trauma (including den-tal treatment).

**Systemic anaphylaxis** is an acute-onset (type I) generalized and poten-tially fatal reaction to various allergens (e.g. penicillin, peanuts, bee sting, latex). Clinically it may pesent with pallor, swelling (e.g. facial angioedema), rash (e.g. urticaria), itching, respiratory difficulty (laryngeal oedema or asthma), cyanosis, peripheral vasodilatation, ↓ BP, ↑HR, arrhythmias, shock, abdominal pain, vomiting, or diarrhoea.
Management of anaphylaxis is an emergency (discussed in Chapter 6).

## Autoimmune diseases

Autoimmune diseases result from the formation of antibodies that target host antigens (autoantibodies). The fundamental cause is unclear. *Organ-specific autoimmune diseases* (e.g. Graves' disease (hyperthyroidism), Addison's disease [hypoadrenalism], type I diabetes, pernicious anaemia, pemphigus, pemphigoid, etc.) are caused by organ or cell-specific autoantibodies → primarily type II hypersensitivity reactions.

*Collagen (or connective tissue, or rheumatoid) diseases* (rheumatoid arthritis, lupus erythematosus, systemic sclerosis, Sjögren's syndrome, polymyositis/dermatomyositis and mixed connective tissue disease) are due to non organ-specific autoantibodies → to type II or III hypersensitivity reactions. Raynaud's phenomenon (see pages 25 and 136) is often associated.

The immunopathogenesis of autoimmune conditions is not as clearcut as the above distinction implies and several other immune mechanisms (e.g. complement activation) may be in process.

**Systemic lupus erythematosus (SLE)** is due to the formation and inadequate removal of ICs → widespread vasculitis and multi-system disease. Antinuclear antibodies (ANA) are detected in most patients. Anti-double-stranded DNA, rheumatoid factor (RF), and other antibodies may also be present. Typically, young women are affected and present with fever, malaise and, more characteristically, joint pains and skin rash (e.g. photosensitivity, or the well-known 'butterfly' rash over the cheeks—erythematous eruption with white raised margins). Other features may result from involvement of the kidneys (→ hypertension or renal failure), heart (→ pericarditis or endocarditis), blood (→ anaemia, leucopenia, thrombocytopenia), CNS (→ neurological or psychiatric disease), etc. Oral lesions may mimic those of lichen planus. Treatment is with NSAIDs, systemic steroids (for the acute phases) and immunosuppressive agents such as azathioprine, chloroquine or methotrexate. Dental management may be complicated by anaemia, bleeding tendency, risk of infective endocarditis, Sjögren's syndrome, renal disease, steroid therapy, and adverse effects of immunosuppressants (e.g. oral ulceration).

**Systemic sclerosis (scleroderma)** is characterized by fibrosis of the subcutaneous tissues → progressive stiffening of the skin, GI tract and other organs (lungs, heart, kidneys, etc.). Calcinosis, Raynaud's phenomenon, Esophageal involvement, Sclerodactyly and Telangiectasia may be seen (CREST syndrome). Anti-centromere antibodies are detected in most patients. Mask-like restriction of facial movement and narrowing of the eyes and the mouth produce the characteristic facies. Stiffening of the tongue, involvement of the TMJ, resorption of the mandibular angle and widening of the periodontal ligament are also common features. The disease has a poor prognosis and treatment is rarely effective.

## Diseases of possible immunopathogenesis

Many disorders have associated immune changes, but the exact role of these in the aetiopathogenesis is unclear. Some have already been discussed; others are mentioned here.

**Behçet's syndrome**—a multi-system disease (basically a vasculitis), typically with oral and genital ulcers, and uveitis.

**Wegener's granulomatosis**—a vasculitis, presenting primarily with granulomatous lesions in the respiratory tract (including the nose, paranasal tissues and occasionally the gingivae) and necrotizing glomerulonephritis.

**Polyarteritis nodosa**—is another vasculitis → multi-system disease.

# Neurological disorders I

❶ Neurological disorders may give a false impression of low intelligence.

## Congenital neurological disorders

*Cerebral palsy* is cerebral damage around the time of birth (primarily due to hypoxia) manifesting with disordered movement and posture (spastic is the most common type), and about 50% of patients have associated problems such as learning disability, epilepsy, defects of vision, hearing or speech, or emotional disturbances. Patients may also suffer from swallowing problems, drooling, TMJ subluxation, malocclusion, or ↓ manual dexterity → ↑ dental disease. There is no effective treatment.

*Huntington's chorea* is an autosomal dominant condition affecting men and presenting in early middle age with progressive dementia and irregular dance-like involuntary movements. Oral hygiene is often poor and patients often sustain facial injuries from falls. There is no effective treatment and prognosis is poor.

*Spina bifida* is a neural tube defect associated with deficiency of folic acid during pregnancy. Myelomeningocele is the most severe form and may be associated with paraplegia, faecal and/or urinary incontinence, meningitis risk and, occasionally, brain abnormalities. There is no effective treatment. Patients often become latex allergic.

## Epilepsy

Epilepsy is an episodic abnormal electrical activity of the brain. It affects primarily young people.

*Generalized seizures* include tonic-clonic, absence, myoclonic and atonic types. They are usually 1°, but may be 2° (see below). Prodromal features (mood or behavioural changes) [the aura] may precede a seizure and can last for several hours.

*Tonic-clonic* (grand mal) epilepsy is characterized by loss of consciousness (LOC) and generalized tonic spasm into an extended position. Within <1 min, the tonic phase is followed by a clonic phase with repetitive jerking movements of the trunk and limbs. There may be tongue-biting or urinary incontinence. Recovery is within a few minutes and may be followed by headache, confusion or sleepiness.

If seizure lasts >5 min, the patient has entered 'status epilepticus', which constitutes an emergency as it may result in respiratory embarrassment and brain hypoxia and damage.

*Absence* (petit mal) presents with sudden arrest of movement, speech and attention, following which, patient carries on where they left off.

*Myoclonic jerks* typically resemble those seen in many normal individuals just before they fall asleep, but can happen at any time and may result in the patient falling to the ground.

*Partial seizures* are the result of 'misfiring' of a certain part of the brain → localized motor or sensory symptoms, or psychomotor manifestations. They may be 1° (cryptogenic) but, more often, an intracranial cause can be identified (2° partial seizures; see below). Partial seizures may also be divided into simple (focal symptoms or signs alone) or complex (if there is LOC). Complex partial seizures can be differentiated from generalized seizures by the presence of focal symptoms or an aura (usually a brief hallucination) at the onset. Limb paralysis (Todd's palsy) following the seizure is also a sign of partial seizure.

*Jacksonian epilepsy* involves the motor cortex and presents with unilateral seizures. Temporary limb weakness (Todd's palsy) often follows.

*Temporal lobe epilepsy* presents with hallucinations, confusion and amnesia.

▶2° Seizures may be due to cerebral space-occupying lesions (SOL), vascular defects, trauma, infections, neurofibromatosis, cerebral palsy, anoxia, metabolic abnormalities, drug withdrawal, or febrile illnesses (*febrile convulsions;* common in young children and rarely of significance).

*Management considerations*

For the management of fits in the dental surgery see page 292. Epileptics may sustain oral and maxillofacial injuries during a fit.

Some drugs, fatigue, starvation, stress or infection may precipitate fits. There is no evidence that lidocaine in LA can cause fits. Several drugs, e.g. antidepressants, however, may be epileptogenic and are contraindicated.

Antiepileptic drugs include phenytoin and carbamazepine in particular. Phenytoin has adverse effects, including gingival swelling. Other anticonvulsants (e.g. carbamazepine, valproate, lamotrigine) have fewer adverse effects. Management of patients may also be complicated by other associated handicaps (e.g. learning impairment) or psychiatric disorders.

## Multiple sclerosis (MS)

MS is an immunologically mediated (possible viral aetiology) disorder seen in young adults and is characterized by plaques of demyelination in the CNS. Presentation and progression of MS is highly variable. The cranial nerves are often affected, resulting in visual disturbances and other sensory deficits, trigeminal neuralgia or facial paralysis. Remissions are common, but eventually some disablement occurs in most patients. There is no effective treatment: corticosteroids or interferon may help.

## Parkinson's disease

Parkinson's disease is due to degeneration of dopaminergic neurones of the substantia nigra → rest tremor, rigidity and bradykinesis (slow movements). There is often drooling of saliva and the face is expressionless, but this should not be misinterpreted as an impaired cognitive state. The term 'parkinsonism' refers to a similar syndrome resulting usually from use of drugs such as neuroleptics (antipsychotics). Treatment of both forms is with L-dopa or other dopamine agonists. Anticholinergics help reduce the tremor.

# Neurological disorders II

## Stroke or cerebrovascular accident

CVA is acute brain damage due to ischaemic infarction or cerebral bleeding, manifesting with focal CNS symptoms. The commonest scenario is a unilateral *cerebral infarct* → contralateral hemiplegia (initially flaccid, but later spastic—see UMN lesions [page 37]) with some sensory loss and dysphasia. Coma and death are common. The cause of the infarction is either *cerebral thrombosis* due to atherosclerosis, or, more often, *embolism* by a thrombus arising from the heart (usually due to AF) or the carotid artery. *Transient ischaemic attack* is when symptoms resolve in <24 h. Less frequently, CVA is due to *intracerebral haemorrhage* → a unilateral expanding lesion, exerting pressure and damaging part of the brain.

↑ BP, ↑ age, diabetes, smoking, obesity, AF, prosthetic heart valves, previous history of coronary or peripheral artery disease and TIA are risk factors for CVA, and should be addressed in prevention management. Carotid ultrasound can detect many patients at risk of CVA. Aspirin with dipyridamole and/or other antiplatelet drugs (e.g. clopidogrel) should be used. Oral anticoagulation (warfarin) is necessary if there is AF or heart valve disease. In the acute phase following a stroke, aspirin ± thrombolysis may be beneficial, but haemorrhage must first be excluded. Reduction of disability is the main long-term concern.

Dental management may be complicated by communication difficulties, facial palsy, impaired mobility, associated diseases, and bleeding tendency.

## Intracranial bleeds

*Subarachnoid haemorrhage* is spontaneous bleeding into the subarachnoid space, usually resulting from rupture of berry aneurysms. It presents with sudden excruciatingly severe headache and vomiting, frequently followed by collapse and coma. Neck stiffness may also develop. Treatment is an emergency—often surgical (aneurysm clipping or evacuation) or may be medical (BP control, rest, analgesia and vasodilators).

*Subdural haemorrhage* is bleeding between the dura and arachnoid from veins connecting cortex and venous sinuses. This may occur spontaneously or following minor trauma, especially in anticoagulated patients. Typical presentation is with ↑ intracranial pressure (ICP) and fluctuating neurological changes → gradual deterioration of level of consciousness, often resembling stroke. Surgical evacuation of clot via burr holes is usually curative.

*Extradural haemorrhage* is bleeding between the dura and the skull usually from the middle meningeal artery following skull fracture. Worsening headache, vomiting, focal neurological signs, and deterioration of level of consciousness (↓ Glasgow Coma Scale [GCS]) at any stage following head injury (even days after apparent initial recovery) are all signs of ↑ ICP, and should raise suspicion of extradural haemorrhage. Prognosis, if clot is evacuated early, is good to excellent (if artery is ligated [by a neurosurgeon]).

## Infections of the nervous system

*Bacterial meningitis* is most often caused by *Neisseria meningitidis* (meningococcus), which is carried in the nasopharynx and may spread to the meninges via the bloodstream or occasionally as a result of maxillofacial trauma. Other causes of bacterial meningitis include *Haemophilus influenzae* (primarily affecting unvaccinated toddlers) and *Streptococcus pneumoniae* (usually affects adults, elderly people and the immunocompromised). Clinically, there are signs of meningism (headache, neck stiffness and photophobia) and frequently also ↑ ICP (↑ BP, ↓ pulse, vomiting, fits and ↓ consciousness) and septicaemia (variable rash). Refer immediately for lumbar puncture (contraindicated if ↑ ICP, as it can precipitate brain herniation and death by coning of the brain stem). Start blind antibiotic treatment based on most likely cause; mortality is low with prompt treatment, but permanent neurological damage may occur.

*Viral meningitis* is usually mild and self-limiting.

*Encephalitis* is most commonly caused by herpes simplex virus (HSV) (herpetic encephalitis) and may present with meningism, signs of ↑ ICP, and a variety of neurological and personality changes. The disease may be fatal without heroic doses of aciclovir.

*Brain abscess* is usually 2° to ear, sinus or pulmonary infection, but may also occur as a complication of head trauma or infective endocarditis. *Staphylococcus aureus* is the usual culprit. Periodontal pockets and periapical infections have also been associated with brain abscesses.

## Brain tumours

Brain tumours may be 1° (particularly in children [see page 185]) or 2° (particularly in adults; typically from breast or lung carcinomas). Presentations can be extremely variable depending on site(s) affected. Raised intracranial pressure (↑ ICP) is common. Acoustic neuromas cause symptoms and signs related to cranial nerve VIII, but also V, VII, IX and X. Pituitary tumours are discussed on pages 210–211. Benign 1° tumours are often successfully removed, but may leave permanent disabilities. Prognosis of malignant brain tumours is poor.

# Neurological disorders III

## Syncope

Syncope is a transient LOC resulting from ↓ cerebral blood flow. Causes include vasovagal syncope or fainting (an autonomic reflex precipitated by pain or psychological factors, such as fear of a needle, and producing vasodilatation, bradycardia and LOC), postural hypotension, cardiac arrhythmias, aortic stenosis, severe coughing, etc. Recovery is swift, if the patient is laid flat immediately. Failing this, the patient may have a seizure.

## Hypoxic encephalopathy

Hypoxic encephalopathy results from persistently ↓ oxygenation of the brain caused by head trauma, severe hypotension (shock), airways obstruction, or complication of GA. Cerebral hypoxia causes loss of consciousness in <1 min and, if prolonged for >3 min, dilated pupils, coma, irreversible brain damage and finally, death.

## Cranial nerve neuropathy

Cranial nerve neuropathy may present as focal sensory or motor defects (see Chapter 2), or multiple defects affecting several cranial nerves (polyneuropathies) (e.g. bulbar palsy—weakness of muscles supplied by the medulla [nerves IX–XII inclusive]) often in association with peripheral neuropathies.

Facial paralysis, sensory loss and/or other impairments of cranial or peripheral nerves may be due to CVA, head injury, maxillofacial or cranial trauma or surgery, or tumours of the base of skull or maxillofacial region (e.g. antral or parotid), local infection (e.g. osteomyelitis, mastoiditis, middle ear infection), inflammatory disease affecting nervous tissue (multiple sclerosis, AIDS, neurosyphilis, sarcoidosis, Lyme disease, connective tissue disease, Behçet's syndrome, Guillain–Barré syndrome [immunologically mediated polyneuropathy, usually following viral infection], herpes zoster [e.g. affecting the geniculate ganglion—Ramsay–Hunt syndrome]), Bell's palsy (acute-onset LMN facial paralysis; usually associated with HSV infection; prednisolone and aciclovir may help, although most patients recover spontaneously).

Peripheral neuropathy may also be caused by systemic disorders such as diabetes, vitamin $B_{12}$ or thiamine deficiency (e.g. alcoholism), and heavy metal intoxication (e.g. mercury—not a problem for dental patients or staff, if adequate standards of mercury hygiene are applied).

## Facial pain and headache

The differential diagnosis of facial pain and headache is discussed on Chapter 7. Common causes include (see also Table 7.5):

### Tension headache

Bilateral constant ache or band-like pressure. Caused by tension of frontal, occipital or temporal muscles. Worse in the evening, better on vacation. Reassurance and simple analgesics are usually adequate.

### Migraine

Unilateral throbbing headache with nausea, vomiting and photophobia. Caused by arterial dilatation. Often precipitated by alcohol, tyramine-containing foods (e.g. chocolate) or drugs (nitroglycerin, contraceptives, etc.). Attacks may respond to NSAIDs with anti-emetics, but 5HT receptor agonists (zolmitriptan, sumatriptan, etc.) are more effective. Prophylaxis is with propranolol, pizotifen or amitriptyline.

### Migrainous neuralgia (cluster headaches)

Pain localized usually around one eye. Episodes last 15 min to 3 h and may recur several times a day, or at a regular time every day. Attacks may respond to oxygen or a 5HT receptor agonist.

### Trigeminal neuralgia

Severe unilateral lancinating pain involving a trigeminal branch. Usually affecting older women. Trigger zones may exist. Cause may be a tortuous cerebral blood vessel compressing the trigeminal ganglion. Treatment is with carbamazepine, surgery to the trigeminal nerve branches or intracranial neurosurgery.

### Atypical (psychogenic) facial pain

A continuous dull ache usually affecting the maxillary region in the absence of any abnormal findings clinically or on investigation. Treatment is mainly with cognitive behavioural therapy and antidepressants.

# Psychiatry

**Classification** of psychiatric disorders should ideally be based on aeti-ology, but this is not usually fully understood. A broad classification into organic (i.e. with demonstrable pathology) and functional (e.g. schizo-phrenia, mood disorders) is often used but is rather misleading, as there is growing evidence of biological and/or anatomical changes underlying most functional disorders.

Functional disorders are often divided into psychoses (characterized by delusions, hallucinations, abnormal behaviour and lack of insight; include schizophrenia and bipolar affective disorder) and neuroses (with symp-toms that are an exaggeration of normal). Some also distinguish mental illnesses from personality, developmental, and behavioural disorders, which are not usually preceded by normal functioning.

All this nomenclature can be confusing and occasionally misleading, therefore, the simplest way to classify phychiatric disorders is according to clinical presentation. A brief outline of the most important conditions, based on the International Classification of Diseases (ICD), is as follows:

## Classification of psychiatric disorders

- Organic disorders
  - Delirium
  - Dementia (e.g. vascular dementia and Alzheimer's disease)
- Mental disorders due to psychoactive substance (e.g. alcohol) use
- Schizophrenia, and related psychotic disorders
- Mood (affective) disorders
  - Bipolar affective disorder (mania with or without depression)
  - Depressive disorder
- Neuroses
  - Generalized anxiety disorder
  - Panic disorder (panic attacks)
  - Phobic disorders (e.g. agoraphobia, social phobia, specific phobia)
  - Obsessive-compulsive disorder (OCD)
  - Post-traumatic stress disorder
  - Dissociative (conversion) disorders
  - Somatoform disorders (somatization disorder, hypochondriasis, persistent pain disorder)
- Behavioural disorders
  - Eating disorders (anorexia nervosa and bulimia nervosa)
  - Sleep disorders (e.g. insomnia)
  - Sexual dysfunction and gender identity disorders (paraphilias)
- Childhood behavioural and emotional disorders (autism, contact disorder, attention-deficit and hyperactivity disorder [ADHD], etc.)
- Personality disorders (e.g. antisocial or psychopathic personality)

**Aetiology** of psychiatric disorders includes:
- Predisposing factors (heredity, traumatic early life events, personality)
- Precipitating factors (significant life events prior to disease onset)
- Perpetuating (maintaining) factors, that allow the disorder to persist

**Examination** should include mental state examination (see Chapter 2) and general examination (neurological system in particular). None of the findings are specific to one condition; suicidal ideation and impaired cognitive state for instance may be seen in any psychiatric disorder.

**Management** of psychiatric disorders may include hospitalization (sometimes compulsory), pharmacotherapy (antipsychotics, antidepressants, mood-stabilizers, anxiolytics, etc.), electroconvulsive therapy (ECT), psychological therapy (counselling, behavioural therapy, cognitive therapy, individual or group psychotherapy), and social rehabilitation.

*Hospitalization* of psychiatric patients is rarely indicated. Inpatients who suffer delirium (e.g. following an operation), and are considered to be a risk to themselves or others, may, in the UK, be detained under section 5(2) of the Mental Health Act 1983.

If alcohol is the cause, patients may be detained under common law.

*Antipsychotic (neuroleptic) drugs* are used in the treatment of schizophrenia, delirium, psychoactive substance use, and mania. Their main therapeutic effect is antidopaminergic action. *Typical* antipsychotics (haloperidol, chlorpromazine, etc.) are usually used for inpatients, if acutely agitated or delirious. Their side-effects include antimuscarinic symptoms (blurred vision, xerostomia, urinary retention, constipation), drowsiness, and postural hypotention. The most feared effect is neuroleptic malignant syndrome (hyperthermia, rigidity, and autonomic instability [eratic pulse and BP, and sweating]), which needs urgent intensive care. Long-term use may lead to extrapyramidal effects (parkinsonism, restlessness, orofacial dystonias, facial tardive dyskinesias). *Atypical* antipsychotics (clozapine, olanzapine, risperidone, quetiapine, etc.) can cause drowsiness, dizziness, hypotension, xerostomia, etc. but are less likely to cause serious adverse effects.

*Antidepressants* are used primarily in depression, but they are also useful in the treatment of neuroses. Most commonly used are tricyclic antidepressants (TCAs; amitriptiline, nortriptiline, dothiepin, etc.) and selective serotonin re-uptake inhibitors (SSRIs; fluoxetine, paroxetine, citalopram, sertaline, etc.). TCAs may cause sedation, postural hypotension, arrhythmias, and peripheral antimuscarinic effects (blurred vision, xerostomia, urinary retention, constipation). SSRIs may cause sexual dysfunction, nausea and vomiting. Monoamine oxidase inhibitors (MAOIs) are less commonly used now.

*Mood-stabilizers* are primarily used in the prophylaxis of bipolar affective disorder. Lithium is usually the first choice. Common side-effects include dehydration, xerostomia, impaired taste and tremor. Long-term lithium therapy requires regular monitoring of renal and thyroid function. Carbamazepine (an anticonvulsant) is a useful alternative.

*Anxiolytics* are used in the treatment of anxiety disorders (benzodiazepines), insomnia (temazepam or zopiclone), convulsions (diazepam or clonazepam), alcohol withdrawal (diazepam or chlordiazepoxide), or as premedication in general anaesthesia (temazepam) and when sedation with amnesia is desired (midazolam). They can be highly addictive and should only be used in short-term courses.

*ECT* is urgent treatment primarily for major depressive episodes.

# Important psychiatric disorders I

## Organic brain disorders

*Delirium* is an acute organic brain disorder presenting with agitation, confusion, ↓ consciousness, persecutory delusions, and transient illusions and hallucinations. Causes include alcohol or drug intoxication, systemic or CNS infections, endocrine abnormalities, electrolyte imbalance, hypoglycaemia, hypoxia, head injury, postoperative state (especially at night time), etc. Management involves investigation for and treatment of the underlying cause, reassuring nursing, haloperidol and/or temazepam.

*Dementia* is a chronic progressive deterioration of mental function characterized primarily by an impaired cognitive state (↓ memory, concentration and orientation). Language, mood, behaviour, intelligence, insight and other aspects of mental state are also affected, but consciousness is not ↓. The two main acutes of dementia are Alzheimer's disease (common over the age of 65; characterized by global atrophy of the brain; short-term memory loss; deteriorating intellectual function and personality), and vascular or multi-infarct dementia (resulting from multiple cerebral infarcts associated with arteriosclerosis and ↑ BP; stepwise deterioration of cognitive state with focal neurological features; personality and insight are usually not affected until late). Other causes include Lewy body dementia, multiple sclerosis, Huntington's disease, Parkinson's disease, endocrine abnormalities, hepatic failure, renal failure, vitamin deficiency (e.g. thiamine in alcoholics), head injury, AIDS-related dementia, neurosyphilis, other CNS infections, etc.
Oral neglect is typical and, despite ↑ need of dental care, patients are often unable to cooperate with treatment under LA.

## Psychoactive substance use (see also Chapters 1 and 5)

Substances that may be misused includes alcohol, tobacco, cannabis, opioids (e.g. heroin), hypnotics, cocaine, amphetamines, hallucinogens (e.g. LSD and ecstasy), and volatile solvents (Table 4.16). Psychiatric abnormalities may be related to acute intoxication with one of these (e.g. delirium, convulsions, or coma), psychological or physical dependence (inability to function without substance), withdrawal symptoms (for alcohol, these include anxiety, tremor, insomnia and, eventually convulsions and/or delirium tremens), and long-term effects on mental functioning and behaviour (e.g. dementia and other psychiatric disorders).

*Alcoholism* is discussed in Chapter 1. The oral and maxillofacial surgeon is commonly faced with the management of alcoholics as inpatients. Alcohol withdrawal symptoms may further complicate an already difficult postoperative management following major head and neck surgery.

►Remember that the main concern at this stage is a smooth postoperative recovery and not treatment of the addiction, which can be dealt with at a later date. It is important to prevent serious withdrawal symptoms giving regular chlordiazepoxide, while some consultants allow the patients small amounts of alcohol. Administration of thiamine is also necessary.

**Table 4.16** Current popular club drugs

| Street name | Constituents | Effects | Comments |
|---|---|---|---|
| Cat | Methcathanone | A cocaine like high with hallucinations similar to mescaline | Analogue of methamphetamine |
| China White | Beta hydroxide methyl fentanyl | 6000 times as potent as pure natural heroin | Analogue of fentanyl |
| Crack | Cocaine | Produces euphoria | Commonly abused |
| Double Stack or PMA | Paramethoxy amphetamine | Fails to produce the pleasurable MDMA effects and users take more of the drug seeking the high. Causes a dramatic rise in body temperature in excess of 109° and death occurs from hyperthermia | Analogue of methamphetamine |
| DXM | Dextro methorphan | Produces hallucinations and a heavy 'stoned' feeling in users | Often passed off as Ecstasy at clubs and Raves. Also found in many OTC cold remedies |
| Ecstasy | MDMA | Resembles methamphetamine, but unlike it, can also produce hallucinations and a pronounced feeling of emotional closeness to others | The most sought after club drug. Abused at Rave dance parties |
| EVE | MDE | Does NOT produce the feeling of emotional closeness of Ecstasy | Analogue of Ecstasy |
| GBL | Gamma-butyrolactone | Taken alone or especially when mixed with alcoholic it produces a stupor, vomiting and coma | Related to GHB and sold over the internet to avoid laws against GHB |
| GHB, Super-G, Liquid-G, Liquid Ecstasy | Gamma hydroxy-butyric acid | Taken alone or especially when mixed with alcoholic it produces a stupor, vomiting and coma | Originally thought to be a human growth hormone and abused by body builders till banned by FDA in 1991 |

**Table 4.16** Contd.

| Street name | Constituents | Effects | Comments |
| --- | --- | --- | --- |
| Ice | Methamphetamine | Produces a 10-h stimulating high | A smokable form of methamphetamine; similar effect to crack cocaine |
| Nexus—or 2C-B | 4-bromo-2,5-dimethoxy phenethylamine | Produces strong Ecstasy-like feelings of closeness. Highly sought after for sexual enhancement properties. Less powerful hallucinations than DOB | Phenylethylamine analogue of the powerful hallucinatory drug DOB (4-bromo-2,5-dimethoxyam phetamine) |
| Rohypnol | Flunitrazepam | When mixed with alcohol often used as a 'date rape' or sexual predator drug | Analogue of valium but ten times more powerful |
| Special K | Ketamine | Produces hallucinations and stupor and is highly addictive though hallucinatory effect lasts only 1 h | Analogue of PCP |
| YABA | Methamphetamine | Produces a 10-h stimulating high | An ultra pure form of methamphetamine often combined with caffeine |

# Important psychiatric disorders II

## Schizophrenia

Schizophrenia is a common psychotic disorder that affects ~1% of the population. The boundaries between the 'self' and the outside world are broken → abnormal thoughts, beliefs and perceptions. Onset is in early adulthood, and diagnosis is based on first-rank symptoms including delusional perception ('I saw a dog outside my house and then I knew I was God's chosen one'), characteristic auditory hallucinations (patient's thoughts are audible, running commentary of patient's actions, patient been discussed in third person), thought alienation (insertion, withdrawal or broadcasting) and passivity phenomena (made feelings or acts). In chronic schizophrenia, 'negative' (depressive) symptoms usually predominate. Other mental state abnormalities are noted, but intelligence is spared, at least in early stages. Management involves antipsychotic drugs (usually phenothiazines such as chlorpromazine), hospitalization (for acute psychotic episodes) and social rehabilitation.

## Bipolar affective disorder

Bipolar affective disorder is defined by at least one episode of mania, characterized by mood elevation, ↑ activity, ↓ sleep, pressured speech, grandiose ideas, disinhibited and irresponsible behaviour, and other mental state abnormalities. Manic episodes may lead to exhaustion, or have devastating social consequences, and are prevented if lithium is taken regularly. Depressive episodes may occur in the interim period.

Dental treatment should not be attempted during manic episodes (as indeed any acute psychotic episode); patients can be aggressive.

## Depression

Depression is common with ~1 in 5 women and 1 in 10 men affected at some point. Possibly, a much higher proportion experiences depressive symptoms at some point, but these are likely to have a predominantly non-biological aetiology. Symptoms include low mood, tiredness, ↓ energy and activity, ↓ appetite, disturbed sleep (early morning wakening particularly), loss of interest, anhedonia (not getting any pleasure from things once enjoyed), low self-esteem, feelings of guilt, worthlessness and hopelessness, and often, suicidal ideation. Mental state examination may reveal abnormalities such as general neglect, poor eye contact, slowness and poverty of speech, nihilistic thoughts (patient is to blame for everything), poor concentration, etc. Anxiety may be associated.

*Dental aspects* of depression include ↑ incidence of TMJ dysfunction and atypical facial pain. Certain oral complaints may be delusional, including halitosis, oral dysaesthesiae (burning mouth or glossodynia), disturbed taste sensation, discharges and dry mouth (although the latter may be due to antidepressant therapy).

## Anxiety disorders

Anxiety disorders may be associated with a variety of oral manifestations such as bruxism, lip chewing, TMJ dysfunction, a complaint of dry mouth, and several hypochondriacal features (e.g. cancer phobia). It must be remembered though, that stress may have a much greater effect on health (possibly through neuroimmunological mechanisms) than once appreciated. Dental treatment may generate anxiety, and specific phobias related to dentistry exist. A calm, confident, sympathetic and reassuring manner helps, as do preoperative anxiolytics and painless procedures.

## Eating disorders

Eating disorders affect primarily adolescent girls preoccupied with an overvalued idea to be thin → self-induced starvation, vomiting and purging, abuse of appetite suppressants and excessive exercise. In *anorexia nervosa* this behaviour leads to significantly ↓ body weight as well as cardiovascular complications, anaemia, endocrine abnormalities (e.g. amenorrhoea) and hypokalaemia. In *bulimia nervosa* weight is not ↓ due to intermittent compensating uncontrolled bingeing. GI complications and dental caries are common. Sialosis, angular cheilitis and erosion of teeth are seen in both conditions.

USEFUL WEBSITES
http://www.emedicine.com
http://health.nih.gov/

# Special care groups

# Children

## Consent

- At age 16 years (18 in Australia/USA/Canada), a young person is regarded as an adult and can be presumed to have capacity to consent to treatment if competent.
- In the UK, children under the age of 16 years may also have capacity to consent if they have the ability to understand the nature, purpose and possible consequences of the proposed investigation or treatment, as well as the consequences of non-treatment.
- Where a child under 16 years old is deemed not competent to consent, a person with parental responsibility or defined guardianship (e.g. their mother or guardian) may authorize investigations or treatment, which are in the child's best interests.
- For the conditions to judge 'best interest', see below in the section on learning disabilities.
- Generally, however, formal assent to treatment from a legal parent or guardian is sought for treatment of all children under 16 or 18 years.

## Health

- Always enquire about genetic and developmental conditions and take a good family history and immunization history.
- Respiratory infections are very common in young children and should be excluded before a GA is given.

## Oral health

From national surveys in the UK, the levels of caries in 5-year-old children are not improving and may be worsening (especially in disadvantaged groups and deprived areas) with some improvements in 12-year olds. A high proportion of caries remains untreated. Caries risk varies with diet and oral care, and may be greater in socioeconomically disadvantaged people.

## Clinical considerations

*General anaesthetics* in children under the age of 3 years, need to be given by a paediatric-trained anaesthetist.

*Paediatric clinics and wards* are separate from adult, and certain procedures are different. Care is usually shared with the paediatric team. There is a general consensus that white coats should be avoided in paediatric wards. Try to see and examine the child in the presence of their parent/guardian and a paediatric nurse.

*Drug doses* should be reduced according to age and/or body weight or body surface area. Always consult the relevant drug formulary (e.g. BNF [UK] or PDR [USA]) before prescribing for a child.

# Pregnant patients

During pregnancy, because of the danger of miscarriage and teratogenicity, particularly in the 1st trimester, it is important to avoid or minimize exposure to trauma and to:
- drugs (Table 5.1);
- radiography (see Chapter 3);
- infections;
- alcohol and tobacco;
- mercury.

## Oral health care considerations
- Pregnancy is the ideal opportunity to start preventive dental education.
- Drugs and radiation should be avoided whenever possible.
- Most dental treatment is best carried out in the 4th–6th month of pregnancy (2nd trimester).
- In the 3rd trimester, avoid GA because of the liability of vomiting and do not lay the patient supine, as this may cause hypotension.
- Pregnancy may predispose to:
  - pregnancy gingivitis;
  - pregnancy epulis.
- Drugs that pass in breast milk are contraindicated during breast-feeding.
- Dentists are advised not to undergo treatments on pregnant women that involve removing or placing amalgam.

**Table 5.1** Drugs used in dentistry, which may be contraindicated in pregnancy or lactation

| Drugs to avoid | 1st trimester | 2nd and 3rd trimesters | Close to delivery | During lactation[a] |
|---|---|---|---|---|
| Aminoglycosides | | Avoid | | |
| Anticoagulants[b] | Avoid | | Avoid | Avoid |
| Antifibrinolytics | Avoid | Avoid | Avoid | |
| Aspirin | | | Avoid | Avoid |
| Atropine | | | | Avoid |
| Barbiturates | | Avoid | | |
| Benzodiazepines[c] | | Avoid | Avoid | Avoid |
| Chloral hydrate | | | | Avoid |
| Corticosteroids[d] | | Avoid | Avoid | Avoid |
| Co-trimoxazole | | | Avoid | |
| Danazol | Avoid | Avoid | Avoid | Avoid |
| Diflunisal | | | | Avoid |
| Erythromycin | | | | Avoid |
| Etretinate | Avoid | Avoid | Avoid | |
| Gentamicin | | Avoid | | |
| Mefenamic acid | | Avoid | Avoid | |
| Metronidazole | Avoid | | | Avoid |
| Opioids[e] | | | Avoid | |
| Penicillin | | | | Avoid |
| Phenothiazines | | | | Avoid |
| Rifampicin | | | Avoid | |
| Sulphonamides | | Avoid | Avoid | Avoid |
| Tetracyclines | | Avoid | Avoid | Avoid |
| Tricyclics | | Avoid | Avoid | |

[a] These and other drugs enter the breast milk and could in theory harm the infant.
[b] Oral anticoagulants.
[c] If these are necessary, use a short-acting drug, e.g. temazepam.
[d] Systemic corticosteroids.
[e] Including related compounds, e.g. codeine, dihydrocodeine, pentazocine and pethidine.

# Older persons

Owing to the increase in life expectancy and fall in birth rate in the developed world, the numbers of older persons are increasing, with people aged 60 years or over now forming a much larger part of the population than children. There has also been a large increase in the number of people aged >85 years.

## Health

Demographic changes have consequences for healthcare services. Particular problems include:

*Cardiovascular diseases* such as ischaemic heart disease and hypertension. Socially disadvantaged groups and people from black and Asian ethnic communities are particularly vulnerable.

*Mental health problems* Under-detection of mental illness in older people is widespread, due to the nature of the symptoms and the fact that many older people live alone. Depression is under-diagnosed in people aged 65 and over, particularly in residents in care homes.

*Diabetes* Socially disadvantaged groups and people from black and Asian minority ethnic communities are particularly vulnerable.

*Malnutrition* may be due to a diet of 'tea and toast'.

*Polypharmacy* In the UK, 36% of older people take four or more medicines. Depression, apathy and the physical effects of ageing, such as arthritis, and failing eyesight and memory decrease compliance.

## Oral health care considerations

*Access* to dental services can be difficult. Older persons often struggle with stairs and may rely on wheelchairs or walking frames that necessitate ramps and wide doorways. Domiciliary visits may be necessary; however, treatment options may be limited in the home environment.

*Patient management* Older persons especially need treating with patience and respect. Treatment is best carried out with the patient sitting upright. Local anaesthetics carry less risk than GA.

## Dental aspects

There is an increase in the numbers of elderly people with a natural dentition, but this brings with it potential management problems dealing with worn dentitions, root caries, periodontal disease and patients becoming edentulous at older ages. Xerostomia can exacerbate caries, denture and mucosal problems. Marking of dentures with the patient's name can prevent mix-ups in hospitals or residential care homes.

## Social considerations

Retirement and old age can bring with them loss of income, poverty, loss of social status, and consequent negative impacts on health.

Older people living alone or with elderly relatives may need arrangements to be made for home care while recovering from surgery.

# Patients with learning disabilities

- Learning disability has been defined as 'a significant impairment of intelligence and social functioning acquired before adulthood'.
- Over one million people in the UK have learning disabilities—with about 200 000 being classed as severely affected.

## Health

- Physical impairments (such as heart defects) and epilepsy are common in people with learning disabilities.
- Psychiatric and behavioural problems (such as schizophrenia and autism) are more common.

## Social

Over the past 15 years in the UK there has been a move away from people with learning disabilities living in institutions to community-based dwelling. This has had implications for education and provision of medical and dental services.

## Consent

- Some patients with learning disabilities, no matter how well the facts about treatment are explained to them are incapable of understanding them or the implications of the treatment decision they are being asked to make. Such patients are regarded as not competent to give consent. For a person 'to be competent' or 'to have the capacity to consent' they must be able to reason and weigh the risks and benefits and consequences of their decision.
- If a patient is unable to communicate adequately they are regarded as not competent.
- If a health professional believes a patient lacks the capacity to consent they cannot give or withhold consent to treatment on behalf of that patient, but they may carry out an investigation or treatment judged to be in that patient's best interest as approved by the patients guardian, which in some cases may be court-appointed.

### Principle of best interest

In deciding what actually is in the patient's best interests you should take into account:

- treatment options, prognosis, complexity and cost of treatment;
- any evidence of the patient's previous preferences;
- knowledge of the patient's background;
- views of family members.

## Oral health

- When comparing children and adults with and without learning disabilities, the prevalence of caries is similar. However, rates of untreated caries and of extractions are higher in those with learning disabilities.
- Levels of gingivitis and periodontal disease are higher in people with learning disabilities than in the general population.

## Clinical considerations

- The emphasis should be on preventing disease and promoting good oral health, by establishing comprehensive prevention programmes including good oral hygiene, non-cariogenic diet, fissure sealants, topical fluoride applications, and consideration for use of antimicrobial mouth rinses (e.g. chlorhexidine).
- The management of patients with learning disabilities will depend on the severity of the disability, with a minority of patients requiring examination and treatment under conscious sedation or GA.

# Patients from minority ethnic groups

Western countries are becoming more diverse due to extensive migration patterns. In the UK, the minority ethnic population grew by 53%, from 3.0 million in 1991 to 4.6 million in 2001. Most of the minorities in the UK are Asian and Muslim. Many people in the UK belonging to cultural and ethnic minority groups were born in the UK, with second and third generation status being common. Thus many people from cultural and ethnic minorities are well acculturated.

## Health

Certain conditions have different prevalence and mortality rates in different ethnic groups. For example:

*Violence:* Black and minority ethnic (BME) people are more likely to be victims of harassment, violence, and robbery. Afro-Caribbeans tend to be victims of serious crimes.

*Diabetes:* South Asian and Caribbean populations have lower rates of type I diabetes, but much higher rates of type II diabetes. The higher rates of diabetes are also linked to renal and coronary heart disease.

*Tuberculosis:* There is a high incidence in people coming from endemic areas and new immigrants from South Asia and Africa, and a high mortality among people born in Ireland.

*Coronary heart disease:* Mortality rates are high in South Asian and white populations, and lower in Caribbean populations.

*Sickle cell anaemia:* The prevalence is high in African and Caribbean populations.

*HIV disease:* An increased incidence of HIV disease is seen in people from high prevalence areas, which can affect children and adults.

## Oral health

### Barriers to care may include

- Cost
- Language
- Mistrust of dentist (perceived unnecessary treatment)
- Anxiety
- Hygiene concerns
- Cultural misunderstandings

### Periodontal disease

Aggressive periodontitis is more common in Afro-Caribbean children, but chronic periodontitis is more common in South Asian adults.

### Caries levels

There is some evidence that there are higher caries levels in the deciduous dentition of children from some ethnic minorities in the UK (particularly Asian children, and when the mother does not speak English), but that this difference disappears in the permanent dentition. However, the caries levels in the deciduous teeth of Afro-Caribbean children are lower than in the UK population as a whole.

Adult dental health may be better among Asian, Bangladeshi, black African, black Caribbean, Indian, Pakistani, Chinese and Vietnamese groups.

### Oral cancer

The use of betel and chewing tobacco in certain Asian groups leads to an ↑ incidence of submucous fibrosis, leucoplakias and oral cancer.

# Asylum seekers and refugees

## Health concerns

The health problems of asylum seekers are:
- Communicable diseases in the early phase of entry to the country, e.g.
  - TB;
  - hepatitis A, B, C;
  - HIV;
  - parasitic infections.
- Effects of war and torture, e.g.
  - amputated limbs;
  - sexual assault;
  - malnutrition;
  - prolonged periods in camps;
  - dental torture;
  - mental disorders.

## Social considerations

Social isolation and poverty have a compounding negative impact on mental health, leading in later phases to:
- depression;
- panic attacks;
- stress-related effects (such as increased susceptibility to infection).

### Access barriers

In the UK, access to medical treatment is free for those in the process of seeking asylum, but many have difficulty obtaining it, the main barriers being:
- Language. It is important for the services of a trained advocate or interpreter to be available unless you speak the same language as the patient. Refugees may bring a family member or friend to interpret. Though this may help in obtaining background information, it may result in inaccurate interpreting and also make it difficult to discuss sensitive issues. Language issues complicate the process of informed consent.
- Time and continuity of care.
- Information on health services.

# Drug abusers

**Substances used include:** alcohol, tobacco, amphetamines, cannabis, cocaine, heroin, volatile substances.

## Reasons for use

- Peer pressure
- Enjoyment
- Alleviate poor quality of life
- Alleviate feelings of personal inadequacy
- Social and economic

## Classification of drug use

Spectrum from occasional use through regular use, to dependence, addiction and tolerance.

## Trends in drug use

Accurate data on illicit drug use are unavailable, but trends indicate a significant rise in amphetamine and Ecstasy use since the 'Rave' culture began in the 1980s, although the use of Ecstacy may have peaked. Probably 2/3 of secondary school pupils have experimented with drugs of abuse. Alcohol and tobacco in particular are widely abused by young and old alike. The use of 'crack' cocaine, especially by Afro-Caribbean communities is increasing, as are volatile substances in 12–16 year olds.

## Health

- Problems for delivery of care, including anti-social behaviour.
- IV drug abusers have a tendency to be needle-phobics and are at increased risk of blood-borne viruses, TB and sexually transmitted infections.
- Alcoholics may have liver dysfunction, with a bleeding tendency and impaired drug metabolism.
- Poor diet and poor oral care behaviours.

## Social considerations

Drug abuse can lead to anti-social behaviour, conflict with the police, employers and families, crime, violence, and homelessness.

## Clinical considerations (see also Chapter 4)

General considerations are:
- irregular attendance
- high prevalence of dental/maxillofacial trauma
- possibility of drug interactions
- high levels of untreated dental disease including caries, advanced periodontal disease (due to poor oral hygiene/diet) and oral malodour
- increased risk of microbial endocarditis
- potential drug-seeking behaviour

In addition, drugs can cause dehydration, and xerostomia may be relieved by frequent intake of sugary drinks.

*Alcoholism* is often associated with an increased risk of infection and haemorrhage, neglected dentition, maxillofacial and dental trauma, periodontal disease, implant failure and erosion due to acidic beverages and gastro-oesophageal disorders.

*Smoking* is linked to chronic airways disease, ischaemic heart disease and various cancers. Tobacco and alcohol can both contribute to malodour, and have a synergistic effect in causing oral cancer. Smoking predisposes to tooth staining, periodontal disease, candidosis, dry socket, keratoses and implant failure.

*Drug withdrawal* can lead to rebound dental pain that was previously suppressed. Methadone, which is used to manage opioid withdrawal, is cariogenic and erosive and leads to sugar cravings. It is now available in sugar-free form.

# Prisoners

### Demographics

The prison population tends to differ from the general population in that:

- Most inmates are aged 15–34 years.
- >95% are men.
- Levels of educational attainment are often low.
- Levels of previous unemployment are often high.

### Health

Prisoners are atypical in health compared with the general population, having a higher incidence of mental problems, drug misuse and promiscuity. As a consequence, blood-borne infections such as hepatitis B, C and HIV, and TB and STDs are more common.

### Clinical considerations

*Oral health needs*

- Levels of untreated caries in prisoners is about 4 times greater than in people in the general population from similar social backgrounds.
- Poor oral hygiene and high rates of smoking lead to increased levels of periodontal disease.
- There is a high incidence of facial and dental trauma from violence.

*Management*

Consider cross-infection control implications of communicable diseases.

USEFUL WEBSITES
http://www.bsdh.org.uk/guidelines.html
http://www.iadh.org

# Chapter 6

# Emergencies

# Emergency kit

Emergencies should be prevented where possible but, in any event, all staff must be trained in their management and should have an emergency kit readily available. Most emergency drugs (EXCEPT adrenaline/epinephrine) are best given IV (but usually slowly) if possible, as this allows for rapid action but, in primary care settings, IM injections will suffice.

This kit should contain:

*Always*
- Oral airway (e.g. a face mask with an Ambu 300 bag)
- Apparatus for giving oxygen at 10–15L/min
- Aspirator
- Alcohol wipes, tourniquet, syringes, needles and IV cannulae
- Sugar, such as glucose solution or Lucozade, or Hypostop, for oral use
- Drugs for injection:
  - Glucagon 1 mg for IM injection (or 20% sterile glucose [dextrose monohydrate] solution for IV injection)
  - Adrenaline (epinephrine) solution 1 in 1000 (1 mg/mL) for IM injection
  - Hydrocortisone sodium succinate 100–500 mg for IM/IV injection (needs to be made up in sterile water)
  - Diazepam 10 mg for IM/IV injection
  - Chlorpheniramine 10–20 mg for IM/IV injection
- Other drugs
  - Salbutamol inhaler (100 microgram/puff)
  - Glyceryl trinitrate sublingual tablets (500 microgram) or spray (400 microgram/puff)
  - Aspirin 300 mg tablets
- Glucometer device with BM sticks (for blood glucose assay)

*If appropriate training has been completed, additional kit may include:*
- Defibrillator (e.g. automated external defibrillators; AED)
- Intubation kit
- Crystalloid and colloid solution for IV fluids
- Sodium bicarbonate solution 50 mL of 8.4% for IV injection
- Flumazenil 500 microgram (5 mL) (Anexate) for IV injection
- Morphine 5–10 mg for SC/IM/IV injection
- Cyclizine 50 mg for IM/IV injection
- Atropine 3 mg for IM/IV injection

AEDs have simplified the process of defibrillation. ECG interpretation and charging of the machine in preparation to shock are automated. The use of such machines should be within the capabilities of all health care staff and it is quite appropriate for reception, administrative and secretarial staff to be trained in their use. Every emergency ambulance in the UK carries a defibrillator and the ambulance service should be involved at the earliest opportunity as part of a dual response. When attempted defibrillation is delayed, the chances of successful resuscitation are greatly enhanced if basic life support (BLS) is performed.

▶▶The most important tool you will have in any emergency is your brain, which operates best if you remain calm. This is important with the conscious patient (as it helps them to calm down as well), but even more so with the unconscious patient (easier said than done!). Knowledge and practice of procedures can do wonders for your confidence and efficacy. Make sure you keep up to date with drug doses and procedures (e.g. attend resuscitation training, at least annually).

# Collapse

**Causes** of collapse include (Table 6.1):
- Syncope
  - Vasovagal syncope (fainting)
  - Postural hypotension
  - Bradycardia (e.g. heart block)
  - Aortic stenosis
  - Severe coughing
- Hypoglycaemia
- Shock
  - Anaphylaxis
  - Acute heart failure
  - Haemorrhage
  - Sepsis
- MI or cardiac arrest
- Stroke
- Corticosteroid insufficiency
- Epilepsy
- Drug reaction
- Hysteria

## Management

In any emergency, you should adopt a standard well-tested initial approach (primary survey), which first addresses Airway, Breathing and Circulation (ABC).
- *Airway*: Assess and establish a patent airway (e.g. clear airway or intubate), while protecting the cervical spine (if history of injury).
- *Breathing*: Listen (with examiner's ear near patient's nose) and feel for breathing, while looking for chest expansion. Give $O_2$ or, if in respiratory arrest, ventilate.
- *Circulation*: Check the pulse and BP.
  - If in shock, treat depending on cause (e.g. IV colloids for hypovolaemic shock, IV antibiotics for septic shock).
  - If in cardiac arrest, resuscitate (see page 276).

The next step following ABC is 'D' (disability), which consist of a quick assessment of neurological status, primarily by checking level of consciousness (see Glasgow Coma Scale; GCS—page 558).

Once the airway, breathing and circulation are supported, the cause of the collapse should be identified and corrected, if possible. The dentist should be aware of the patient's medical history, in which case, the cause is often obvious. If not, a quick history should be obtained from a third party or the patient's notes.

The commonest cause of collapse in dental practice is fainting and postural hypotension. It is therefore generally advisable to treat patients flat (supine), especially if giving injections or undertaking surgery, which will prevent collapse from vasovagal syncope or postural hypotension. If loss of consciousness occurs in the supine position, or the patient does not quickly resume consciousness when placed in the supine position, then seriously consider other possible causes.

Hypoglycaemia is the next most common cause of collapse in dental practice. If in doubt, a BM stick should give a rapid diagnosis. Glucose should be given in these cases, preferably orally if the patient is not unconscious but otherwise IV. If anaphylaxis or corticosteroid insufficiency are suspected, IV or IM hydrocortisone may be given, and, in any event, are very safe in the short term.

The most common and important causes of collapse will be discussed in the next few sections. In addition, two more causes must be mentioned:

**Stroke** (cerebrovascular accident [CVA]) usually occurs in elderly patients (see page 234). Atherosclerosis is the main cause, but hypertension during a stressful situation (e.g. dental treatment) may precipitate it. Hemiplegia, aphasia, or loss of consciousness may be features. All you can do at this stage is maintain the airway and summons medical help.

**Hysteria** may develop in a susceptible individual because of the stress associated with a visit for health care. Hyperventilation, crying, etc. make the diagnosis obvious, but patients may collapse. Be calm and reassuring. Breathing with a paper bag around the mouth and nose may prevent respiratory alkalosis, but could also further upset the patient.

In unconscious patients, follow the basic principles of ABC.

**Table 6.1** Summaries of management of collapse in dentistry

| Cause | Clinical features | Precipitating factors | Management |
|---|---|---|---|
| Faint | Dizziness, weakness, nausea, pallor, cold moist skin (clammy), pulse initially slow and weak | Anxiety, pain, fatigue, fasting, high temperature | Lower patient's head (lay them flat). Recovery is usually rapid—within seconds (± smelling salts) |
| Hypoglycaemia | Drowsiness, disorientation, irritability, aggression, warm moist skin, pulse full and rapid | Lack of food, too much insulin | Lay patient flat<br>Give glucose orally (4 sugar or dextrose lumps or glucose drink) or intravenously (50 mL 50% sterile glucose)<br>Get medical assistance |
| Cardiac arrest | Loss of consciousness, cessation of respiration, absence of arterial pulses, pallor or cyanosis | MI, hypoxia, anaesthetic overdose | Summon medical assistance<br>Lay patient flat on hard surface<br>Give blow to sternum<br>Start cardiopulmonary resuscitation |
| Stroke | Loss of consciousness, hemiplegia | Hypertension | Maintain airway |
| Corticosteroid insufficiency | Loss of consciousness, pulse weak and rapid, falling BP | Stress or trauma in patients on steroids | Lay patient flat<br>Give methylprednisolone 500 mg or hydrocortisone 500 mg IV<br>Give oxygen<br>Summon medical assistance |

| | | |
|---|---|---|
| Epilepsy | Loss of consciousness, widespread jerking, sometimes incontinence | Some drugs, starvation, menstruation | Lay patient in head injury position<br>Stop them damaging themselves<br>Maintain airway<br>If not recovered in 5 min, give diazepam 0.1 mg/kg IV or midazolam 2 mg IV every minute |
| Anaphylaxis | Loss of consciousness, cold clammy skin, pulse weak and rapid, oedema/urticaria/wheeze, falling BP | Exposure to allergen, e.g. penicillin | Lay patient flat<br>Give 1 mL 1:1000 adrenaline IM. Give hydrocortisone sodium succinate 200–500 mg IM or IV or methylprednisolone 500 mg IV.<br>Give oxygen<br>Summon medical assistance |
| Suspected drug reaction | Variably confusion, drowsiness, fits or loss of consciousness | Drugs | Lay patient flat<br>Maintain airway<br>Summon medical assistance |
| Hysteria | Often a female patient. Variable hyperventilation, crying, etc. | Anxiety | Exclude organic reactions (above)<br>Reassure |

# Fainting

*Precipitating factors*

- Anxiety
- Sight of a needle—a common precipitant
- Pain
- Fatigue
- Fasting
- High room temperature

*Prevention*

- Ensure the patient eats before treatment under local analgesia
- Adopt a reassuring manner and do not cause undue anxiety
- Keep instruments (particularly any sharps) out of patient's view
- Lay the patient supine *before* any injections
- Do not cause the patient pain

*Clinical features*

- Dizziness
- Weakness
- Nausea
- Pallor
- Cold and moist (clammy) skin
- Slow and thin pulse initially (becomes faster later)
- Loss of consciousness (LOC)

*Management*

- Immediately lay the patient flat on their back with the legs raised. Unless laid flat, a fainting patient may develop cerebral hypoxia and then convulse.
- Loosen the patient's collar.
- If he/she does not recover immediately, check the blood glucose, summons assistance, give oxygen (10–15 L/min) and check the pulse.
  - If pulse is slow, this may suggest a vasovagal attack, which might respond to 300 microgram atropine IV.
  - If pulse is absent, this is cardiac arrest (see page 276).
- If he/she recovers, observe for 15 min.

## Postural hypotension

Rapidly bringing a patient upright from lying down may produce postural hypotension, particularly:

- after prolonged periods lying down;
- in the elderly;
- in those on anti-hypertensives, tricyclic antidepressants or atropinics.

Paradoxically, the converse may occur late in pregnancy if, when the patient lies down the gravid uterus inhibits venous return to the heart by compressing the inferior vena cava (supine hypotensive syndrome). Prevent this by positioning the patient slightly sideways in the dental chair.

# Chest pain

There are many causes of chest pain, but severe pain may indicate myocardial ischaemia (angina or MI). The causes and clinical presentation of IHD have been discussed in Chapter 4.

## Angina
*Management*
- Stop the procedure
- Reassure and calm the patient
- Keep the patient upright
- Give sublingual GTN 0.5 mg (1 tablet or 2 puffs of spray)
- Give oxygen (10–15 L/min)
- If pain is not relieved in 5 min, repeat GTN, and ask patient to chew 300 mg aspirin
- If pain is not relieved, or if there is sweating, nausea, vomiting, breathlessness, arrhythmia, or LOC, consider treating as MI (see below); summons assistance; if cardiac arrest, resuscitate; if already in hospital, take blood for FBC, U&Es, and cardiac enzymes; admit to hospital urgently for consideration of thrombolysis
- If pain is relieved, observe for 15 min and discharge.

## Myocardial infarction
*Management*
- Stop the procedure
- Reassure and calm the patient
- Keep patient upright (lay the patient flat only if he/she is hypotensive)
- Call immediately for medical assistance
- Give sublingual GTN 0.5 mg (1 tablet or 2 puffs of spray)
- Give oxygen(10–15 L/min)
- Give 300 mg of aspirin to chew
- If trained, give 5–10 mg morphine IV (as analgesic) + 50 mg cyclizine IV (as anti-emetic)
- If cardiac arrest, resuscitate
- Admit to hospital urgently for consideration of thrombolysis
- If already in hospital, take blood for FBC, U&Es, and cardiac enzymes.

# Acute heart failure

Unfortunately, both fluid overload and anaemia (from blood loss during and/or after operation) are common following major head and neck surgery, and often remain unrecognized for a considerable time, straining the heart and tipping susceptible individuals into heart failure. The dentist may then be faced with the management of acute heart failure. An MI should be considered, and a systemic infection (e.g. UTI or respiratory infection) or arrhythmia (e.g. AF), may be associated and further complicate management. These conditions have been discussed more extensively on Chapter 4.

*Clinical features*
- Tachycardia
- ↑ Respiratory rate
- Dyspnoea and orthopnoea
- Respiratory crackles
- Distress

*Management*
- Reassure and calm the patient
- Sit patient upright
- Give oxygen (15 L/min)
- Do an ECG (look for arrhythmia or signs of MI)
- Take blood for FBC, U&Es, and cardiac enzymes
- Order an urgent CXR (look for cardiomegaly and signs of pulmonary oedema [e.g. bilateral shadowing and effusion at costophrenic angles])
- Get advice from, or refer to, medical team
- Give 40–80 mg furosemide IV
- Give 5 mg of morphine SC/IM/IV + 50 mg cyclizine IV
- Give GTN or an ACE inhibitor, unless hypotensive
- If in AF and heart rate >120 bpm, give 250 mg digoxin by slow IV infusion and repeat as necessary (avoid if MI)
- If anaemic, organize urgent blood transfusion (give blood slowly and with furosemide to avoid overload [unless hypotensive]).

# Cardiac arrest

*Causes*
The commonest cause of cardiac arrest, especially outside hospital, is ventricular fibrillation (VF), which usually follows an MI. VF necessitates urgent defibrillation. Electromechanical dissociation (EMD) of the heart is less common and may result from hypovolaemia, hypothermia, pulmonary embolism, drug intoxication (e.g. general anaesthetic), electrolyte imbalance, etc.

*Recognition*
- Sudden loss of consciousness
- Absent arterial pulses (carotid or femoral)
- Gasping or absent respiration (after 15–30 s)
- Pupils begin to dilate (after about 90 s)

▶ Assessment should be simultaneous with management.

## Management

*Basic life support* (see front cover)
- Approach with care
- Shake the patient gently and shout: 'Are you alright?'
- Give precordial thump, if arrest is witnessed (and certain)
- Call for assistance:
  - If in general practice—from another colleague and an ambulance
  - If in hospital—the resuscitation team and a defibrillator
- Clear and maintain the airway (head tilt and chin lift [or jaw thrust])
- Look, feel and listen for breathing (up to 10 s); give two effective breaths (up to 5 attempts, looking for rising of chest wall), using a face mask (deliver air with mouth-to-mask technique, or better using an Ambu bag, ideally, connected to an oxygen delivery device)
- Check carotid pulse (up to 10 s)
  - If pulse present, continue with 10–15 breaths/min
  - If pulse absent or inadequate, place on a firm surface and start cardiopulmonary resuscitation (CPR; external cardiac compression [two finger breadths above xiphisternum and ~5 cm deep] plus artificial ventilation, at a rate of 15:2 [whether one or two rescuers] aiming for ~100 compressions/min)

▶ In small children, aim for 1 finger breadth above xiphisternum, 2–3 cm compressions using only one hand (or two fingers in infants), and a 5:1 compression-to-breath ratio.

*Advanced life support* (see back cover)
In hospital, the resuscitation team should arrive and take over within 1–2 min. By now, and while you were 'buying' the patient time with your basic life support (ABC and CPR), the patient should be connected to an ECG monitor and a defibrillator should be available.

Advanced life support includes:
- continuing CPR
- treatment of potentially reversible causes
- intermittent (as necessary) defibrillation. The provision of automated external defibrillators (AEDs) or shock advisory defibrillators (SADs) allows appropriately trained clinical staff to defibrillate safely and effectively after relatively simple training.
- administration of drugs, such as IV adrenaline, atropine, lignocaine, 8.4% sodium bicarbonate (to combat acidosis), etc.

# Respiratory obstruction

Respiratory obstruction may involve part of the airways or it may be complete, particularly if it involves the upper airways, and this rapidly leads to cerebral hypoxia and, after ~3 min, to brain damage and death.

Respiratory obstruction in relation to dental surgery occurs mainly through:
- Mechanical obstruction by an object (foreign body) in the airways
- Pressure on the airways
- Bronchospasm in obstructive airways disease (COPD and asthma)

## Mechanical obstruction by an object in the airways

### Causes and prevention
- Unfortunately, it is only too common that inlays, crowns and endodontic instruments continue to be dropped into the airways. Use of rubber dam reduces these mishaps.
- It is also a relatively common error to collect extracted teeth in a swab and then by mistake use that swab again postoperatively, transferring removed teeth or root fragments back into the mouth. Only use clean swabs for postoperative haemostasis.

### Management of objects that cannot be accounted for
If material such as a crown, an extracted tooth, or a broken burr cannot be found lying free in the mouth, it can either be:
- within the body (in the oral tissues, respiratory tract, or GI tract), or
- outside the body.

The following procedures are advisable:
- Check the mouth and throat carefully.
- Check the area around the patient.
- Check in the aspirator's tubing and container.
- If the object cannot be found, take plain radiographs of the neck, chest and abdomen (two views of each at right angles).
- Direct bronchoscopy may well be more successful than chest radiography in locating (and removing) an inhaled foreign body (usually identified in the right bronchial tree) before it results in abscess formation and/or collapse of the lung distal to the obstruction.

### Management of upper airways obstruction

*If patient is conscious:*
- Encourage his/her own efforts to cough the object out.
- Do not perform blind finger sweep, as this may impact the foreign body further.
- Young children should be held upside down. Back blows or chest thrusts may assist in retrieving the object.

▶ Do not slap the back of a patient sitting upright, as this might actually cause the object to fall further into the respiratory tract. However, if obstruction is complete (e.g. object between vocal cords), this may partially free the airways.

- Older children and adults may benefit from the Heimlich manoeuvre or abdominal thrust (Fig. 6.1).

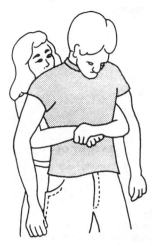

**Fig. 6.1** The Heimlich manoeuvre: The operator grabs one fist with the opposite hand and rapidly presses inwards and upwards

*If patient is unconscious:*
- Lay him/her supine and with head below chest as much as possible, and perform abdominal thrust from above.
- If object is not retrieved, a cricothyroid puncture is necessary.

### Management of a swallowed object
Swallowed objects mostly pass uneventfully with the faeces, but plain radiographs of the abdomen are indicated.

## Pressure on the airways
*Causes*
- Laryngeal oedema (trauma, infection, insect bite, or acute angioedema)
- Impacted middle third facial fracture
- Tongue falling into the pharynx (e.g. in bilateral mandibular fracture)
- Bleeding into, or infection of, fascial spaces of the neck
- Malignancy involving the neck

*Management*
If the cause cannot be treated, tracheotomy may become necessary (see Chapter 11).

**Obstructive airways disease** is discussed on page 280.

# Obstructive airways disease

## Acute asthmatic attack

*Precipitating factors*

- Infection
- Allergen
- Anxiety
- Cold
- Exercise
- Some drugs (e.g. NSAIDs)

*Recognition*

- Acute dyspnoea
- Wheeze
- Cough
- Use of accessory muscles of respiration
- If severe: difficulty speaking
- If life-threatening: exhaustion, confusion, ↓ pulse and BP, silent chest and cyanosis

*Investigations*

- Peak expiratory flow
  - If <50% of expected: severe attack
  - If <30% of expected: life-threatening attack
- Pulse oximetry
- Arterial blood gases
- CXR

*Management*

*If in general dental practice*

- Reassure and calm the patient
- Keep the patient upright
- Give 2–4 puffs salbutamol inhaler (usually patient's own), preferably with a spacer or give salbutamol 5 mg via oxygen-driven nebulizer
- Give oxygen (10–15L/min)
- If attack does not resolve within 5 min,
  - Give corticosteroids (40 mg prednisolone PO or 200 mg hydrocortisone IM/IV)
  - Call for assistance; refer urgently to local hospital's Medical Admissions Unit

*If in hospital*

- Reassure and calm the patient
- Give 2.5–5 mg nebulized salbutamol or 5–10 mg nebulized terbutaline with $O_2$
- Give 200 mg hydrocortisone IV
- If attack is severe:
  - Add 500 microgram nebulized ipratropium
  - Seek assistance of medical team, which may suggest:
  - 250–500 mg aminophylline given slowly IV over 20 min
- If attack is life-threatening, admission in an Intensive Treatment Unit (ITU) for assisted ventilation is indicated.

## Exacerbation of COPD

*Recognition*
- Dyspnoea
- Wheeze
- Cough

*Management*
- Reassure and calm the patient
- Give oxygen, but with care (<30% $O_2$, especially if type II respiratory failure [see page 146])
- Give nebulized salbutamol ± ipratropium and IV steroids as above
- Perform relevant investigations as above
- Request urgent physiotherapy to clear sputum
- Take sputum sample for microscopy (M), and culture and sensitivity (C + S)
- Consider giving antibiotics (e.g. amoxicillin)
- If severe, involve the medical team.

# Diabetic emergencies

Collapse in a diabetic is usually due to abnormal blood glucose levels (usually hypoglycaemia) (Table 6.2), but other causes (e.g. faint or cardiac arrest) should also be considered.

## Hypoglycaemia

### Causes
- Failure to take food (e.g. keeping the patient waiting at lunch time!)
- Overdose of insulin (or drugs, including alcohol)
- Excessive exercise
- Excessive stress or anxiety

### Recognition
- Warm and sweaty skin
- Rapid bounding pulse
- Anxiety, irritability, or agitation
- Tremor
- Followed by:
  - Confusion
  - Drowsiness
- If not promptly treated:
  - Loss of consciousness
  - Convulsions
  - Coma

### Management
- Take a blood sample
  - For rapid diagnosis—by a BM stick
  - For laboratory measurement of blood glucose—by venepuncture (but you will have to act before the result is known)
- Give glucose as soon as possible
  - If conscious: give glucose drink orally
  - If unconscious: give oxygen (10–15 L/min), and 50 mL of 20% dextrose IV (followed by a saline flush, as dextrose is irritant for the veins) or 1 mg glucagon IM (if no IV access), then oral glucose when patient arouses
- Then, give Hypostop (sublingual carbohydrate gel) to keep blood glucose level up.

## Diabetic ketoacidosis

### Causes
- Poor control of blood glucose (inadequate insulin)
- Infection
- Surgery
- Vomiting

### Recognition (see also page 200)
- Dry skin and mouth (dehydration)
- Rapid weak pulse and ↓ BP

- Hyperventilation and acetone breath
- Vomiting and abdominal pain
- Polyuria and polydipsia
- Confusion and lethargy
- Slow decline into coma, if untreated

### Investigations
- Take blood to check plasma glucose and electrolytes
- Take arterial blood to check for ↓ pH and bicarbonate
- Take a urine sample to check for glucosuria and ketonuria

### Management
- Start aggressive rehydration with 0.9% saline, starting at a rate of 1 L/h
- Give at least 10 U of soluble insulin (e.g. Actrapid)
- As the blood glucose level starts normalizing:
  - Use 5% dextrose instead of normal saline
  - Start insulin infusion according to sliding scale (based on regular blood glucose measurements)
  - Give potassium (20–40 mmol/L of IV fluid), unless serum $K^+$ >5.5 mmol/L
- Involve the medical team.

⚠ Never give insulin to treat coma in a diabetic, unless there is absolutely no question that it is caused by hyperglycaemia.

**Table 6.2** Collapse in a diabetic[a]

| | Hypoglycaemia | Hyperglycaemia |
|---|---|---|
| Features | Warm sweaty skin | Dry skin and mouth |
| | Rapid, full pulse | Weak rapid pulse. BP↓ |
| | Dilated pupils | Increasing drowsiness |
| | Anxiety or irritability later | (± acetone on breath) |
| | Confusion and disorientation | Vomiting, hyperventilation |
| | Rapid onset of coma | Slow decline into coma |
| Management | Take blood (for glucose level) | Take blood (for glucose level) |
| | Immediately give glucose 25 g orally (or 4 sugar lumps, or sugary liquids) if conscious. If unconscious, immediately give either 50 ml 20% sterile dextrose IV or glucagon 1 mg IM and then oral glucose or Hypostop when patient arouses | Put up an IV infusion of 8.4% bicarbonate |
| | | Obtain medical opinion |

[a] There may be other causes.

# Adrenal crisis

*Causes*

Many patients are on, or have been treated with, corticosteroids and often appear healthy. Exogenous steroids suppress the hypothalamo-pituitary–adrenal (HPA) axis. Such patients lack the capacity to respond with the normal physiological output of endogenous corticosteroids in response to the stress of:

- operation;
- infection;
- trauma;
- severe vomiting.

*Prevention* is with adequate steroid 'cover' (see page 208).

*Recognition*

Acute adrenal insufficiency (Addisonian crisis) may present with:

- Nausea (with or without vomiting)
- Weakness
- Hypotension
- Weak and rapid pulse
- Confusion
- Hypoglycaemia
- Collapse (may resemble a faint, but hypotension that does not respond to lying the patient flat)
- Coma (if untreated)

*Management*

- Lay the patient flat, with the legs raised.
- Summons medical assistance.
- Give 200 mg hydrocortisone IV or 500 mg methylprednisolone IV (slowly).
- Give oxygen (10–15 L/min)
- Take blood for glucose and electrolyte estimation.
- Put up an intravenous infusion:
  - Initially give colloid solution and monitor BP.
  - When BP stable, continue with normal saline or dextrose-saline.
- Give glucose (orally or IV), if there is hypoglycaemia.
- Determine and deal with the underlying cause once BP has been stabilized. Control of pain and infection are particularly important.
- Steroid supplementation (100 mg hydrocortisone at 6-hourly intervals) must be continued for at least 3 days after the BP has returned to normal.

# Anaphylaxis

*Causes*

Anaphylaxis is a type I or acute hypersensitivity immunological reaction involving rapid release of IgE in response to various allergens including drugs (e.g. penicillin, codeine, aspirin, GA), latex, foods (e.g. peanuts) and insect bites (see pages 228 and 230). The commonest offender is penicillin.

Anaphylaxis is more likely to occur after parenteral use of the drug, and can arise between 1 and 30 min after drug administration.

Anaphylaxis is more liable to occur in patients known to be allergic to the particular, or a related, drug, or with any allergies including asthma, eczema or hay fever. However, it may develop even in the absence of a prior history of allergy to the drug, or even, occasionally, in the absence of any known previous exposure to the drug.

*Prevention*

Always take a good medical history, including drugs and allergies. Avoid potential allergens, but be aware of what people may call allergy. Cephalosporins are a common alternative to penicillins, but many authorities discourage their use in patients allergic to penicillin, as there may be a crossover hypersensitivity to cephalosporins as well. Although this association may have been overstated, it is preferable to be cautious, especially if there is a genuine history of anaphylaxis to penicillin.

When giving any injection (particularly intramuscularly), have the patient lying flat; he/she is then unlikely to faint. If the injection is given to the standing patient, there may be a delay in distinguishing anaphylaxis from a simple faint (although the latter has a more rapid onset). Furthermore, collapsing patients can damage themselves as they fall.

*Recognition*

- Feeling of itchiness, paraesthesiae, nausea ± abdominal pain
- Weak and rapid pulse
- Acute hypotension
- Wheezing (bronchoconstriction ± laryngeal oedema)
- Facial swelling (angioedema of lips, tongue and eyelids)
- Cold and clammy skin
- Urticarial rash
- Collapse
- Circulatory and respiratory failure, coma and death may result

*Management* (remember: ABC plus drugs; Table 6.3)

- Lay patient flat with legs raised.
- Maintain the airways.
- Give oxygen (10–15 L/min).
- Summons expert help.
- Give immediately:
  - 0.5 mg (0.5 mL) of 1 in 1000 adrenaline IM, repeated every 5 min according to pulse, BP and respiration (IV preparations [10 times more dilute] may only be given if pulse disappears)

- • 10–20 mg chlorphenamine IM/IV (continued for 24–48h)
  - • 200 mg hydrocortisone IM/IV or 500 mg methylprednisolone IV (action is delayed and only prevents late deterioration)
- • Give 0.9% saline IV according to BP.
- • Be prepared to do CPR if necessary.
- • Patient may need further expert management, possibly in intensive care.

**Table 6.3** Drug treatment of anaphylaxis

|  | Comments | Route | Dose |
|---|---|---|---|
| Adrenaline | 1 in 1000 solution used (contains 1 mg/mL) Give IM rather than SC. Some patients carry aerosolized adrenaline | IM | 0.5–1.0 mL of a 1 in 1000 solution |
| Methylprednisolone | This is effective more rapidly than hydrocortisone but is more expensive. Is already in solution | IV | 500 mg |
| or Hydrocortisone | Only advantage of hydrocortisone sodium phosphate over sodium succinate is that phosphate is already in solution Hydrocortisone sodium phosphate may cause transient paraesthesia after IV injection Effect quicker by IV than IM use, but still takes 2–4 h (persists 8 h) | IV | 100–500 mg slowly |

# Drug reactions

**Local anaesthetics** are the main cause of adverse drug reactions in dentistry.

Lidocaine is a very safe drug if administered properly, but problems may arise if >200 mg of lidocaine without adrenaline or >500 mg of lidocaine with adrenaline are administered, or if the LA is given intravascularly. In these cases, ↑ levels of LA may reach the CNS resulting in disorientation, agitation, or occasionally, collapse and fits. The effects are usually transient, but typically last for several minutes.

*Prevention* is by using recommended doses for LAs and using aspirating syringes especially when inferior dental block injections are given.

*Management* is by stopping the drug and the procedure, giving oxygen, laying the patient flat and reassuring them. If patient is not improving or shows sign of deterioration with loss of consciousness and fits, summon medical help urgently and try to get IV access.

▶ When the patient has recovered, explain what has happened; be frank and do not label them as allergic to the LA!

**General anaesthetics** may cause dangerous adverse reactions, particularly in the CNS (see Chapter 9 for more details).

**Conscious sedation agents** such as benzodiazepines can severely depress the respiratory centre (see Chapter 9). Flumazenil (up to 1 mg IV over 10 min) should be given in cases of respiratory arrest due to this group of drugs.

**Opiates** may also depress the respiratory centre. The antidote is 0.8–2 mg of naloxone IV  (or SC/IM if no IV access) repeated every 2–3 min, until respiration is restored.

**Antibiotics** may also cause acute adverse effects, which are usually allergic in nature (see previous section).

**Oral anticoagulants (warfarin)** may be enhanced by various drugs, occasionally → excess anticoagulation producing very ↑ INR ± bleeding. Such drugs can include:
- Analgesics
  - Aspirin and other NSAIDs
  - Paracetamol/acetaminofen
- Antimicrobials
  - Ampicillin and amoxicillin
  - Sulphonamides (co-trimoxazole)
  - Metronidazole
  - Prolonged therapy with penicillins, erythromycin, cephalosporins, rifamycin
  - Azole antifungals (miconazole)
  - Ritonavir

The ↑ bleeding tendency may have to be corrected by administration of vitamin K or fresh frozen plasma (see Chapter 4).

**Many other drugs** used in dentistry may, less often, cause serious adverse effects that may require urgent attention. Some of these are discussed on Chapter 7.

*Immediate management* in most cases involves the following steps:

- Stop the drug immediately
- Reassure and calm the patient
- Lay the patient flat
- Give oxygen
- Give hydrocortisone 200 mg IM or IV
- Summons medical assistance.

# Bleeding

Life-threatening acute haemorrhage from oral or perioral vessels is very uncommon, but severe haemorrhage may follow damage to larger vessels (see Chapter 11). Patients who have had radical neck dissections (e.g. those with malignancy) may occasionally have acute life-threatening haemorrhage from erosion of the carotid artery under an infected neck flap. Implant placement may hazard the lingual or other arteries.

*Manifestations* of bleeding include:
• rising pulse rate
• falling BP
• collapse.

*Investigations* include:
• *Haemoglobin.* Shortly after haemorrhage no abnormality is found, but the haemoglobin level falls over a few hours as there is haemodilution.
• *Haematocrit* (packed cell volume, PCV) also falls.
• *Central venous pressure (CVP)* falls, and is more sensitive to blood volume loss than is the BP (see Chapter 10).
• Urine output is ↓ (and if the BP remains low, acute renal failure may supervene).

*Management*
• Prevent further blood loss by direct pressure over wound (see also Chapter 4).
• Take blood sample for haemoglobin levels, grouping and cross-matching.
• Set up an IV infusion (see Chapter 10).
• Transfuse to restore blood volume if indicated (see Chapters 4 and 10).

# Epilepsy

A grand mal epileptic convulsive episode is a sequence of:

Aura → Tonic phase → Clonic phase → Recovery

Epileptics vary one from another in the frequency and severity of fits and also individually have good and bad 'phases'.

Fits may be *precipitated by*:
- withdrawal of anticonvulsant medication;
- epileptogenic drugs, such as:
  - alcohol
  - tricyclics or other antidepressants such as fluoxetine
  - phenothiazines
  - local anaesthetics (if given IV)
  - enflurane
  - methohexitone (and other IV anaesthetics);
- fatigue;
- infection;
- stress;
- starvation or hypoglycaemia;
- menstruation;
- flickering lights.

### Management
- Stop the procedure.
- Lay the patient in the recovery (head injury) position (see Chapter 11).
- Clear the airways.
- Protect the patient from hurting him/herself. Move equipment and furniture away.

Most fits resolve spontaneously within 5 min; failing this, treat as status epilepticus.

## Status epilepticus

Status epilepticus is recurrent seizures, occurring without recovery of consciousness between fits. This involves high mortality and morbidity if not rapidly controlled, especially in the elderly.

### Management
- Maintain airways.
- Give oxygen (10–15 L/min).
- Control seizures with an anticonvulsant such as:
  - 10–20 mg diazepam IM/IV over 2–4 min for adults (or rectal diazepam for young children), or
  - 4 mg lorazepam IV (more prolonged action), or
  - 100 mg phenytoin IV over at least 2 min.
- Request medical assistance.
- Try to identify and treat any obvious cause:
  - Do a BM stick—even if uncertain, give 50 mL of 20% dextrose IV.
  - If in hospital take blood for glucose, U&Es, $Ca^{2+}$.
  - If the patient is alcoholic, give 250 mg thiamine IV.

- Connect pulse oximeter and, if available, ECG.
- Start infusion of IV fluids (0.9% saline) and monitor BP.
- If status epilepticus continues or returns, the patient will need expert management, ideally by an anaesthetist (urgent GA and ventilation may be necessary).
- Following recovery patients should be investigated for the cause of the status epilepticus (if not a known epileptic, suspect intracranial lesion).

# Psychiatric emergencies

A psychiatric emergency can generate tensions among and between staff and patient and relatives, and often leads to a crisis out of all proportion to the patient's clinical state. Most mentally ill patients can be persuaded to accept help voluntarily. If the patient is acutely disturbed, decisive action is indicated. If the patient is mute, amnesic, withdrawn or depressed there is usually less urgency (unless there is suicidal ideation).

Cases that dental clinicians are most likely to encounter are primarily related to alcohol or other drugs.

## Management

- Try to make contact with the patient. A disturbed or violent person is often incorrectly treated, as if he/she had no intelligence or awareness of his/her surroundings. Such patients may well comprehend what is being said to them, even though they cannot respond, or respond adversely.
- Do not press questions, but offer an explanation of the situation.
- Tell the patient where he/she is and what is happening.
- Where possible, call the duty psychiatrist.
- If the patient is considered a danger to him/herself or others and refuses help, compulsory detention in hospital is usually required (sectioning).

*Compulsory admission or detention of patients (sectioning)*

Depending on the law, it may be wise to compulsorily detain or admit to hospital patients if:

- they are suffering from a mental disorder of a such nature or degree to warrant detention under observation for at least a limited period;
- to be detained is
  - in the interest of the patient's own health or safety, and/or
  - with a view to the protection of other persons;
- informal admission is not appropriate in the circumstances of the case.

In the UK, under the 'Mental Health Act 1983', a voluntary inpatient that is suddenly at danger because of a compromised mental state (e.g. postoperative delirium) can be detained for up to 72 h against their will, following the recommendation of the doctor in charge of their care (this may be a maxillofacial or other consultant). Sectioning of an outpatient (or an inpatient for >72 h) requires the involvement of psychiatric services. Alcohol-related problems do not qualify under the Mental Health Act for sectioning; in an emergency, you may have to act (detain patient) under common law.

## Management of specific psychiatric emergencies

*Acute alcohol withdrawal syndrome* occurs in about 50% of patients who misuse alcohol when they abruptly stop alcohol consumption. It usually presents with anxiety, tremor, restlessness, tachycardia, ↑ BP, nausea, sweating, and occasionally, hallucinations. Symptoms peak at ~24 h and subside after ~48 h. After this period a minority of patients may develop *delirium tremens*, which is characterized by coarse tremor, confusion, agitation, delusions, hallucinations, tachycardia and fever.

*Management* of alcohol withdrawal is usually with chlordiazepoxide (30–50 mg PO qds the first day, gradually reducing the dose with an aim to stop at ~1 week). Alcoholics are likely to be malnourished and, especially in the post-operative period, should have parenteral vitamin complex injection (Pabrinex). This is particularly important as thiamine deficiency may result in the development of Wernicke's encephalopathy (disorientation, ataxia, nystagmus) or Korsakoff's psychosis (retrograde and anterograde memory impairment—not really a psychosis). If the patient is not in a state to cooperate, you may have to detain them under common law.

*Acute psychosis* (delusions, hallucinations, odd behaviour, lack of insight, etc.) may present in a known schizophrenic or manic patient, or may be part of a delirious state (see 'Organic brain disorders', page 240). Administration of an antipsychotic such as 25 mg chlorpromazine IM, together with calm and reassuring nursing, are usually adequate. If patient remains anxious, consider a benzodiazepine. Contact the psychiatrist on call (except if cause is obviously organic) as sectioning procedures may have to be initiated.

*Acute depression* will not respond to antidepressants as emergency treatment (antidepressants take 2–3 weeks to come into effect). The psychiatrist has to be called for urgent assessment, possible sectioning and perhaps, ECT (see Chapter 4).

*Actively suicidal patients* need urgent assessment. Talk to the patient openly about the risk, and encourage them to do the same by showing empathy and establishing good rapport. If the patient appears to be at risk, contact the on-call psychiatrist urgently and make sure a nurse accompanies the patient at all times. If the patient tries to leave hospital, take away his/her clothes (and explain why). Do not interfere physically if possible. Actively suicidal patients almost invariably need admission to hospital, compulsory if need be. It is worth noting that most of the cases of deliberate self-harm are associated with a psychiatric disorder.

*Disorientated elderly patients* are best managed if a close relative is constantly with them. Do not isolate the patient and, at night-time, leave a low light on. Stop all sedatives as these ↑ confusion. If agitated and psychotic, chlorpromazine may have some benefit. Try to treat any identifiable causes such as hypoxia or electrolyte imbalance (although the postoperative state, especially at night, is the commonest cause in a maxillofacial ward). If the patient is uncooperative or attempts to leave the ward or hospital, discuss with your consultant regarding possible sectioning.

*Psychoactive drug reactions* are common in psychiatric patients. If your patient is on *haloperidol* (another antipsychotic drug), be alert of the serious side-effects that may occur, such as acute dystonic reaction (which necessitates 5–10 mg of procyclidine IM). If your patient is on *lithium*, be alert to recognize signs of lithium toxicity (course tremor, ataxia, disorientation, dysarthria, nystagmus and renal impairment), which is an indication for urgent medical admission.

USEFUL WEBSITES
http://www.resus.org.uk/pages/cpatpc.htm#summ
http://en.wikipedia.org/wiki/Medical_emergency

# Oral diseases

# The teeth

## Tooth eruption and development (Table 7.1)

- There is a wide variation in the timing of tooth eruption.
- Where eruption is delayed this is most often because of a local obstruction, e.g. impaction.
- Delayed eruption is usually uncomplicated, unless by pericoronitis (virtually restricted to lower third molars), caries or cyst formation.

## Teething

- Tooth eruption can cause 'teething'—mild gingivitis and soreness and, as a consequence, irritability, disturbed sleep, dribbling, reduction of amount eaten, increased fluid intake, cheek flushing and a perioral rash.
- Many infant illnesses are incorrectly blamed on teething.
- Teething does not cause high fever or convulsions: these are usually the result of coincidental systemic disease (usually infections).
  An acutely sore mouth coinciding with tooth eruption is usually viral stomatitis, frequently herpetic.

**Table 7.1** Tooth development

|  | Tooth | Tooth germ fully formed | Calcification begins | Calcification of crown complete | Appearance in oral cavity | Root complete |
|---|---|---|---|---|---|---|
| Deciduous | Incisors | 17th week fetal life | 4 months fetal life | 2–3 months | 6–9 months | 1–1.5 years after appearance in oral cavity |
|  | Canines | 18th week fetal life | 5 months fetal life | 9 months | 16–18 months |  |
|  | 1st molars | 19th week fetal life | 6 months fetal life | 6 months | 12–14 months |  |
|  | 2nd molar | 19th week fetal life | 6 months fetal life | 12 months | 20–30 months |  |
| Permanent | Incisors | 30th week fetal life | 2–4 months (upper lateral incisor 10–12 months) | 4–5 years | Lower 6–8 years<br>Upper 7–9 years | 2–3 years after appearance in oral cavity |
|  | Canines | 30th week fetal life | 4–5 months | 6–7 years | Lower 9–10 years<br>Upper 11–12 years |  |
|  | Premolars | 30th week fetal life | 1.5–2.5 years | 5–7 years | 10–12 years |  |
|  | 1st molars | 24th week fetal life | Birth | 2.5–3 years | 6–7 years |  |
|  | 2nd molars | 6th month | 2.5–3 years | 7–8 years | 11–13 years |  |
|  | 3rd molars | 6th year | 7–10 years | 12–16 years | 17–21 years |  |

**Other disorders of the teeth** (See Table 7.2.)

**Table 7.2** Disorders of the teeth

| Symptom or sign | Teeth usually affected | Most common causes | Less common causes | Least common causes |
|---|---|---|---|---|
| Late eruption | Any | Genetic variance; impacted teeth | Hypopituitarism; hypothyroidism; cleidocranial dysplasia | Various genetic disorders; irradiation; cytotoxic drugs |
| Missing teeth | Third molars; lateral incisors; second premolars | Genetic variance; impacted teeth; extracted teeth | Ectodermal dysplasia; cleidocranial dysplasia; Down syndrome | Various genetic disorders |
| Extra teeth | Usually anteriorly, often in maxilla | Genetic variance; supernumerary; retention of deciduous precursors | Cleidocranial dysplasia; pre-deciduous dentition (natal teeth) | Various genetic disorders |
| Malpositioned teeth | Canines; second premolars | Crowding; supernumeraries | Abnormal muscle action (e.g. cerebral palsy); cleft palate | Scarring; various genetic disorders |
| Malformed teeth | Second premolars; maxillary incisors | Infected precursor (Turner teeth); trauma to developing tooth | Intra-uterine infections; genetic variance | Various genetic disorders; irradiation; cytotoxic drugs |
| Discoloured teeth | Any; often the maxillary incisors | Extrinsic stain (drugs, smoking); caries; trauma (dead tooth); root treatment | Tetracycline; fluorosis; osteogenesis imperfecta; amelogenesis imperfecta; dentinogenesis imperfecta | Kernicterus; porphyria |
| Painful teeth | Any | Caries (pulpitis) | Trauma; abrasion, erosion, attrition | Irradiation; trigeminal herpes zoster; neoplasms |
| Premature loosening of teeth | Any | Exfoliating primary teeth; chronic periodontal disease | Trauma | Neoplasms; juvenile periodontitis; other forms of severe periodontitis; hypophosphatasia; Ehlers–Danlos syndrome; hyperthyroidism; histiocytosis; Papillon–Lefèvre syndrome |

# Caries prevention

The main methods of preventing caries are dietary counselling and use of fluorides.

## Use of fluorides

Recommendations about the use of fluorides depend on the level of fluoride in the water supply. In the UK, water is either fluoridated to 1 part per million (ppm) or non-fluoridated. The local dental public health department or water-company can provide information on this.

### Fluorides for home use

Fluoride toothpaste

The main fluoride agents in toothpaste are sodium monofluorophosphate and sodium fluoride (NaF). The effect of the fluoride toothpaste prevents caries while the action of the toothbrush removes plaque.

- Recommendations for adults:
  - Teeth should be brushed twice daily and always at night.
  - Use a 1000–1500 ppm fluoridated toothpaste.
- Recommendations for children:
  - Teeth should be brushed twice daily and always at night.
  - Primary teeth should be brushed as soon as they erupt.
  - Use a 1000 ppm fluoride toothpaste. The use of low fluoride toothpastes (i.e. 500–600 ppm) is only justified for children who are at low risk of caries or living in an area with fluoridated water.
  - Apply a small pea-sized piece of toothpaste to the brush (brushing should be supervised in young children).
  - Toothbrushes should have soft bristles and small heads.

Fluoride mouthrinses

Fluoride mouthrinses are effective over and above that of toothpaste alone. Any patient with a high caries risk will benefit from fluoride mouthrinsing, but this should not be recommended to children <6 years, as they are unable to spit and eject.
The 2 main strengths available are:

- 0.05% NaF—for daily use
- 0.2% NaF—for weekly use.

Fluoride supplements

Supplements are no longer used routinely because:

- they have only a small additional benefit over fluoride toothpaste;
- they have been linked to a higher risk of enamel fluorosis;
- compliance with a daily regimen is often problematic.

However, fluoride supplements may be considered for medically or physically compromised children. The daily doses shown are for children living in areas without fluoride in the water:

- 6 months to 3 years—0.25 mg F
- 3 years to 6 years—0.5 mg F
- 6 years and over—1.0 mg F

### Professionally applied fluoride

#### Gels and varnishes

Dentists, hygienists and therapists can apply fluoride gels and varnishes to the teeth of people with a high caries risk. Varnish is more commonly used than gel but, due to the high concentration of fluoride (22 600 ppm), varnish must be applied sparingly—particularly in children. Regular 3 or 4-monthly applications are recommended.

#### Relative effectiveness of methods of delivering fluoride

The evidence for the effectiveness of fluoride described above has come from systematic reviews (Table 7.3).

**Table 7.3** Relative caries reduction effects of the different methods of fluoride application

| Methods | Caries preventive fraction (%) |
| --- | --- |
| Varnish | 46 |
| Gel | 28 |
| Mouthwash | 26 |
| Toothpaste | 24 |

## Dietary counselling to prevent caries

Dietary advice should be tailored to an individual patient's needs and personal circumstances, but general recommendations should include:
- Reducing the frequency and amount of non-milk extrinsic sugars (NMES), i.e. sucrose, glucose, glucose syrup, etc.
- Where possible, NMES consumption should be restricted to mealtimes, limiting the frequency to a maximum of 4 times per day.
- Consumption of intrinsic sugars (i.e. those in fruits and vegetables) and starchy foods should be increased to 5 pieces of fruit/vegetables per day.

# An ABC of oral symptoms and signs

The most common oral complaints and their possible causes are listed below (the symbol * indicates commoner causes). Detailed discussion of these conditions can be found in standard textbooks. This section is primarily aimed at helping formulate a differential diagnosis.

## Anaesthesia

See under 'Paraesthesia and sensory loss' (page 311).

## Blisters

- Immune-mediated skin diseases (see Table 7.4)
  - *Pemphigoid (usually mucous membrane pemphigoid)
  - Pemphigus
  - Erythema multiforme
  - Dermatitis herpetiformis
  - Linear IgA disease
  - Epidermolysis bullosa (including acquired)
  - Lichen planus
- Infections
  - Herpes simplex
  - Herpes zoster-varicella
  - Herpangina
  - Hand, foot, and mouth disease
- Others
  - Burns
  - Angina bullosa haemorrhagica
  - Superficial mucoceles
  - Cysts
  - Abscesses
  - Drugs
  - Amyloidosis
  - Paraneoplastic disorders

## Burning mouth

- Drugs
  - Captopril and other ACE inhibitors
- Organic causes
  - Erythema migrans (geographical tongue)
  - Diabetes
  - Candidosis
  - Deficiency states
    —Vitamin $B_{12}$ or B complex deficiency
    —Folate deficiency
    —Iron deficiency
- Psychogenic
  - *Cancerophobia
  - Depression
  - Anxiety states
  - Hypochondriasis

**Table 7.4** Differentiation and management of the more common vesiculobullous disorders

|  | Pemphigus* | Mucous membrane pemphigoid | Erythema multiforme | Dermatitis herpeti-formis[d] |
|---|---|---|---|---|
| Incidence | Rare | Uncommon | Uncommon | Rare |
| Age mainly affected Sex mainly affected | Middle age | Late middle age | Young adults | Middle age |
| Geographic and predisposing factors | People from around mediterranean | — | Infections (herpes/mycoplasma), drugs | Gluten |
| Oral manifestations | Erosions; blisters rarely persist; Nikolsky sign positive | Blisters (sometimes blood-filled); erosions; Nikolsky sign may be positive | Swollen lips; serosanguinous exudate; large erosions anteriorly; occasional blisters | Blisters; ulcers |
| Cutaneous manifestations | Large flaccid blisters sooner or later | Rare or minor | Target or iris lesions may be present[c] | Pruritic vesicular rash on back and extensor surfaces |
| Histopathology | Acantholysis; intra-epithelial bulla | Subepithelial bulla | Subepithelial bulla | Subepithelial bulla |
| Direct immuno-fluorescence | Intercellular IgG in epithelium | Subepithelial/BMZ[a]; C3; IgG | Subepithelial IgG[b] | Subepithelial IgA |
| Serology | Antibodies to epithelial intercellular cement in most | Antibodies to epithelial basement membrane in few | — | Antibodies to reticulin or endomysium in some |
| Other investigations or features | — | — | — | Biopsy of small intestine |
| Usual treatment | Immuno-suppressants | Topical steroids or tacrolimus | Aciclovir/steroid | Gluten-free diet, sulphapyridine, dapsone |

* vulgaris. There are several other forms with oral lesions. Paraneoplastic pemphigus is associated with transitional epithelium antibodies. IgA pemphigus is associated with IgA antibodies. Oral lesions are less common in pemphigus vegetans.

[a] BMZ = basement membrane zone.

[b] Non-specific findings.

[c] Rarely bullous.

[d] And linear IgA disease.

**Cacoguesia** (unpleasant taste in the mouth)
- Oral infections
  - Chronic periodontitis
  - Acute ulcerative (necrotising) gingivitis
  - Chronic dental abscess
  - Dry socket
  - Pericoronitis
  - Candidosis
  - Sialadenitis
- Habits
  - Smoking
  - Drugs
  - Foods
- Xerostomia
  - Drugs (see Chapter 8)
  - Sjögren's syndrome
  - Irradiation damage
- Psychogenic
  - Depression
  - Anxiety states
  - Psychoses
  - Hypochondriasis
- Drugs (see Chapter 8)
- Starvation
- Respiratory disease
  - Chronic sinusitis
  - Chronic tonsillitis
  - Oro-antral fistula
  - Lung or pharyngeal tumours or infections
- Pharyngeal pouch
- Gastro-oesophageal reflux disease (GORD)
- Frontal lobe tumours
- Liver disease
- Renal disease

**Discharges**
- Dental disease
  - *Chronic dental abscess
  - Pericoronitis
  - Dry socket
  - Cysts
  - Oro-antral fistula
  - Osteomyelitis
  - Osteoradionecrosis
- Salivary gland disorders
  - Sialadenitis
  - Mucocele
- Psychogenic
  - Depression
  - Hypochondriasis
  - Psychosis

## Dry mouth

- Diuretics
- Drugs with anticholinergic effects
  - Atropine and analogues
  - Antidepressants; tricyclic antidepressants, serotonin agonists, or noradrenaline and/or serotonin re-uptake blockers
  - Antihistamines
  - Anti-emetics
  - Phenothiazines
  - Antimigraine agents
  - Antihypertensives
  - Muscarinic receptor antagonists (for treatment of overactive bladder)
  - Lithium
- Drugs with sympathomimetic actions
  - Decongestants
  - Bronchodilators
  - Appetite suppressants
  - Amphetamines
  - Ecstasy
- Other drugs
  - Alpha receptor antagonists (for treatment of urinary retention)
  - Benzodiazepines
  - Dideoxyinosine
  - Hypnotics
  - Opioids and drugs of abuse
  - Cytokines
  - Cytotoxic drugs
  - Histamine H2 antagonists
  - Proton pump inhibitors
  - Protease inhibitors
  - Radioiodine
  - Retinoids
  - Skeletal muscle relaxants
- Dehydration
  - Inadequate fluid intake
  - Uncontrolled diabetes mellitus
  - Diabetes insipidus
  - Diarrhoea
  - Vomiting
  - Severe haemorrhage
  - Drugs causing dehydration (e.g. alcohol, lithium, diuretics, dideoxy-inosine)
- Psychogenic
  - Anxiety states
  - Depression
  - Hypochondriasis
- Salivary gland disease
  - Sjögren's syndrome
  - Irradiation damage
  - Sarcoidosis

- HIV
- HCV
- Salivary gland aplasia
- Ectodermal dysplasia
- Dysautonomia

## Dysarthria
- Oral disease
  - *Painful lesions
  - Loss of mobility of the tongue or palate
  - Cleft palate
  - Tongue piercing
  - Badly fitting prostheses
- Neurological disorders
  - Multiple sclerosis
  - Parkinsonism
  - Cerebrovascular accident
  - Bulbar palsy
  - Hypoglossal nerve palsy
  - Cerebral palsy
  - Myopathies
  - Dyskinesias
- Alcohol
- Drugs
  - Phenothiazines
  - Levodopa
  - Butyrophenones
  - Phenytoin
- Severe xerostomia

## Dysphagia
- Oral disease
  - *Inflammatory, traumatic, surgical or neoplastic lesions (of tongue, palate or pharynx)
- Xerostomia
- Oesophageal disease
  - Foreign bodies
  - Stricture
  - Carcinoma
  - Systemic sclerosis
  - Pharyngeal pouch
- Neurological disorders
  - Stroke
  - Bulbar palsy
  - Syringobulbia
  - Achalasia
  - Myopathies
- Psychogenic
  - Hysteria

## Facial palsy

- Neurological disease
  - *Bell's palsy (usually HSV or other herpes virus infection)
  - Stroke
  - Cerebral tumour
  - Moebius syndrome
  - Multiple sclerosis
  - Trauma to facial nerve or its branches
  - Leprosy
  - Ramsay–Hunt syndrome
  - Guillain–Barré syndrome
  - HIV
  - Lyme disease
- Middle ear disease
  - Cholesteatoma
  - Mastoiditis
- Parotid trauma or malignancy
- Others
  - Melkersson–Rosenthal syndrome
  - Sarcoidosis (Heerfordt syndrome)
  - Myopathies

## Facial swelling

- Inflammatory
  - *Oral infection
  - Cutaneous infection
  - Insect bite
- Traumatic
  - Oedema or haematoma associated with surgery or injury
  - Surgical emphysema
- Immunological
  - Allergic angioedema
  - Hereditary angioedema
  - Crohn's disease
  - Orofacial granulomatosis (OFG)
  - Melkersson–Rosenthal syndrome
  - Cheilitis granulomatosis
  - Sarcoidosis
- Endocrine and metabolic
  - Cushing's syndrome (Cushing's disease or systemic corticosteroid therapy)
  - Myxoedema
  - Acromegaly
  - Obesity
  - Nephrotic syndrome
- Superior vena cava (SVC) syndrome (obstruction of SVC, e.g. by bronchial carcinoma)
- Cysts
- Neoplasms

- Foreign body
- Congenital (e.g. lymphangioma)

**Halitosis**
- Oral infections
  - *Chronic periodontitis
  - Acute ulcerative (necrotising) gingivitis
  - Oral abscess
- Dry socket
- Nasal and pharyngeal infections, tumours or foreign bodies
- Xerostomia
- Foods
  - Garlic
  - Curries and spices
  - Onions
  - Durian
- Habits
  - Tobacco use
  - Alcohol
  - Solvent abuse
  - Amphetamines
- Drugs
  - Chloral hydrate
  - Nitrites and nitrates
  - Dimethyl sulphoxide
  - Cytotoxic drugs
  - Phenothiazines
- Psychogenic
- Systemic disease
  - Respiratory tract tumours or infections
  - Hepatic cirrhosis and liver failure
  - Renal failure
  - Diabetic ketosis
  - Gastrointestinal disease
  - Inborn errors of metabolism such as trimethylaminouria

**Hyperpigmentation**
*Generalized (difuse)*
- *Racial
- Foods
- Drugs
  - Amiodarone
  - Antimalarials (e.g. chloroquine)
  - Minocycline
  - Oral contraceptive pill
  - Phenothiazines
  - Phenytoin
  - Zidovudine
- Tobacco use
- Betel use
- Post inflammatory (e.g. lichen planus)

- Endocrinopathies
  - Addison's disease
  - ACTH therapy
  - Nelson's syndrome
  - Inappropriate ACTH production
- Others
  - Albright syndrome
  - Neurofibromatosis
  - Haemochromatosis
  - Exposure to heavy metals (e.g. iron, lead)
  - Laugier–Hunziker syndrome

### Localized (small macules)
- *Amalgam tattoo
- Ephelis
- Lentigo
- Naevus
- Melanoma
- Peutz–Jegher syndrome
- Kaposi's sarcoma
- Epithelioid angiomatosis
- Varicosity (common in lower lip vermilion)

## Loss of taste
- Anosmia
  - *Upper respiratory tract infections
  - Naso-ethmoidal fracture
- Neurological disease
  - Cerebrovascular disease
  - Multiple sclerosis
  - Bell's palsy
  - Fractured base of skull
  - Posterior cranial fossa tumour
  - Cerebral metastasis
  - Trigeminal neuropathy
- Psychogenic
  - Anxiety states
  - Depression
  - Psychosis
- Drugs (e.g. penicillamine)
- Irradiation
- Xerostomia
- Zinc or copper deficiency

**Pain** (see also Table 7.5 and Fig. 7.1)

**Table 7.5** Differentiation and management of important types of facial pain[a]

|  | Idiopathic trigeminal neuralgia | Atypical facial pain | Migraine | Migrainous neuralgia |
|---|---|---|---|---|
| **Age (years)** | >50 | 30–50 | Any | 30–50 |
| **Sex** | F > M | F > M | F > M | M > F |
| **Site** | Unilateral, mandible or maxilla | ± Bilateral, maxilla | Any | Retro-orbital |
| **Associated features** | — | ± Depression | ± Photophobia; ± nausea; ± vomiting | ± Conjunctival infection; ± lacrimation; ± nasal congestion |
| **Character** | Lancinating | Dull | Throbbing | Boring |
| **Duration of episode** | Brief (seconds) | Continual | Many hours (usually day) | Few hours (usually night) |
| **Precipitating factors** | ± Trigger areas | None | ± Foods ± stress | Alcohol ± stress |
| **Usual treatments** | Carbamazepine | Antidepressants CBT[b] | Analgesics; Sumatriptan | Sumatriptan; oxygen |

[a] Most oral pain is caused by local disease.
[b]CBT= cognitive behavioural therapy.

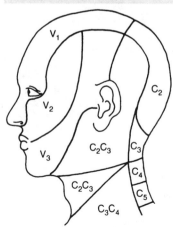

**Fig. 7.1** Sensory nerve supply to the head and neck
V= Trigeminal          C= Cervical

- Diseases of the teeth and supporting tissues
  - *Pulpitis
  - Periapical periodontitis
  - Lateral (periodontal) abscess
  - Acute ulcerative (necrotising) gingivitis
  - Periocoronitis
  - Dry socket
- Diseases of the jaws
  - Fracture
  - Osteomyelitis
  - Infected cyst
  - Malignant neoplasm
  - Neuralgia-inducing cavitational osteonecrosis (NICO)
- Diseases of the maxillary antrum
  - Acute sinusitis
  - Malignant neoplasm
- Diseases of the salivary glands
  - Acute sialadenitis
  - Calculi or other obstruction to duct
  - Severe Sjögren's syndrome
  - Malignant neoplasms
- Diseases of the eyes
  - Glaucoma
- Psychogenic pain
  - Atypical facial pain
  - Oral dysaesthesia (burning mouth and glossodynia)
  - TMJ pain-dysfunction syndrome
  - Other painful symptoms which may be associated with anxiety or depression
- Vascular disorders
  - Migraine
  - Migrainous neuralgia
  - Temporal arteritis (giant cell arteritis)
- Neurological disorders
  - Trigeminal neuralgia
  - Malignant neoplasms involving the trigeminal nerve
  - Multiple sclerosis
  - Herpes zoster (including post-herpetic neuralgia)
  - Bell's palsy (occasionally)
  - Severe unilateral neuralgia with conjunctival tearing (SUNCT)
- Referred pain
  - Angina or MI
  - Lesions in the neck or chest (including lung cancer)

## Paraesthesia and sensory loss

- Peripheral causes
  - *Surgical damage to nerves (including local analgesic injections)
  - Fractures of the jaws
  - Osteomyelitis
  - Pressure by a lower denture on the mental nerve

- Neoplasms in antrum or nasopharynx
- Tumour deposits in mandible or pterygomandibular space
- Intracranial disease
  - Multiple sclerosis
  - Tumours
  - Syringobulbia
  - Surgical treatment of trigeminal neuralgia
  - Cerebrovascular disease
- Psychogenic
  - Hyperventilation syndrome
  - Hysteria
- Drugs
  - Acetozolamide
  - Labetalol
  - Sulthiame
- Benign trigeminal sensory neuropathy
- Tetany
- Some connective tissue diseases

## Pigmentation

See 'Hyperpigmentation' (Page 308)

## Purpura

- *Trauma
- Platelet and vascular disorders
  - Thrombocytopenia (especially autoimmune, drugs, and leukaemia)
  - Thrombasthenia
  - Von Willebrand's disease
  - Scurvy
  - Ehlers–Danlos syndrome
  - Chronic renal failure
- Viral infections
  - Infectious mononucleosis
  - Rubella
  - HIV
- Amyloidosis
- Localized oral purpura (angina bullosa haemorrhagica)

## Red areas

### Generalized redness

- *Atrophic candidosis
- Scarlet fever
- Avitaminosis B (rarely)
- Iron deficiency
- Pernicious anaemia
- Irradiation mucositis
- Chemotherapy-induced mucositis
- Mucosal atrophy
- Plasmacytoid gingivostomatitis
- Polycythaemia

### Localized red patches
- *Denture-related stomatitis
- Median rhomboid glossitis
- Geographic tongue
- Pyogenic granuloma
- Giant cell granuloma
- Contact allergies
- Erythroplasia
- Purpura (see above)
- Telangiectases
- Haemangioma (purple)
- Chemical burn
- Lichen planus
- Lupus erythematosus
- Kaposi's sarcoma
- Epithelioid angiomatosis
- Varicosity (common in lower lip vermilion)
- Mucositis

## Sialorrhoea
- Painful oral lesions
- Foreign bodies
- Oesophageal obstruction
- Drugs
  - Cholinergic drugs (as used in myasthenia gravis)
  - Buprenorphine
- Heavy metal poisoning
- Rabies

▶ The term sialorrhoea may also be given to *drooling* of saliva as a result of poor neuromuscular coordination, as in infants, those with learning disability, Parkinsonism, or facial palsy.

## Trismus
- Extra-articular causes (primarily muscle spasm)
  - Infection and inflammation near masticatory muscles
  - TMJ pain-dysfunction syndrome
  - Fractured condylar neck
  - Trauma (e.g. by injection) to medial pterygoid muscle
  - Fibrosis (including systemic sclerosis, post-irradiation and submucous fibrosis)
  - Tetanus
  - Tetany
  - Invading neoplasm
  - Myositis ossificans
  - Coronoid hypertrophy (or fusion to zygomatic arch)
  - Hysteria
- Intra-articular causes
  - Internal derangement (anterior disk displacement)
  - Dislocation
  - Intracapsular fracture
  - Arthritides
  - Ankylosis

## Ulcers

- Physical causes
  - *Trauma (from teeth, prostheses, iatrogenic, or artefactual)
  - Chemical, electrical, thermal, or radiation burns
- Neoplastic
  - Squamous cell carcinoma
  - Other (e.g. antral) tumours
- Recurrent aphthous stomatitis (RAS)
- Drugs (drug toxicity or hypersensitivity reactions)
  - Cytotoxics (e.g. methotrexate)
  - NSAIDs
  - Nicorandil
  - Several other drugs (see Chapter 8)
- Necrotizing sialometaplasia
- Eosinophilic ulcer

*Ulcers associated with systemic disease*

- Cutaneous disease
  - Erosive lichen planus
  - Pemphigus
  - Pemphigoid
  - Erythema multiforme
  - Dermatitis herpetiformis
  - Linear IgA disease
  - Chronic ulcerative stomatitis
  - Epidermolysis bullosa
  - Graft versus host disease (GVHD)
- Blood disorders
  - Anaemia
  - Neutropenia (e.g. cyclic neutropenia)
  - Chronic granulomatous disease
  - Leukaemia
  - Myelodysplastic syndromes
  - Hypereosinophilic syndrome
- Gastrointestinal disorders
  - Coeliac disease
  - Crohn's disease
  - Ulcerative colitis
- Connective tissue diseases and vasculitides
  - Lupus erythematosus
  - Behçet's syndrome
  - Sweet's syndrome
  - Reiter's syndrome
  - Polyarteritis nodosa
  - Wegener's granulomatosis
  - Giant cell arteritis
- Infective diseases
  - Herpes simplex
  - Varicella zoster virus (chickenpox, herpes zoster)
  - Cytomegalovirus
  - Epstein–Barr virus (EBV)

- Coxsackie viruses
- ECHO viruses
- HIV
- Acute ulcerative (necrotising) gingivitis
- Tuberculosis
- Syphilis
- Gonorrhoea
- Histoplasmosis
- Blastomycosis
- Paracoccidioidomycosis
- Cryptococcosis
- Leishmaniasis

## White patches

- Developmental
  - Leucoedema
  - White sponge naevus
  - Other rare syndromes
- *Frictional (including cheek biting)
- Infective
  - Thrush
  - Chronic hypertrophic candidosis
  - Some papillomas (viral warts)
  - Hairy leucoplakia (EBV-associated, usually in HIV patients)
  - Syphilitic keratosis
- Pre-neoplastic or neoplastic lesions
  - Smoker's keratoses (e.g. smoker's palate)
  - Idiopathic keratosis
  - Dysplastic (dyskeratotic) lesions
  - Actinic cheilitis
  - Verrucous carcinoma
  - Early invasive carcinoma
- Lichen planus
- Lupus erythematosus
- Skin grafts
- Chronic renal failure
- Chemical burns

## Xerostomia

See 'Dry mouth' (page 305)

## Oral complaints that are often psychogenic

- Dry mouth
- Sore or burning mouth
- Bad taste or disturbed taste
- Atypical facial pain
- Atypical odontalgia
- Paraesthesias and anaesthesia
- TMJ pain-dysfunction syndrome
- Non-existent discharges
- 'Gripping' dentures
- Vomiting or nausea caused by dentures
- Supposed sialorrhoea
- Non-existent lumps
- Multiple complaints (the 'syndrome of oral complaints')

⚠ It is essential to exclude organic causes.

# Disorders by site

To help with differential diagnosis, the various sites are listed here alphabetically, along with possible disorders that may involve them.

## Antrum and nose

### Discharge from nose
- Common cold
- Allergic rhinitis
- Sinusitis
- Foreign body
- Malignant disease
- Rarely, CSF rhinorrhoea

### Pain
- Trauma (mid-facial fractures)
- Sinusitis (usually acute, but occasionally chronic)
- Psychogenic (e.g. atypical facial pain)
- Malignant disease
  - Squamous carcinoma
  - Other neoplasms
- Fungal infections (rarely)

### Swelling
- Fibro-osseous lesion (e.g. fibrous dysplasia)
- Malignant disease

### Radioopacity
- Bleeding from injury
- Antral mucocele (common incidental finding)
- Neoplasia
- Infection

## Gingiva

### Red areas
- Chronic gingivitis (restricted to the gingival margins)
- Desquamative gingivitis
  - Lichen planus
  - Mucous membrane pemphigoid
  - Pemphigus
- Erythroplasia
- Infections
- Plasma cell gingivitis
- Crohn's disease
- Sarcoidosis
- Orofacial granulomatosis
- Neutropenia
- Leukaemia
- Carcinoma
- Wegener granulomatosis
- Kaposi sarcoma

*Bleeding*
- Periodontal disease
  - *Chronic gingivitis
  - Chronic periodontitis
  - Acute ulcerative (necrotising) gingivitis
- Haemorrhagic diseases
  - Platelet and vascular disorders
  - Leukaemia
  - HIV
  - Idiopathic thrombocytopenic purpura
  - Hereditary haemorrhagic telangiectasia
  - Ehlers–Danlos syndrome
  - Scurvy
  - Angiomas
- Clotting defects
  - Liver disease
  - Obstructive jaundice
  - Haemophilia
  - von Willebrand's disease
- Drugs
  - Anticoagulants
  - Aspirin
  - Cytotoxics
  - Sodium valproate

*Swelling*
*Generalized*
- *Chronic 'hyperplastic' gingivitis
- Drugs
  - Phenytoin
  - Ciclosporin
  - Calcium channel blockers such as nifedipine or diltiazem
- Hereditary gingival fibromatosis
- Leukaemia
- Mucopolysaccharidosis
- Mucolipidosis
- Hypoplasminogenaemia
- Wegener's granulomatosis
- Scurvy

*Localized*
- *Abscesses
- Cysts
- Pyogenic granulomas
- Fibrous epulis
- Giant cell lesions
- Other benign or malignant neoplasms
- Foreign bodies
- Wegener's granulomatosis
- Sarcoidosis
- Amyloidosis

*Ulcers*
- Traumatic
- Acute ulcerative (necrotising) gingivitis
- Immunodeficiency
  - Acute leukaemia
  - HIV
  - Agranulocytosis
- Hypoplasminogenaemia
- Other causes of mouth ulcers

## Lips

*Angular stomatitis (cheilitis)*
- Candidosis
- Staphylococcal, streptococcal or mixed infections
- Ariboflavinosis (rarely), iron, folate or $B_{12}$ deficiency
- Crohn's disease
- Orofacial granulomatosis (OFG)
- Anaemia
- HIV
- Diabetes
- Down syndrome

*Bleeding*
- *Trauma
- Cracked lips
- Midline fissure
  - Idiopathic (possibly smoking or weather related)
  - Crohn's disease and OFG
  - Down syndrome
  - HIV
- Acute erythema multiforme
- Angiomas

▶ Underlying haemorrhagic disease inevitably aggravates any tendency to bleed from labial lesions.

*Blisters*
- *Herpes labialis
  - usually reactivation of latent HSV, or
  - part of 1° HSV infection
- Burns
- Herpes zoster
- Erythema multiforme
- Pemphigus (vulgaris or paraneoplastic)
- Mucoceles
- Impetigo

*Desquamation and crusting*
- *Dehydration, particularly exposure to hot dry winds
- Lip licking
- Chemical or allergic cheilitis
- Erythema multiforme

- Psychogenic or factitious
- Kawasaki's disease
- HIV

### Swellings
*Diffuse*
- Individual or racial variation
- Cosmetic surgical lip augmentation (collagen injections)
- Oedema
  - Trauma
  - Infection
  - Insect bite
  - Contact cheilitis
  - Plasmacytoid cheilitis
- Angioedema
  - Allergic
  - Hereditary
- Erythema multiforme
- Kawasaki's disease
- Cheilitis granulomatosa
  - Idiopathic
  - Crohn's disease
  - OFG
  - Melkersson–Rosenthal syndrome
  - Sarcoidosis
- Cheilitis glandularis
- Lymphangioma
- Haemangioma

*Localized*
- Mucocele
- Fibroepithelial polyp
- Viral wart
- Chancre (1° syphilis)
- Tumour
  - Salivary adenoma or adenocarcinoma
  - Squamous cell carcinoma
  - Basal cell carcinoma
  - Keratoacanthoma
  - Other tumours
- Cyst
- Abscess
- Insect bite

### Ulceration
- Trauma
- Infection
  - Herpes labialis
  - Herpes zoster

- Syphilis (chancre)
- Aphthae
- Behçet's syndrome
- Deep fungal infections
- Leishmaniasis
- Squamous cell carcinoma
- Burns
- Lupus erythematosus
- Erythema multiforme (and Stevens–Johnson syndrome)
- Pemphigus
- Lichen planus
- Haematological disorders

### White lesions
- *Keratoses
  - Most commonly actinic keratosis
- Carcinoma
- Lichen planus
- Lupus erythematosus
- Fordyce's spots
- Scars
- Vitiligo

## Neck (swellings)
### Cervical lymph nodes
- Infections
  - *Lymphadenitis (2° to dental, oral, pharyngeal, tonsillar, face or scalp infections)
  - Infectious mononucleosis (EBV)
  - HIV
  - Cytomegalovirus
  - Human herpesvirus-6
  - Tuberculosis or other mycobacterial infections
  - Syphilis
  - Cat scratch disease
  - Brucellosis
  - Toxoplasmosis
- Other inflammatory/immune conditions
  - Connective tissue diseases
  - Crohn's disease and OFG
  - Sarcoidosis
  - Kawasaki disease (mucocutaneous lymph node syndrome)
  - Kikuchi–Fujimoto disease
  - Kimura's disease
  - Angiolymphoid hyperplasia with eosinophilia
- Tumours
  - 2° carcinoma (oral, nasopharyngeal, skin, thyroid, lung or stomach origin)
  - Lymphomas
  - Leukaemias
- Drugs (e.g. phenytoin)

*Salivary glands swellings* (see below).

*Others*

*Side of the neck*
- Actinomycosis
- Fascial space infections
- Branchial cyst (lymphoepithelial cyst)
- Epidermoid cyst (previously sebaceous cyst)
- Pharyngeal pouch
- Cystic hygroma
- Carotid tumours

*Mid-line of the neck*
- Thyroglossal cyst
- Thyroid tumours or goitre
- Deep ranula
- Ludwig's angina
- Dermoid cyst

## Palate

*Lumps*
- Developmental
  - *Unerupted teeth
  - Torus palatinus
  - Cysts
- Inflammatory
  - Abscesses
  - Cysts
  - Necrotizing sialometaplasia
- Neoplasms
  - Oral or antral carcinoma
  - Salivary tumours (e.g. adenocystic carcinoma)
  - Fibrous overgrowths (fibroepithelial polyps)
  - Papillomas
  - Kaposi's sarcoma
  - Lymphomas
  - Other tumours
- Others
  - Foreign bodies
  - Adenomatoid hyperplasia

*Redness*
- *Denture-related stomatitis (candidosis)
- Erythroplasia
- Purpura
- Pemphigus [early lesions]

## Salivary glands

*Dry mouth* (see page 305).

*Swellings*
- Inflammatory
  - *Mumps
  - Ascending sialadenitis
  - Recurrent sialadenitis
  - HIV
  - Cytomegalovirus
  - Actinomycosis
  - Toxoplasmosis
  - Tuberculosis
- Granulomatous
  - Sarcoidosis (e.g. Heerfordt's syndrome)
- Immune-mediated/lymphoproliferative
  - Sjögren's syndrome
  - Mikulicz disease (lymphoepithelial lesion)
  - Mikulicz syndrome (part of other granulomatous or lymphoproliferative disorders)
  - Haematological malignancy
- Sialosis (salivary gland hyperplasia)
  - Alcoholism
  - Obesity
  - Diabetes mellitus
  - Anorexia nervosa or bulimia nervosa
- Deposits (e.g. amyloidosis, haemochromatosis)
- *Duct obstruction
  - Retention mucocele
  - Sialolithiasis
  - Ranula
  - Sialocele (e.g. following partial parotidectomy)
- Drug-associated
  - Chlorhexidine
  - Phenylbutazone
  - Iodine compounds
  - Thiouracil
  - Catecholamines
  - Sulphonamides
  - Phenothiazines
  - Methyldopa
- Benign neoplasms
  - Pleomorphic salivary adenoma (PSA)
  - Warthin's tumour (cystadenolymphoma)
  - Ductal adenoma
  - Oxyphil adenoma
  - Other monomorhic adenomas
- Malignant neoplasms
  - Mucoepidermoid carcinoma
  - Adenoid cystic carcinoma
  - Malignant PSA
  - Acinic cell carcinoma

- SCC
- Adenocarcinoma not otherwise specified (NOS)

## Pain

*Common causes*
- *Mumps
- Stones or other causes of obstruction

*Uncommon causes*
- Sjögren's syndrome
- Acute sialadenitis
- Recurrent sialadenitis
- Gustatory sweating (following parotid surgery)
- Salivary gland malignant tumours
- Drug-associated
  - Antihypertensives
  - Cytotoxics (e.g. vinca alkaloids)

## TMJ

### Ankylosis
- Trauma
- Infection
- Inflammatory
  - Juvenile rheumatoid arthritis (RA)
  - RA
  - Ankylosing spondylitis

### Dislocation
- Yawning (subluxated joint)
- Trauma
- Phenothiazines (rarely)
- Hysteria (rarely)

### Limitation of mouth opening
See 'Trismus' (page 313).

### Pain
- Trauma (e.g. condylar fracture)
- TMJ pain-dysfunction syndrome
- Internal derangement
- Infection
  - Following penetrating injury
  - Haematogenous (e.g. gonococcus)
- Non-infective inflammation
  - Traumatic arthritis
  - RA (especially juvenile)
  - Osteoarthritis
  - Gout
  - Psoriatic arthropathy
- Neoplasms
  - Benign (e.g. osteoma)
  - Malignant (1° or metastases)

## Tongue

### Swellings or lumps

*Localized*

- Congenital
  - Lingual thyroid
  - Hamartomas
- Inflammatory
  - Postoperative infection
  - Insect bite
- Traumatic
  - Oedema
  - Haematoma
- Neoplastic
  - *Fibrous lump (fibroepithelial polyp)
  - Papilloma (viral wart)
  - Carcinoma
  - Granular cell tumour
  - Mucosal neuroma (usually a feature of multiple endocrine neoplasia type IIa)
- Foreign body
- Cyst

*Diffuse*

- Congenital
  - Down syndrome
  - Mucopolysaccharidoses
- Endocrine
  - Cretinism (congenital hypothyroidism)
  - Acromegaly
- Inflammatory
  - Postoperative infection
  - Insect bite
  - Angioedema
- Traumatic
  - Oedema
  - Haematoma
- Neoplastic
  - Lymphangioma
  - Haemangioma
- Amyloidosis
- Cyst

### Sore tongue

*With obvious lesions*

- Any cause of oral ulceration (see above)
- *Geographical tongue
- Median rhomboid glossitis (smoking-associated candidosis)

*With generalized redness and depapillation (glossitis)*

- Anaemia
- Candidosis (rarely)

- Avitaminosis B (very rarely)
- Post-irradiation

*With no physical abnormality*
- Anaemia
- Psychogenic
  - Depression
  - Anxiety
  - Cancerophobia

# Management of oral disorders

Management of common acute oral disorders is outlined in Table 7.6.
Management of other oral disorders is outlined in Table 7.7.

**Table 7.6** Management of the more common acute oral problems

| Disorder | Management |
|---|---|
| Acute pulpitis | Open pulp chamber (or extract); extirpate pulp (arrange endodontics); analgesia |
| Acute apical periodontitis | Open pulp chamber for drainage and relieve occlusion (or extract); ± antimicrobials[a], analgesia |
| Acute apical abscess | Incise and drain if pointing; open pulp chamber for drainage; relieve occlusion (or extract); analgesia ± antimicrobials[a] |
| Acute pericoronitis | Relieve or extract opposing tooth if traumatizing operculum; caustics to operculum ± antimicrobials (if recurrent, arrange extraction) ± hot saline mouth baths |
| Acute ulcerative gingivitis | Oral debridement; mouthwashes of hydrogen peroxide, antimicrobial (metronidazole), periodontal care |
| Lateral periodontal abscess | Incise and drain ± extraction or antimicrobials; hot saline mouth baths, analgesia |
| Acute bacterial sialadenitis | Determine cause (usually duct obstruction or xerostomia); antimicrobials (flucloxacillin); ± drainage |
| Acute fascial space infections | Drain pus, remove cause, high-dose antimicrobials, hydration, admit patient |
| Acute candidosis | Determine cause; antifungals (nystatin, miconazole; amphotericin, fluconazole) |
| Acute viral stomatitis | Symptomatic treatment mainly is available:<br>(a) Reduce fever; give paracetamol/acetoaminophen elixir<br>(b) Analgesia<br>(c) Maintain fluid intake<br>(d) Sedation if required (promethazine)<br>(e) Maintain oral hygiene (mouthwashes of chlorhexidine 0.2%)<br>(f) Soft diet<br>(g) ± antivirals, e.g. aciclovir (particularly useful in the immunocompromised for herpetic infections |
| Acute sinusitis (also for oro-antral fistula) | (a) Inhalations<br>± steam; ephedrine hydrochloride nasal drops 1% (not in patients on monoamine oxidase inhibitors) or oxymetazoline or aromatic mixtures such as Karvol® (menthol, chlorbutol cinnamon oil, pine oil, thymol and terpineol) or menthol and eucalyptus, or tinct. benzoin<br>(b) Antimicrobials: amoxycillin, erythromycin<br>(c) Analgesia |
| Dry socket | See 'Alveolar osteitis' (Table 7.7) |

[a] Penicillin if there are no contraindications to this (see Chapter 8) Penicillin or metronidazole are indicated if there are systemic effects, pyrexia, trismus, or severe lymphadenitis.

**Table 7.7** Diagnosis and management of oral diseases (Adapted from Scully C. et al, 2004. Atlas of Oral & Maxillofacial Diseases, Taylor & Francis)

| Condition | Typical main clinical features | Diagnosis | Investigations | Management |
|---|---|---|---|---|
| Abscess (dental) | Pain ± swelling | Clinical mainly | Radiography ± vitality test | Drain either by incision if pointing, or through tooth. Analgesics ± antimicrobials |
| Acanthosis nigricans | Hyperpigmented confluent papillomas mainly in groin/axillae | Clinical plus biopsy | Biopsy, gastroscopy, barium studies Exclude diabetes mellitus and malignancy | Treat underlying cause |
| AIDS | Opportunistic infections (especially fungal and viral), Kaposi's sarcoma, lymphomas, encephalopathy | Confirmed by HIV antibodies or RNA | HIV antibodies and viral load CD4 lymphocyte count | Highly active anti-retroviral therapy (HAART). Prophylaxis/treatment of infections |
| Acromegaly | Increasing prognathism and hand size, headaches, tunnel vision, lethargy, weight gain | Enlarging pituitary fossa Increased growth hormone | Lateral skull radiography, growth hormone assays, visual fields, CT/MRI | Treatment of pituitary adenoma |
| Actinic cheilitis | See Cheilitis | | | |
| Actinomycosis | Purplish indurated swelling(s) over mandible or neck | Clinical plus microbiology 'Sulphur granules' | Pus for microscopy and culture | Drainage, Antimicrobial: penicillin or tetracycline for 4 weeks+ |
| Acute bacterial sialadenitis | Painful salivary swellings ± fever and/or trismus | Clinical plus bacteriology | Pus for culture and sensitivity | Antimicrobial: flucloxacillin |

**Table 7.7** Contd.

| Condition | Typical main clinical features | Diagnosis | Investigations | Management |
|-----------|-------------------------------|-----------|----------------|------------|
| Acute necrotizing ulcerative gingivitis | Interdental papillary ulceration and bleeding, halitosis, pain | Clinical mainly | Smear may help Consider excluding HIV | Antimicrobial: penicillin or metronidazole. Oral hygiene improvement. Mechanical debridement |
| Addison's disease | Weakness, lassitude, loss of weight, hyperpigmentation | Clinical plus low blood pressure, hyponatraemia, hyperkalaemia, reduced cortisol and increased ACTH | BP, electrolytes, 24-h cortisol Synacthen test | Corticosteroids |
| Adenoid cystic carcinoma | Firm salivary swelling | Clinical plus investigations | Biopsy and radiography | Surgery |
| Agammaglobulinaemia | Recurrent pyogenic infections, especially respiratory and cutaneous | Reduced immuno-globulins | Serum immunoglobulins | Immunoglobulin replacement Antimicrobials |
| Albright's syndrome | Fibrous dysplasia, precocious puberty, hyperpigmentation, endocrine disease | Clinical plus investigations | Radiography ± bone biopsy | ± Surgery ± calcitonin |
| Alveolar osteitis (dry socket) | Empty painful extraction socket, halitosis | Clinical | Radiography to exclude fracture or foreign body | Debridement, saline or chlorhexidine irrigations, obtundent dressing ± antimicrobial |
| Amalgam tattoo | Grey to black pigmented area(s) usually over the mandible | Clinical | ± Radiography. Biopsy if any doubt | Reassurance |

| | | Clinical plus investigations | Radiography and biopsy | Surgery |
|---|---|---|---|---|
| Ameloblastoma | Slow growing swelling, usually in mandible | Clinical plus investigations | Radiography and biopsy | Surgery |
| Amyloidosis | Macroglossia, ulcers, petechiae | Clinical plus investigations | Biopsy | Dimethyl sulphoxide or carboxy-pyrrolidine-oxo-hexanoyl pyrrolidine carboxylic acid (CPHPC) |
| Angioedema [see also hereditary angioedema] | Facial or labial swelling | Clinical | C1 esterase inhibitor, IgE, C3 and C4 levels | Antihistamines/corticosteroids |
| Angular cheilitis | See Cheilitis | | | |
| Aphthae | Recurrent oral ulcers only | Clinical | Full blood picture. Exclude underlying systemic disease (e.g. coeliac disease) | Corticosteroids topically, Amlexanox, topical tetracycline (doxycycline) |
| Atypical facial pain | Persistent dull ache typically in one maxilla in a woman | Clinical | Clinical and radiographic exclusion of organic disease | Reassurance, tricyclic antidepressants, SSRIs |
| Bacillary angiomatosis | Resembles Kaposi's sarcoma | Clinical and investigations | Biopsy | Antimicrobials (erythromycin or doxycycline) |
| Bell's palsy | Lower motor neurone facial palsy only | Clinical | Consider excluding middle ear lesion, HSV, Lyme disease, cerebellopontine angle tumour, diabetes, hypertension, HIV | Corticosteroids systemically. Protect cornea. Aciclovir, valaciclovir or famciclovir may be indicated |
| Behçet's syndrome | Recurrent oral and genital ulceration, other systemic features | Clinical | Full blood picture, white cell count and differential | Colchicine, thalidomide, steroids, rebamipide or azathioprine may be indicated |
| Black hairy tongue | Black hairy tongue | Clinical | — | Reassurance. Brush tongue ± tretinoin |

**Table 7.7** Contd.

| Condition | Typical main clinical features | Diagnosis | Investigations | Management |
|---|---|---|---|---|
| Bourneville–Pringle disease | Papules or nodules around nose/mouth, subungual fibromas, ash leaf patches | Clinical plus cerebral radio-opacities | Skull radiography, Biopsy skin lesions | Anticonvulsants |
| Bruton's syndrome | See Agammaglobulinaemia | | | |
| Bruxism | Attrition and sometimes masseteric hypertrophy | Clinical | — | Occlusal splint ± botulinum toxoid |
| Bulimia nervosa | Recurrent self-induced vomiting | Clinical | Full blood picture, electrolytes | Reassurance. Psychiatric care. Restoration of dental erosions |
| Burning mouth syndrome | See Glossodynia | | | |
| Calculus, salivary | Recurrent salivary swelling ± pain at mealtimes | Clinical ± investigations | Radiography/sialography | Surgery ± lithotripsy |
| Cancrum oris | Chronic ulceration | Clinical ± investigations | Consider biopsy Consider immune defect | Debridement. Antimicrobial. Improve nutrition |
| Candidosis | White or red persistent lesions | Clinical ± investigations | Smear plus culture Consider immune defect | Antifungal (nystatin, amphotericin, fluconazole or itraconazole) |
| Carcinoma | Ulcer, lump or red or white lesion | Clinical plus investigations | Biopsy. Chest and jaw radiography | Surgery ± radiotherapy |

| | | | | |
|---|---|---|---|---|
| Chancre | Single, painless indurated ulcer usually on lip or tongue | Clinical | Syphilis serology ± biopsy | Antimicrobial: penicillin |
| Cheek-chewing | Shredded or keratotic lesions around occlusal line and/or on lower labial mucosa | Clinical | — | Avoid habit |
| Cheilitis, actinic | Soreness and/or keratosis on lower lip Sun exposure | Clinical | — | Avoid exposure. Bland UV protecting creams. ± Laser excision ± Imiquimod ± retinoids ± 5-fluorouracil cream |
| angular | Soreness of commissures | Clinical | Haematological screen Denture assessment | Denture modification/replacement Oral and denture hygiene Antifungal: miconazole |
| glandularis | Lip swelling | Clinical plus investigations | Biopsy | Intralesional steroids ± surgery |
| granulomatosa | See orofacial granulomatosis | | | |
| Cherubism | Slowly enlarging swellings over mandible or maxillae | Clinical plus investigations | Radiography + biopsy | Reassurance |
| Child abuse syndrome | Various injuries inconsistent with history | Clinical ± radiography | Photographs + radiography | Protect child from further abuse |
| Chronic granulomatous disease | Recurrent pyogenic infections, cervical lymphadenopathy | Clinical plus investigations | Assay neutrophil phagocytosis and killing of bacteria | Antimicrobials Bone marrow transplantation |
| Chronic mucocutaneous candidosis | Persistent mucocutaneous candidosis | Clinical plus investigations | Assay T-cell function. Biopsy + fungal culture | Antifungals (fluconazole or itraconazole) |

**Table 7.7** Contd.

| Condition | Typical main clinical features | Diagnosis | Investigations | Management |
|---|---|---|---|---|
| Cicatricial pemphigoid | See Mucous membrane pemphigoid | | | |
| Cleidocranial dysplasia | Patent fontanelles, clavicles can approximate | Clinical plus radiographs | Radiography of skull and clavicles | Remove supernumary teeth/cysts |
| Coeliac disease | Loose stool, malabsorption, loss of weight/failure to thrive | Clinical plus jejunal villous atrophy Tissue transglutaminase | Gliadin or endomysial antibodies, transglutaminase + small bowel biopsy | Gluten-free diet |
| Condyloma acuminata | Warts (condylomas) | Clinical | Biopsy | Surgery, podophyllum or interferon or imiquimod |
| CREST syndrome | Raynaud's phenomenon, changing facial appearance. Mucosal telangiectases ± Sjögren's syndrome | Clinical plus investigations | Clinical + anti-centromere antibodies + radiographs | Immunosuppressives |
| Crohn's disease | Loose stool, malabsorption, abdominal pain ± orofacial granulomatosis | Clinical plus investigations | Barium meal and follow-through | Sulfasalazine or corticosteroids or tacrolimus or infliximab |
| Cyclic neutropenia | Recurrent pyogenic infections | Clinical plus neutropenia | Serial neutrophil counts | Antimicrobial, colony-stimulating factor |
| Denture-induced hyperplasia | Hyperplasia close to denture flange | Clinical | — | Ease denture flange; excise hyperplasia |

| | | | | |
|---|---|---|---|---|
| Denture-related stomatitis | Erythema in denture-bearing area | Clinical | Fungal culture | Leave denture out at night stored in antifungal ± use topical antifungals |
| Dermatitis herpetiformis | Pruritic rash mainly on extensor surfaces | Clinical plus investigations Small bowel biopsy | Lesional biopsy + small bowel biopsy + gliadin antibodies | Gluten-free diet Dapsone or sulphapyridine or sulphamethoxypyridozine |
| Dermatomyositis | Proximal limb and trunk weakness plus heliotrope rash | Clinical plus investigations | Serum creatine kinase and aldolase Electromyography Skin/muscle biopsy | Systemic corticosteroids, other systemic immunosuppressants and acetylsalicyclic acid |
| Dermoid cyst | Submental swelling | Clinical plus investigations | Radiography | Surgery |
| Desquamative gingivitis | Erythematous desquamating gingivae | Clinical plus biopsy | Biopsy | Topical corticosteroids, improve oral hygiene |
| Diabetes mellitus | Polyuria, polydipsia | Hyperglycaemia | Blood sugar (fasting) Glucose tolerance test | Diet or insulin ± oral hypoglycaemic agent |
| Discoid lupus erythematosus | See Lupus | | | |
| Dry mouth | See Sjögren's syndrome | | | |
| Dry socket | See Alveolar osteitis | | | |
| Ectodermal dysplasia | Dry thin hair, dry skin, fever, hypodontia | Clinical | Radiography for hypodontia | Restorative dentistry |
| Ephelis | See Freckles | | | |

**Table 7.7** Contd.

| Condition | Typical main clinical features | Diagnosis | Investigations | Management |
|---|---|---|---|---|
| Epidermolysis bullosa | Blisters at sites of trauma | Clinical plus histology | Biopsy | Protect against trauma Vitamin E ± phenytoin |
| Epiloia | See Bourneville–Pringle disease | | | |
| Epulis | | | | |
| congenital | Firm nodule on gingiva | Clinical | Consider excision biopsy | Excise if no resolution |
| fibrous | Firm nodule on gingiva | Clinical | Excision biopsy | Excise |
| fissuratum | Firm leaflike swellings | Clinical | Consider excision biopsy | Change denture. Excise |
| giant cell | Purplish swelling in premolar area | Clinical plus investigations | Exclude hyperparathyroidism | Surgery |
| in pregnancy | Soft swelling typically on anterior gingivae | Clinical | Pregnancy test Consider excision biopsy | Leave or excise |
| Erythema | | | | |
| migrans | Desquamating patches on tongue | Clinical | — | Reassurance |
| multiforme | Oral ulcers, swollen lips. Target lesions | Clinical | Consider biopsy | Corticosteroids, aciclovir if herpes-induced |
| nodosum | Tender red lumps on shins | Clinical plus investigations | Biopsy ± serum for immune complexes | Treat underlying cause |
| Erythroplakia [erythroplasia] | Red velvety patch | Clinical plus histology | Biopsy | Excise |
| Exfoliative cheilitis | Exfoliation of lips | Clinical | — | Topical tacrolimus or pimecrolimus |
| Facial arthromyalgia | TMJ pain, click, limitation of movement | Clinical | Radiography ± arthroscopy | Reassurance, occlusal splint, anxiolytics or antidepressants |
| Familial fibrous dysplasia | See Cherubism | | | |

| | | | | |
|---|---|---|---|---|
| Familial white folded gingivostomatitis | White persistent lesions in mouth, rectum, vagina | Clinical plus family history | ± Biopsy | Reassurance |
| Felty's syndrome | Rheumatoid arthritis, splenomegaly, neutropenia | Clinical plus investigations | Full blood picture, RF, erythrocyte sedimentation rate | Salicylates |
| Fibroepithelial polyp | Firm pink polyp | Clinical | Excision biopsy | Excision |
| Fibroma, leaf | See Fibroepithelial polyp | | | |
| Fibromatosis, gingival | Firm pink gingival swellings | Clinical | Excision biopsy | Excision |
| Fibrous dysplasia | Bony swelling | Clinical plus investigations | Radiographs and biopsy | Excision or await resolution |
| Fibrous lump | See Fibroepithelial polyp | | | |
| Foliate papillitis | Painful swollen foliate papilla | Clinical | — | Reassurance |
| Fordyce spots | Yellowish granules in buccal mucosae or lips | Clinical | — | Reassurance |
| Fragilitas ossium | Spontaneous fractures, blue sclera | Clinical plus investigations | Radiography | Orthopaedic care |
| Freckles (ephelides) | Brown macules | Clinical | Consider biopsy | Reassurance |
| Frey's syndrome | Gustatory sweating | Clinical | Starch-iodine test | Glycopyrrolate |

**Table 7.7** Contd.

| Condition | Typical main clinical features | Diagnosis | Investigations | Management |
|---|---|---|---|---|
| Gardner's syndrome | Osteomas, desmoid tumours, colonic polyps | Clinical plus investigations | Radiography of jaws, colonoscopy | Excision of colonic polyps |
| Geographic tongue | See Erythema migrans | | | |
| German measles | Macular rash, fever, occipital lymphadenopathy | Clinical | Consider serology | Symptomatic |
| Glandular fever | Fever, sore throat, generalized lymphadenopathy | Serology for definitive diagnosis | White cell count and differential, Paul Bunnell test, consider HIV and other serology | Symptomatic, corticosteroids systemically if airways threatened |
| Glossitis | | | | |
| atrophic | Depapillated tongue | Clinical plus investigations | Full blood picture, haematinic assay | Treat underlying cause |
| benign migratory | See Erythema migrans | | | |
| in iron deficiency | Depapillated tongue | Clinical plus investigations | Full blood picture, serum ferritin | Treat underlying cause |
| median rhomboid | See Central papillary atrophy | | | |
| Moeller's in vitamin $B_{12}$ deficiency | Depapillated tongue | Clinical plus investigations | Full blood picture, serum $B_{12}$ | Treat underlying cause |
| Glossodynia | Burning normal tongue | Clinical plus investigations | Full blood picture, haematinic assay, fasting blood glucose | Treat underlying cause where possible ± antidepressants |
| Gorlin–Goltz syndrome (Gorlin's syndrome) | Odontogenic keratocysts, basal cell naevi, skeletal anomalies | Clinical plus investigations | Radiography skull, jaws, chest | Remove cysts ± Etretinate |
| Haemangioma | Blush or reddish swelling | Clinical ± aspiration ± angiography | Empties on pressure | Leave or cryoprobe, laser or sclerosant |

| | | | | |
|---|---|---|---|---|
| Haemophilia | Haemarthroses, ecchymoses, severe bleeding after trauma | Clinical plus investigations | Haemostasis assays | Cover surgery with factor replacement ± antifibrinolytics |
| Hairy leucoplakia | White lesions on tongue | Clinical | HIV serology ± biopsy | HAART (highly active anti-retroviral treatment) |
| Halitosis | Oral malodour | Clinical | Oral/ENT examination and radiography | Treat underlying cause ± deodorants |
| Hand, foot and mouth disease | Oral ulcers, mild fever, vesicles on hands and/or feet | Clinical | — | Symptomatic |
| Heck's disease | Oral papules | Clinical | Biopsy | Observe, interferon or remove |
| Heerfordt's syndrome | Uveitis, parotitis, fever, facial palsy | Clinical plus investigations | CXR. Biopsy, serum angiotensin-converting enzyme, calcium levels | Corticosteroids |
| Hereditary angioedema | Recurrent facial swellings | Clinical plus investigations | C1 esterase inhibitor, C3 and C4 assays | Danazol or stanazolol or C1 esterase inhibitor |
| Hereditary haemorrhagic telangiectasia | Telangiectasia on lips, mouth, hands | Clinical | Full blood picture and haemoglobin | Laser or cryoprobe to bleeding telangiectases |
| Herpangina | Oral ulcers, mild fever | Clinical | — | Symptomatic ± aciclovir, valaciclovir or famciclovir |

**Table 7.7** Contd.

| Condition | Typical main clinical features | Diagnosis | Investigations | Management |
|---|---|---|---|---|
| Herpetic stomatitis | Oral ulcers, gingivitis, fever | Clinical | Sometimes smear or serology | Symptomatic ± aciclovir, valaciclovir or famciclovir |
| Herpes labialis | Vesicles, pustules, scabs at mucocutaneous junction | Clinical | — | Penciclovir or aciclovir cream |
| Herpes zoster | See Shingles | | | |
| Histiocytosis (Langerhans cell) | Osteolytic lesions | Clinical plus investigations | Biopsy Skeletal survey | Depends on type; from no treatment to curettage chemotherapy and irradiation depending on lesion extent |
| Histoplasmosis | Cough, fever and weight loss | Histology | Biopsy + CXR | Fluconazole, itraconazole or amphotericin |
| Hodgkin's lymphoma | Chronic lymph node swelling ± fever | Histology | Biopsy ± lymphangiogram ± MRI | Radiotherapy/chemotherapy |
| Horner's syndrome | Bilateral pupil constriction, ptosis | Clinical | CXR + physical examination | Identify cause |
| HIV | See AIDS | | | |
| Human papillomavirus infections | Warty lesions | Clinical ± investigations | Biopsy | Excise, podophyllum, imiquimod or topical or intralesional interferon |
| Hyperparathyroidism | Renal calculi, polyuria, abdominal pain Brown tumour in jaws | Investigations | Jaw + skeletal radiography, plasma calcium, phosphate and parathyroid hormone, bone scan | Remove parathyroid adenoma |
| Hypo-adrenocorticism | See Addison's disease | | | |

| Condition | Clinical features | Investigation | Details | Management |
|---|---|---|---|---|
| Hypohidrotic ectodermal dysplasia | | See Ectodermal dysplasia | | |
| Hypoparathyroidism, congenital | Tetany, cataracts, enamel hypoplasia | Investigations (may be part of polyendo-crinopathy syndrome) | Plasma parathormone, calcium phosphate levels | Calcium, vitamin D |
| Hypophosphatasia | Anorexia, bone pain, weakness | Clinical plus investigations | Plasma calcium phosphate and alkaline phosphatase levels | Calcium, vitamin D |
| Idiopathic midfacial granuloma syndrome | Ulceration | Histology | Biopsy, anti-neutrophil cytoplasmic antibody (ANCA) | Chemotherapy |
| Impetigo | Facial rash, blisters, often golden yellow | Microbiology | Culture and sensitivity | Antimicrobial: penicillin |
| Infectious mononucleosis | | See Glandular fever | | |
| Kaposi's sarcoma | Purplish macules or nodules | Histology | Biopsy, HIV serology | Chemotherapy or radio-therapy, HAART |
| Kawasaki disease | Lymphadenopathy, conjunctivitis, dry lips, strawberry tongue, desquamation, cardiomyopathy/myocarditis | Clinical mainly | Full blood picture, erythrocyte sedimentation rate, electro-cardiogram | Symptomatic |
| Keratoconjunctivitis sicca | | See Sjögren's syndrome | | |

**Table 7.7** Contd.

| Condition | Typical main clinical features | Diagnosis | Investigations | Management |
|---|---|---|---|---|
| Keratosis | | | | |
| frictional | White lesion | Clinical | ±biopsy | Try to eliminate cause |
| smoker's | White lesion in palate | Clinical | ±biopsy | Try to eliminate cause |
| verrucous | Raised or warty white lesion | Clinical and histology | Biopsy | Excise if dysplastic, stop tobacco use |
| sublingual | White lesion in floor of mouth and ventrum of tongue | Clinical and histology | Biopsy | Excise if dysplastic, stop tobacco use |
| Langerhans cell histiocytoses | See Histiocytosis | | | |
| Leishmaniasis | Mucocutaneous ulceration, lymphadenopathy | Clinical and histology | Biopsy | Pentamidine, meglumine or stibogluconate |
| Leprosy | Hypo- or hyperpigmented patches, lymphadenopathy, neuropathy | Clinical and histology | Biopsy | Dapsone or clofazimine |
| Letterer–Siwe disease | See Histiocytosis | | | |
| Leucopenia | Recurrent infections | Blood picture, biopsy | Full blood picture, bone marrow biopsy | Antimicrobial |
| Leukaemia | Anaemia, bleeding tendency, infections, lymphadenopathy | Blood picture, biopsy | Full blood picture + film, bone marrow biopsy | Chemotherapy |
| Leucoplakia | See Keratosis and see Hairy leucoplakia | | | |
| Lichen planus | Mucosal white or other lesions. Polygonal purple pruritic papules on skin | Clinical and histology | Biopsy ± immunofluorescence | Corticosteroids or tacrolimus or pimecrolimus topically, stop tobacco use |

| | Clinical features | Diagnosis | Investigations | Management |
|---|---|---|---|---|
| Lichenoid lesions: drug-induced | Mucosal white lesions. Polygonal purple pruritic papules on skin | Clinical and histology | Biopsy | Corticosteroids topically, stop taking drug Consider replacing restorations |
| Linear IgA disease | Mucosal vesicles or desquamative gingivitis | Clinical and histology | Biopsy ± immunofluorescence | Dapsone ± sulfapyridine, gluten free diet |
| Localized oral purpura | Blood blisters only in mouth | Clinical | Platelet count, biopsy may be needed to differentiate from pemphigoid | Reassurance ± deflate blisters |
| Ludwig's angina | Tender brawny submandibular swelling, fever | Clinical | Pus for culture and sensitivity | Drainage, antimicrobials: penicillin in high dose ± tracheostomy |
| Lupus erythematosus | Arthralgia, fever, rash, lymphade-nopathy, lichenoid mucosal lesions | Clinical plus investigations | Antibodies to double-stranded DNA | Corticosteroids, antimalarials |
| Lyme disease | Acute arthritis—mainly knee, rash ± facial palsy | Clinical plus serology | Serology | Antimicrobials |
| Lymphadenitis acute | Tender swollen lymph nodes | Clinical plus investigations | Temperature, examine drainage area White cell count and differential | Depends on cause |
| chronic | Chronically enlarged lymph nodes | Clinical plus investigations | Temperature, examine drainage area White cell count and differential. CXR. Consider biopsy ± HIV testing | Depends on cause |

**Table 7.7** Contd.

| Condition | Typical main clinical features | Diagnosis | Investigations | Management |
|---|---|---|---|---|
| Lymphangioma | Swelling but empties on pressure | Clinical | — | Leave or surgery, cryotherapy, laser therapy or sclerosant |
| Lymphoma | Wide spectrum. Swollen lymph nodes, fever, weight loss | Clinical plus histology | Biopsy. Radiography | Chemotherapy ± radiotherapy |
| Lymphosarcoma | See Lymphomas | | | |
| McCune–Albright syndrome | See Albright's syndrome | | | |
| Maffucci's syndrome | Enchondromatosis plus cavernous haemangiomas | Clinical plus investigations | Radiography | Reassurance |
| Masseteric hypertrophy | Masseter enlarged on both or occasionally one side | Clinical | ±MRI | Symptomatic Rarely surgery ± botulinum toxoid |
| Measles | Fever, lymphadenopathy, conjunctivitis, rhinitis, aculopapular rash | Clinical | — | Symptomatic Avoid aspirin |
| Median rhomboid glossitis | Rhomboidal red or nodular and depapillated or white, in midline of dorsum of tongue, just anterior to circumvallate papillae | Clinical and microbiology | Smear of lesion | Antifungals if Candida present Stop smoking |

| | | | |
|---|---|---|---|
| Melanoma | Usually hyperpigmented papule in palate | Clinical plus histology | Biopsy (wide excision) | Surgery |
| Melanotic macules | Hyperpigmented macule | Clinical | Consider biopsy | Reassurance |
| Melkersson–Rosenthal syndrome | Facial swelling, fissured tongue, facial palsy | Clinical plus investigations | Exclude Crohn's disease and sarcoidosis | Reassurance ± salazopyrine ± dapsone ± intralesional steroids |
| Migrainous neuralgia | Nocturnal unilateral retro-ocular pain | Clinical | — | $H_3$ blockers, oxygen, analgesics |
| Molluscum contagiosum | Umbilicated papules | Clinical | Consider HIV infection | Pierce with orangewood stick |
| Morsicatio buccarum | See Cheek chewing | | | |
| Mucoceles | Fluctuant swelling with clear or bluish contents | Clinical | — | Surgery or cryotherapy |
| Mucoepidermoid tumour | Firm salivary swelling | Clinical plus investigations | Biopsy ± radiography | Surgery |
| Mucormycosis | Sinus pain and discharge plus fever and palatal ulceration | Clinical plus investigations | Biopsy. Radiography. Full blood picture Exclude diabetes | Surgery. Antifungals |

**Table 7.7** Contd.

| Condition | Typical main clinical features | Diagnosis | Investigations | Management |
|---|---|---|---|---|
| Mucous membrane pemphigoid | Blisters, mainly in mouth occasionally on conjunctivae, larynx, genitals or skin. Scarring | Clinical and histology | Biopsy + immunostaining | Topical corticosteroids, Pimecrolimus or tacrolimus. Systemic steroids or dapsone or tetracyclimus plus nicotinamide |
| Multiple basal cell naevus syndrome | See Gorlin–Goltz syndrome | | | |
| Multiple myeloma | Bone pain, anaemia, nausea, infections, amyloidosis | Clinical plus investigations | Radiography. Serum and urine electrophoresis. Bone marrow biopsy | Radiography and chemotherapy |
| Mumps | Fever, painful swollen salivary gland(s) but no pustular discharge from duct | Clinical mainly | Serology may be helpful | Symptomatic |
| Mycosis fungoides | Variable rash | Clinical plus investigations | Biopsy, Full blood picture Bone marrow biopsy | Topical chemotherapy ± radiotherapy |
| Myelodysplastic syndrome | Ulcers, anaemia, neutropenia, thrombocytopenia | Clinical plus investigations | Full blood picture. Bone marrow biopsy | Chemotherapy. Bone marrow transplantation |
| Necrotizing sialometaplasia | Ulceration in palate | Clinical ± investigations | Biopsy may be indicated | Self-healing |

| | Features | Diagnosis | Investigations | Management |
|---|---|---|---|---|
| Neurofibromatosis | Neurofibromas and skin pigmentation | Clinical usually | Radiography and biopsy may help | Excise symptomatic tumours |
| Noma | See Cancrum oris | | | |
| North American blastomycosis | Chronic oral ulceration, pulmonary involvement | Clinical plus investigations | Biopsy ± CXR | Antifungals: fluconazole, ketoconazole, itraconazole or amphotericin |
| Oral dysaesthesia | See Burning mouth | | | |
| Oral submucous fibrosis | Firm fibrous bands in cheek and/or palate | Clinical. History of betel use | — | Avoid betel and pan. Corticosteroids intralesionally |
| Orf | Umbilicated nodule | Clinical and history | Electron microscopy ± biopsy | Spontaneous resolution |
| Orofacial granulomatosis | Facial swelling, mucosa cobble-stoned, ulcers, angular stomatitis (see also Crohn's disease) | Clinical plus investigations | Exclude Crohn's disease/ sarcoidosis. Biopsy ± allergy testing | Avoid allergens. Reassurance. Corticosteroids intralesionally. Clofazimine, anti-TNF agents or minocycline |
| Osler–Rendu–Weber syndrome | See Hereditary haemorrhagic telangiectasia | | | |
| Osteogenesis imperfecta | See Fragilitis ossium | | | |

**Table 7.7** Contd.

| Condition | Typical main clinical features | Diagnosis | Investigations | Management |
|---|---|---|---|---|
| Osteomyelitis | Pain, swelling, fever | Clinical plus investigations | Radiography. Pus for culture and sensitivity | Drainage. Antimicrobials |
| Osteopetrosis | Anaemia, cranial neuropathies, hepatosplenomegaly | Clinical plus investigations | Radiography, Biopsy | Bone marrow transplant |
| Osteoradionecrosis | See Osteomyelitis | | | |
| Osteosarcoma | Pain, swelling | Clinical plus investigations | Radiography. Biopsy | Surgery ± chemotherapy |
| Paget's disease | Pain, craniofacial neuropathies, cardiac failure | Clinical plus investigations | Radiography, serum alkaline phosphatase, urinary hydroxyproline | Bisphosphonates, acetylsalicylic acid, calcitonin |
| Pain dysfunction syndrome | See Facial arthromyalgia | | | |
| Papillary hyperplasia | Small papillae in palate | Clinical | ±biopsy | Surgery or leave alone |
| Paracoccidioidomycosis | Chronic oral ulceration, pulmonary involvement. Time in Latin America | Clinical plus investigations | Biopsy ± chest radiography | Antifungals: fluconazole, ketoconazole, itraconazole or amphotericin |
| Parodontal abscess | Painful swelling alongside a periodontally involved tooth | Clinical | Radiography, culture pus | Drain. Antimicrobial: penicillin |
| Pemphigoid | See Mucous membrane pemphigoid | | | |

| | | | | |
|---|---|---|---|---|
| Pemphigus | Skin vesicles+bullae. Mouth ulcers | Clinical plus histology | Biopsy. Serology. Immunostaining | Corticosteroids systematically. Consider azathioprine or gold or mycophenolate ± plasmapheresis |
| Periadentitis mucosa necrotica recurrens (Sutton's ulcers) | See Aphthae | | | |
| Periarteritis nodosa | See Polyarteritis nodosa | | | |
| Pericoronitis | Painful swelling of operculum of partially erupted tooth ± trismus ± fever | Clinical | Radiography | Debridement ± antimicrobial. Reduce occlusion. Consider extracting offending tooth |
| Periodontitis (acute apical) | Pain, tenderness on touching tooth | Clinical plus investigations | Radiography ± vitality test | Open tooth for drainage and relieve occlusion (or extract), analgesics ± antimicrobial |
| Perleche | See Cheilitis, angular | | | |
| Phycomycosis | See Mucormycosis | | | |
| Pleomorphic salivary ademona | Firm salivary swelling | Clinical plus investigations | Biopsy ± radiography | Surgery |
| Polyarteritis nodosa | Fever, weakness, arthralgia, myalgia, abdominal pain, hypertension | Clinical plus raised ESR. Histology | Full blood picture, ESR. Biopsy | Systemic corticosteroids |

**Table 7.7** Contd.

| Condition | Typical main clinical features | Diagnosis | Investigations | Management |
|---|---|---|---|---|
| Polycythaemia rubra vera | Headache, thromboses, haemorrhage, splenomegaly | Clinical plus investigations | Haemoglobin, full blood picture, marrow biopsy | Phlebotomy ± chemotherapy |
| Polyps—fibroepithelial | See Fibroepithelial polyp | | | |
| Pulpitis | Toothache | Clinical plus investigations | Radiography ± vitality test | Open tooth for drainage (or extract). Extirpate pulp. Analgesics |
| Pyogenic arthritis | Pain, fever, limited jaw movement, swelling | Clinical mainly | Radiography, culture joint aspirate | Antimicrobial, analgesics |
| Pyogenic granuloma | Swelling, usually on lip, tongue or gum | Clinical | Biopsy (excision) | Excise |
| Pyostomatitis vegetans | Irregular oral ulcers and pustules | Clinical plus investigations | Biopsy. Exclude Crohn's disease and ulcerative colitis | Treat underlying condition |
| Ranula | See Mucocele | | | |
| Recurrent aphthous stomatitis | See Aphthae | | | |
| Recurrent parotitis | Recurrent painful parotid swelling | Clinical | Sialography. Exclude Sjögren's syndrome | Consider duct dilatation or sialadenectomy. Antimicrobials |
| Reiter's syndrome | Arthritis, conjunctivitis, mucocutaneous lesions, urethritis | Clinical mainly | Full blood picture, ESR. Radiography | Tetracycline. Non-steroidal anti-inflammatory drugs |

| | | |
|---|---|---|
| Rheumatoid arthritis | Painful swollen small joints ± deformities Associated with Sjögren's syndrome | Clinical plus investigations Check for xerostomia | Rheumatoid factor; full blood picture, radiography | Salicylates. Non-steroidal anti-inflammatory drugs |
| Rickets | Skeletal deformities, retarded growth, fractures | Clinical plus investigations | Blood calcium, phosphate, alkaline phosphatase. Radiography. Renal function tests | Vitamin D. Calcitonin |
| Rubella | See German measles | | | |
| Rubeola | See Measles | | | |
| Sarcoidosis | Various—especially hilar lymphadenopathy and rashes | Clinical plus investigations | CXR + serum angiotensin-converting enzyme (SACE) | Corticosteroids systemically or other immunosuppresives or TNF blockers (infliximab or etanercept) |
| Scleroderma | Tightening facial and other skin Associated with Sjögren's syndrome | Clinical and serology | Serology Scl-70 antibody | Corticosteriods, immuno-suppressants, antifibrinolytics or vasodilators |
| Scrotal tongue | Fissured tongue | Clinical | — | Reassurance |
| Scurvy | Purplish chronically swollen gingivae | Clinical | White blood cell count. Vitamin C levels | Vitamin C |
| Shingles | Painful facial rash and oral ulcers if affecting maxillary or mandibular division of trigeminal nerve | Clinical | Consider underlying immune defect | Analgesics, ± aciclovir, valaciclovir or famciclovir ± protect cornea |

**Table 7.7** Contd.

| Condition | Typical main clinical features | Diagnosis | Investigations | Management |
|---|---|---|---|---|
| Sialolithiasis | See Calculus, salivary | | | |
| Sialorrhoea | Excess salivation | Clinical | Salivary flow rate | Avoid anticholinesterases, otherwise reassurance or consider atropinics |
| Sialosis | Painless persistent bilateral salivary gland swelling | Clinical plus investigations | Exclude alcoholism, diabetes, bulimia, sarcoidosis, Sjögren's syndrome, liver disease | Remove underlying cause |
| Sinusitis (acute) | Pain especially on moving head | Clinical plus radiography | Radiography | Decongestants, analgesics and antimicrobial |
| Sjögren's syndrome | Autoimmune exocrinopathy. Dry eyes, dry mouth and often a connective tissue disease | Clinical plus investigations | Serology—SS-A (Ro) and SS-B (La) antibodies. Exclude sarcoidosis, HCV, HIV. Consider labial gland biopsy ± salivary flow rate ± sialography ± scintiscan | Artificial tears and saliva. Preventive dentistry, pilocarpine, cevimeline |
| Smoker's keratosis | See Keratosis | | | |
| South American blastomycosis | See Paracoccidioidomycosis | | | |

| | | | | |
|---|---|---|---|---|
| Staphylococcus aureus lymphadenitis | Painful swollen lymph node(s) ± fever | Clinical mainly | Pus for culture and sensitivity | Antimicrobials |
| Stevens–Johnson syndrome | See Erythema multiforme | | | |
| Streptococcal tonsillitis | Sore throat. Tonsillar exudate | Clinical mainly | Throat swab | Antimicrobials |
| Stroke | Hemiplegia usually ± facial palsy | Clinical | — | Physiotherapy |
| Subluxation-TMJ | Limited jaw movement ± pain, condyle palpably displaced | Clinical | — | Reduce. Consider Dautrey operation |
| Surgical emphysema | Swelling that crackles on palpation | Clinical | — | Reassurance. Antimicrobials |
| Tori | Asymptomatic bony lumps | Clinical | — | Reassurance. Surgery if interfering with denture wear |
| Toxic epidermal necrolysis | See Erythema multiforme | | | |

**Table 7.7** Contd.

| Condition | Typical main clinical features | Diagnosis | Investigations | Management |
|---|---|---|---|---|
| Toxoplasmosis | Lymphadenopathy ± chorioretinitis | Clinical plus investigations | Serology | Sulphonamide + pyrimethamine |
| Trigeminal neuralgia | Severe lancinating pain often associated with trigger zone | Clinical mainly | Skull base CT, MRI | Avoid trigger zone. Carbamazepine ± phenytoin, gabapentin, baclofen or clonazepam |
| Tuberculosis | Cough, cervical, lymphadenopathy, weight loss, oral ulceration | Clinical plus investigations | CXR Sputum microscopy and culture Biopsy | Antimicrobials: rifampicin, isoniazid, ethambutol, streptomycin |
| White sponge naevus | See Familial white folded gingivostomatitis | | | |
| Zygomycosis | See Mucormycosis | | | |

USEFUL WEBSITES
http://www.lib.uiowa.edu/hardin/md/dent.html
http://www.uky.edu/~cmiller/

# Therapeutics

# General principles

The following points should be borne in mind with regard to any form of treatment, including drugs:

▶The first principle must be to do no harm.

- Always discuss treatment with the patient, and warn of possible consequences (good and bad), and of possible complications.
- Prescribe only drugs with which you are totally familiar.
- Always check drug doses, contraindications, interactions and adverse reactions in the latest edition of the *British National Formulary (BNF)*, in which is found the *Dental Practitioners' Formulary*, the *Compendium of Pharmaceutical Specialties* (CAN), or the *Physicians Desk Reference* (USA).
- Ensure there is no history of allergy or untoward effect.
- Reduce drug doses in:
  - children,
  - the elderly,
  - liver disease, and
  - kidney disease.
- Avoid drugs, where possible, in pregnancy (see Chapter 5).
- Drug interactions are mainly a problem with GA agents.
- Most drugs can have adverse effects. These are not always frequent or of great significance.

This chapter is not intended to be totally comprehensive, and alternative therapies may well be available. Some drugs and therapies of relevance are not discussed here, but may be mentioned in relevant chapters (particularly Chapters 4, 6, and 9). The term 'contraindication' in this chapter often refers only to a relative contraindication.

Tables 8.1–8.3 outline material relevant to prescribing.

**Table 8.1** Latin abbreviations sometimes used when prescribing. Directions should preferably be in English without abbreviation

| Abbreviation | Latin | English meaning |
| --- | --- | --- |
| a. c. | ante cibum | before food |
| b. d. | bis die | twice daily |
| o. d. | omni die | every day |
| o. m. | omni mane | every morning |
| o. n. | omni nocte | every night |
| p. c. | post cibum | after food |
| p. r. n. | pro re nata | when required |
| q. d. s. | quater die sumendus | to be taken four times daily |
| q. q. h. | quarta quaque hora | every four hours |
| stat | | immediately |
| t. d. s. | ter die sumendus | to be taken three times daily |
| t.i.d. | ter in die | three times daily |

**Table 8.2** Some useful abbreviations in therapeutics

| | |
| --- | --- |
| ACBS | Advisory Committee on Borderline Substances |
| approx. | Approximately |
| BAN | British Approved Name |
| BMI | body mass index |
| BP | British Pharmacopoeia |
| BPC | British Pharmaceutical Codex |
| CD | preparation subject to prescription requirements under The Misuse of Drugs Act |
| CDSM | Committee on Dental and Surgical Materials |
| CPMP | Committee on Proprietary Medicinal Products |
| CRM | Committee on the Review of Medicines |
| CSM | Committee on Safety of Medicines |
| DPF | Dental Practitioners' Formulary |
| e/c | enteric-coated |
| EMEA | European Medicines Evaluation Agency |
| f/c | film-coated |
| HRT | hormone replacement therapy |
| i/m | intramuscular |
| i/v | Intravenous |

**Table 8.2** Contd.

| | |
|---|---|
| INR | international normalized ratio |
| max. | Maximum |
| MCA | Medicines Control Agency, now MHRA |
| MHRA | Medicines and Healthcare products Regulatory Agency |
| m/r | modified-release |
| NCL | no cautionary labels |
| NHS | National Health Service |
| NHS | not prescribable under National Health Service (NHS) |
| NICE | National Institute for Clinical Excellence |
| NP | proper name |
| NPF | Nurse Prescribers' Formulary |
| OTC | over the counter |
| PGD | patient group direction |
| PoM | prescription-only medicine |
| ® | trade mark |
| Rinn | Recommended International Non-proprietary Name |
| s/c | sugar-coated |
| SLS | Selected List Scheme |
| SMAC | Standing Medical Advisory Committee |
| SPC | Summary of Product Characteristics |
| USP | United States Pharmacopeia |
| WD | withdrawn or specially imported drugs |

**Table 8.3** List of Dental Preparations (2004). The following list has been approved by the appropriate Secretaries of State, and the preparations therein may be prescribed by dental practitioners

Aciclovir Cream, BP
Aciclovir Oral Suspension, BP, 200 mg/5 mL
Aciclovir Tablets, BP, 200 mg
Amoxicillin Capsules, BP
Amoxicillin Oral Powder, DPF
Amoxicillin Oral Suspension, BP
Amphotericin Lozenges, BP
Amphotericin Oral Suspension, BP
Ampicillin Capsules, BP
Ampicillin Oral Suspension, BP
Artificial Saliva, DPF

## Table 8.3 Contd.

Artificial Saliva Substitutes as listed below (to be prescribed only for indications approved by ACBS):
AS Saliva Orthana®
Glandosane®
Biotene Oralbalance®
BioXtra®
Saliveze®
Salivix®
Ascorbic Acid Tablets, BP
Aspirin Tablets, Dispersible, BP
Azithromycin Oral Suspension, 200 mg/5 mL, DPF
Benzydamine Mouthwash, BP 0.15%
Benzydamine Oromucosal Spray, BP 0.15%
Carbamazepine Tablets, BP
Carmellose Gelatin Paste, DPF
Cefalexin Capsules, BP
Cefalexin Oral Suspension, BP
Cefalexin Tablets, BP
Cefradine Capsules, BP
Cefradine Oral Solution, DPF
Chlorhexidine Gluconate 1% Gel, DPF
Chlorhexidine Mouthwash, BP
Chlorhexidine Oral Spray, DPF
Chlorphenamine Tablets/Chlorpheniramine Tablets, BP
Choline Salicylate Dental Gel, BP
Clindamycin Capsules, BP
Diazepam Oral Solution, BP, 2 mg/5 mL
Diazepam Tablets, BP
Diflunisal Tablets, BP
Dihydrocodeine Tablets, BP, 30 mg
Doxycycline Capsules, BP, 100 mg
Doxycycline Tablets, 20 mg, DPF
Ephedrine Nasal Drops, BP
Erythromycin Ethyl Succinate Oral Suspension, BP
Erythromycin Ethyl Succinate Tablets, BP
Erythromycin Stearate Tablets, BP
Erythromycin Tablets, BP
Fluconazole Capsules, 50 mg, DPF
Fluconazole Oral Suspension, 50 mg/5 mL, DPF
Hydrocortisone Cream, BP, 1%
Hydrocortisone Oromucosal Tablets, BP
Hydrocortisone and Miconazole Cream, DPF
Hydrocortisone and Miconazole Ointment, DPF
Hydrogen Peroxide Mouthwash, BP
Ibuprofen Oral Suspension, BP, sugar-free
Ibuprofen Tablets, BP
Lidocaine 5% Ointment/Lignocaine 5% Ointment, DPF
Menthol and Eucalyptus Inhalation, BP 1980
Metronidazole Oral Suspension, DPF
Metronidazole Tablets, BP
Miconazole Oromucosal Gel, BP
Mouthwash Solution-tablets, DPF
Nitrazepam Tablets, BP
Nystatin Ointment, BP

**Table 8.3** Contd.

Nystatin Oral Suspension, BP
Nystatin Pastilles, BP
Oxytetracycline Tablets, BP
Paracetamol Oral Suspension, BP
Paracetamol Tablets, BP
Paracetamol Tablets, Soluble, BP
Penciclovir Cream, DPF
Pethidine Tablets, BP
Phenoxymethylpenicillin Oral Solution, BP
Phenoxymethylpenicillin Tablets, BP
Povidone–Iodine Mouthwash, BP, 1%
Promethazine Hydrochloride Tablets, BP
Promethazine Oral Solution, BP
Sodium Chloride Mouthwash, Compound, BP
Sodium Fluoride Oral Drops, BP
Sodium Fluoride Tablets, BP
Sodium Fusidate Ointment, BP
Temazepam Oral Solution, BP
Temazepam Tablets, BP
Tetracycline Tablets, BP
Triamcinolone Dental Paste, BP
Vitamin B Tablets, Compound, Strong, BPC
Zinc Sulphate Mouthwash, DPF

**DPF preparations**

Preparations on the List of Dental Preparations are specified as DPF are described as follows in the DPF. Although brand names have sometimes been included for identification purposes preparations on the list should be prescribed by non-proprietary name.

**Sub-sections**
Amoxicillin Oral Powder
Artificial Saliva,
Azithromycin Oral Suspension 200 mg/5 mL
Carmellose Gelatin Paste
Cefradine Oral Solution
Chlorhexidine Gluconate 1% Gel
Chlorhexidine Oral Spray
Doxycycline Tablets 20 mg
Fluconazole Capsules 50 mg
Fluconazole Oral Suspension 50 mg/5 mL
Hydrocortisone and Miconazole Cream
Hydrocortisone and Miconazole Ointment
Lidocaine 5% Ointment/Lignocaine 5% Ointment
Metronidazole Oral Suspension
Mouthwash Solution-tablets
Penciclovir Cream
Zinc Sulphate Mouthwash

# Prescribing

## General comments

- The legal responsibility for prescribing lies with the doctor/dentist who signs the prescription.
- Prescriptions should be written legibly in ink or otherwise so as to be indelible, should be dated, should state the full name and address of the patient, and should be signed in ink by the prescriber.
- The age and the date of birth of the patient should preferably be stated, and it is a legal requirement in the case of prescription-only medicines (POM) to state the age for children under 12 years.
- Use non-proprietary drug titles whenever possible (generic drugs are usually much cheaper).
- Dose and dose frequency should be stated; in the case of preparations to be taken 'as required' a minimum dose interval should be specified.
- The names of drugs and preparations should be written clearly and not abbreviated, using approved titles only.
- The symbol 'NP' on NHS forms should be deleted if it is required that the name of the preparation should not appear on the label.
- The quantity to be supplied may be stated by indicating the number of days of treatment required in the box provided on NHS forms. In most cases the exact amount will be supplied. This does not apply to items directed to be used 'as required'—the dose and frequency are not given the quantity to be supplied needs to be stated.
- When several items are ordered on one form the box can be marked with the number of days of treatment provided the quantity is added for any item for which the amount cannot be calculated.
- Although directions should preferably be in English without abbreviation, it is recognized that some Latin abbreviations are used (Appendix 5). Some other useful abbreviations are listed on Appendix 1.
- Drug dosage may need modification for use in children, the elderly, and in patients with liver and kidney disorders, various other diseases or on certain drugs (see later in the chapter).
- The following are also important:
  - The unnecessary use of decimal points should be avoided, e.g. 3 mg, not 3.0 mg.
  - Quantities of 1 gram or more should be written as 1 g etc.
  - Quantities less than 1 g should be written in milligrams, e.g. 500 mg, not 0.5 g.
  - Quantities less than 1 mg should be written in micrograms, e.g. 100 micrograms, not 0.1 mg.
  - When decimals are unavoidable a zero should be written in front of the decimal point where there is no other figure, e.g. 0.5 mL, not .5 mL.
  - Use of the decimal point is acceptable to express a range, e.g. 0.5–1 g.
  - 'Micrograms' and 'nanograms' should not be abbreviated. Similarly 'units' should not be abbreviated.
  - The term 'millilitre' (ml or mL) is used in medicine and pharmacy, and cubic centimetre, c.c., or cm$^3$ should not be used.

## Prescribing by dental surgeons

- Until new prescribing arrangements are in place for NHS prescriptions dental surgeons should use form FP10D (GP14 in Scotland, WP10D in Wales) to prescribe only those items listed in the Dental Practitioners' Formulary.
- The Act and Regulations do not set any limitations upon the number and variety of substances that the dental surgeon may administer to patients in the surgery or may order by private prescription—provided the relevant legal requirements are observed the dental surgeon may use or order whatever is required for the clinical situation.
- There is no statutory requirement for the dental surgeon to communicate with a patient's medical practitioner when prescribing for dental use. There are, however, occasions when this would be in the patient's interest and such communication is to be encouraged.

The list of Dental Preparations (2004) is outlined in Table 8.3.

## Prescribing drugs in hospitals

- Prescriptions written by unregistered staff must be authorized (i.e. signed) by a provisionally or fully registered doctor or dentist.
- Some drugs, once formally prescribed by a doctor/dentist, may be given when required (PRN), at the discretion of nursing staff.
- It is reasonable to expect nurses to recognize night sedatives, analgesics and anti-emetics, but where 'when required' drugs are prescribed for other indications, these should be clearly stated in writing.
- Nurses should not be expected to take responsibility for choosing from a selection of prescriptions for similar drugs, different routes of administration and doses without the prescriber specifying the criteria to be considered when making such decisions.
- In some countries, nurses trained and authorized by the authorities to give IV drugs may do so, provided that this does not require them to make entry into the vein; in other words they can give drugs into a drip. The first dose should be given by the dental surgeon, who can then check for adverse reactions.

# Prescribing for special groups

### Prescribing for children

- Doses of all drugs are much lower than for adults. As a rough guide, Table 8.4 can be used, but always check against the recommended dose per unit body weight.
- Oral preparations are invariably preferable to injectable or rectal drugs.
- Tetracyclines are contraindicated < age 7–8 years because of tooth discoloration.
- Aspirin is contraindicated < age of 16 years because of the danger of Reye's syndrome (see below).
- Diazepam may have anomalous effects, causing overactivity rather than sedation.

### Prescribing in pregnancy and during breast feeding

- Because of the danger of damage to the fetus, all drugs should be avoided in pregnancy, unless their use is essential.
- Tetracyclines, retinoids and thalidomide in particular, must be avoided.

For more details see Chapter 5 and Tables 8.26 and 8.27.

### Prescribing for the elderly (see also Tables 8.26–8.29)

- Lower drug doses are almost invariably indicated.
- Compliance may be poor.
- Care should be taken when there is possibility of renal or hepatic dysfunction; this will necessitate reduced doses.

**Table 8.4** Prescribing for children

| Age | Average weight (kg) | Average weight (lb) | Drug dose as percentage of adult dose | Drug dose mg/kg if adult dose = 1mg/kg |
|---|---|---|---|---|
| Over 2 weeks | 3.2 | 7 | 12 | 2 |
| 4 months | 6.5 | 14 | 20 | |
| 1 year | 10 | 22 | 25 | |
| 3 years | 15 | 33 | 33 | 1.5 |
| 7 years | 23 | 51 | 50 | |
| 12 years | 37 | 82 | 75 | 1.25 |

# Drugs and food

- Most oral drugs are best given with or after food.
- However, the following oral drugs should be given at least
  30 min *before* food, as their absorption is otherwise delayed:
  - Aspirin
  - Erythromycin
  - Paracetamol/acetoaminophen
  - Penicillins (some)
  - Rifampicin
  - Tetracyclines (except doxycycline)
- Grapefruit juice disturbs absorption of ciclosporin, calcium channel
  blockers (e.g. nifedipine), or terfenadine. Grapefruit juice and drinks
  that contain grapefruit juice or fresh, canned, or frozen grapefruit, may
  also alter the metabolism of several drugs, increasing the toxicity of
  benzodiazepines, carbamazepine and corticosteroids. Sour orange juice
  (e.g. Seville oranges), real lime juice, cranberry, and tangelos (a hybrid
  of grapefruit), may possibly also have this effect. The effect appears to
  last for at least 3 days following ingestion, and could perhaps be longer
  in some patients.
- Citrus juice improves iron absorption, but may cause some medications to dissolve prematurely in the stomach rather than in the intestine as intended. Therefore, taking drugs with carbonated sodas
  and acid fruit juices is usually not recommended.
- Calcium, in dairy foods and in calcium supplements, chelates tetra-
  cylines, which therefore pass through the body without being
  absorbed. Avoid high-calcium foods (milk products or supplements)
  within 2 h of taking the medication, to minimize this problem.
- Iron, magnesium and aluminium in drugs can impair absorption of
  tetracyclines.
- Iron reduces absorption of quinolones (e.g. ciprofloxacin).
- Aluminium can impair absorption of azole antifungals.
- Phytates in chapattis bind calcium and impair its absorption.
- Warfarin can be antagonized by vitamin K in foods such as liver,
  cabbage, spinach, cauliflower, green tea and broccoli.
- Warfarin activity can be enhanced by:
  - garlic supplements;
  - cranberry juice (*Vaccinium macrocarpon*);
  - some herbal medicines (see below).

# Intramuscular injections

Antimicrobials, corticosteroids, iron preparations, diazepam, diclofenac and various other drugs may be given IM. IM injections can be painful, are contraindicated in patients with a bleeding tendency and can often be avoided in dentistry.

The indications for IM antimicrobials have been greatly reduced since the advent of oral amoxicillin, which gives extremely high blood levels within 1–2 h, and persists for 9–10 h.

Certain analgesics (e.g. diclofenac) are given IM, when oral administration is contraindicated (e.g. when a patient is 'nil by mouth' prior to a GA). However, if IM injection is definitely indicated, check that the:

- correct drug (and solvent) is used; this is particularly important if another person (e.g. a nurse) makes up the drug.
- patient is not allergic to the drug and that the drug is not otherwise contraindicated.
- drug expiry date has not passed.
- patient is lying down beforehand, in case he or she might otherwise faint.

## Technique
### Site of injection (Fig. 8.1)
*Anterolateral aspect of the thigh (the preferred site)*
Larger injections may be given into the vastus lateralis muscle on the anterolateral aspect of the thigh, where there is a large mass of muscle free from important vessels and nerves.
*Outer aspect of the shoulder*
Small injections can be given into the deltoid muscle on the outer aspect of the shoulder. The shirt or blouse must be removed so that you will not inject too low, as there is then a danger of damage to the radical nerve.
*Anterior part of the upper and outer quadrant of the buttock*
Do not inject into the 'bottom' as at that site there is a danger of damage to the sciatic nerve. To find the safest place for an IM injection into the right buttock, place the tip of the left index finger on the anterior iliac spine and the tip of the middle finger, abducted as shown in the diagram, just below the iliac crest. The injection site is then into the gluteal muscles within the triangle formed by fingers and iliac crest.

### Method of injection
The following procedures should be carried out when giving an IM injection:

- The patient should be lying down.
- Swab the site with isopropyl alcohol.
- Allow the area to dry.
- Rapidly pierce the skin and muscle with the needle (size 19 or 20 for large volumes of fluid, sizes 21 or 23 for small volumes).
- Aspirate to ensure the needle is not in a blood vessel.
- Inject slowly.
- Withdraw the needle and swab the area.
- Dispose of the needle into a sharps bin.
- Observe the patient for adverse reactions (30 min in the case of antimicrobials).

▶ Always have resuscitation equipment and drugs readily at hand.

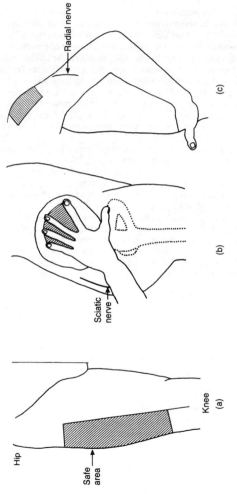

**Fig. 8.1** Sites for intramuscular injection

# Analgesics: general principles

(See also Chapter 9)

- Pain is probably the most important symptom suggestive of oral disease but absence of pain does not exclude disease. Where possible, identify and treat the cause of pain.
- There is considerable individual variation in response to pain, and the threshold is lowered by tiredness, as well as psychogenic and other factors. Try to relieve factors which lower the pain threshold.
- Pain results from tissue damage and the release of chemicals.
- Prostaglandins, as well as potassium, serotonin, bradykinin, substance P, leukotrienes, and thromboxane are involved. Prostaglandins stimulate nerves at the site of injury and cause inflammation and fever.
- Prostaglandin production from arachidonic acid is via an enzymatic pathway involving enzymes termed cyclo-oxygenases (COX).
- COX blockade can cause adverse effects. COX-1 enzymes are constitutive, and blocking also affects the gastrointestinal and renal tracts, and blood platelets.
- COX-2 is inducible and the main enzyme involved in prostaglandin production, lacking the other effects of COX-1.
- Certain drugs such as non-steroidal anti-inflammatory drugs (e.g. aspirin and other NSAIDs) block COX and thus prostaglandin synthesis.
- COX-2 inhibitors (e.g. celecoxib) have less adverse effects than COX-1 inhibitors on stomach, but may be cardiotoxic.
- Try simple analgesics initially, before embarking on more potent preparations, as in the analgesic ladder (Table 8.5); avoid polypharmacy.
- Chronic pain requires regular analgesia (not just as 'required').
- Many of the more potent analgesics (including pentazocine and distalgesic) produce dependence and are now used less frequently.
- Patient-controlled analgesia (PCA) is increasingly used.

**Table 8.5** The analgesic ladder

| Paracetamol/ Acetoaminophen | Paracetamol/Acetoaminophen ± weak opioid (codeine, dihydrocodeine or NSAID) | Paracetamol/ Acetoaminophen + strong opioid (morphine) |
|---|---|---|

# Useful analgesics (Table 8.6)

**Non-steroidal anti-inflammatory drugs (NSAIDs)** are effective against mild to moderate pain. Their anti-inflammatory properties make them particularly suitable for musculoskeletal pain of chronic rheumatic disorders. They are also used for the treatment of transient musculoskeletal pain, although paracetamol/acetaminofen is now preferred, as it has similar efficacy with a more favourable safety record. NSAIDs are a safer alternative to opioids in the treatment of mild to moderate postoperative pain.

▶The anti-inflammatory properties of NSAIDs are erroneously considered by some to be an indication for their use in oral and maxillofacial infections or for the limitation of postoperative oedema. Even if such effects were advantageous, they require at least a few weeks to be demonstrated; therefore, the use of NSAIDs over paracetamol/acetoaminophen in the treatment of transient mild to moderate pain is difficult to justify.

Most NSAIDS are COX-1 inhibitors and can cause peptic ulceration and further deterioration of renal function, if this is already impaired. They also cause fluid retention as well as nausea, diarrhoea or tinnitus, and interfere with antihypertensives, diuretics and warfarin. NSAIDS may worsen asthma. NSAIDs should be avoided in elderly patients. In addition, they should not be taken by patients with:

- peptic ulceration
- alcoholism
- asthma (if they worsen it)
- a bleeding tendency
- renal disease
- certain drug therapy
  - anticoagulants
  - methotrexate
  - digoxin
  - it is possible but unconfirmed, that NSAIDs should not be given to patients taking lithium.

*Aspirin* is a NSAID, which has long been in use and the efficacy and adverse effects are well recognized. Aspirin is a safe analgesic, but readily causes platelet dysfunction, and excessive doses have led to post-extraction bleeding. Its use is now primarily as an antiplatelet agent (at lower doses than those for analgesia).

Aspirin should be avoided in children under the age of 16 years (possible association with Reye's syndrome—a serious liver disease), mothers who are breast-feeding, gastric disease, bleeding tendency, and those allergic to it. Aspirin should not be given to patients taking oral hypoglycaemics, valproic acid or carbonic anhydrase inhibitors.

*Ibuprofen* has analgesic and antipyretic properties similar to other NSAIDs, but less anti-inflammatory properties and GI adverse effects. It has therefore been used extensively for the management of mild to moderate pain of dental origin, even in children, but it may be cardiotoxic.

*Other NSAIDs* with good efficacy and low incidence of adverse effects include naproxen, diclofenac (Voltarol), and diflunisal. Ketorolac and the

COX-2 inhibitors, celecoxib and parecoxib are less likely to cause upper GI bleeding and may be useful in the short-term management of postoperative pain. Rofecoxib has been withdrawn because of cardiotoxicity and there is concern about others.

### Non-anti-inflammatory analgesics

*Paracetamol/acetaminophen* has similar analgesic and antipyretic properties to aspirin, but is less irritant to the stomach. It is the first choice for the management of mild transient pain, especially in children and the elderly. Paracetamol/acetaminophen is hepatotoxic in overdose—or in repeated doses. It may be given in the short term to any patient with a healthy liver, but it should not be given to a heavy drinker or one who has stopped alcohol after chronic intake.

*Nefopam* is a good alternative for moderate pain not responding to other NSAIDs.

**Opioids** are narcotic analgesics, suitable for moderate to severe pain, particularly of visceral origin, widely used to relieve postoperative pain. Opioids are 'Controlled Drugs', all capable of causing addiction, and are therefore not indicated for long-term pain management, except in palliative care, where this drawback is not applicable.

Opioids may cause nausea, vomiting, drowsiness, constipation and urinary retention. In high doses, they may also cause respiratory depression and hypotension. Overdosage is treated with naloxone (see page 288). Opioids are contraindicated in respiratory failure, alcoholism, in those taking monoamine oxidase inhibitors and in patients with head injury, as they interfere with pupillary responses (important for neurological assessment) and suppress respiration (codeine should be less of a problem in these cases). They should also be used with caution in liver disease, kidney disease, and those who are pregnant or breast-feeding.

Avoid prescribing opioids to drug addicts, who, in need of a 'fix', may falsely complain of severe pain or injury. If an addict is admitted to the ward, contact a psychiatrist for management of withdrawal. Other problems in the management of addicts include overdose, behavioural problems (including theft), violence, viral hepatitis, HIV and other infections.

*Morphine* remains the gold standard for the management of severe pain and also produces euphoria, making it useful in palliative care, but adding to its addictive properties. Morphine may be given orally (Oramorph) or as SC/IM/IV injection, usually together with an antiemetic (e.g. cyclizine).

*Codeine* is appropriate for controlling mild to moderate pain, especially in patients with diarrhoea or troublesome cough. It can be very constipating and may occasionally cause dependence. It can be given orally or IM. Small doses are used in compound preparations with paracetamol/ acetaminophen (Co-codamol)—with no significant advantage.

*Fentanyl* is a useful drug in palliative care, used either as a self-adhesive patch (Durogesic) changed every 3 days, or as lozenges to manage breakthrough pain in those already receiving opioids.

**Other groups of drugs** used for their analgesic properties include:
- Tricyclic antidepressants (e.g. amitryptiline), for chronic pain
- Anticonvulsants (e.g. gabapentin), for neuropathic pain (e.g. neuralgia)
- $5HT_1$ agonists (e.g. zolmitriptan), for migraine.

Table 8.6 Analgesics

| Analgesic | Comments | Tablet contains | Route | Adult dose |
|---|---|---|---|---|
| **NSAIDs**[a] | | | | |
| Aspirin | Mild analgesic: Causes gastric irritation Interferes with haemostasis. Contraindicated in bleeding disorders, children, asthma, late pregnancy, peptic ulcers, renal disease, allergy. | 300 or 325 mg | O | 300–600 mg up to 6 times a day after meals (use soluble or dispersible or enteric-coated aspirin) (max 4 g daily) |
| Celecoxib | Analgesic for mild to moderate pain. COX-2 inhibitor. Use only in peptic ulcer or gastrointestinal bleeding. Contraindicated in pregnancy, allergies, Inflammatory bowel disease. May be cardiotoxic. | 100 mg | O | 100–200 mg twice daily |
| Diflunisal | Analgesic for mild to moderate pain Long action: twice a day dose only. Effective against pain from bone and joint. Contraindicated in pregnancy, peptic ulcer, allergies, renal and liver disease. | 250 mg or 500 mg | O | 250–500 mg twice a day |
| Ibuprofen | Analgesic for mild to moderate pain Effective against pain from bone and joint. Contraindicated in peptic ulcer, allergies, Caution in pregnancy, elderly, renal and liver disease. Do not use together with aspirin. May be cardiotoxic. | 200 mg or 400 mg | O | 200–400 mg three times a day |
| **Non-NSAID** | | | | |
| Paracetamol/ acetoaminophen | Mild analgesic: Hepatotoxic in overdose or prolonged use. Contraindicated in liver or renal disease or those on zidovudine. Available with methionine, as co-methiamol to prevent liver damage in overdose. | 500 mg | O | 500–1000 mg up to 6 times a day (max 4 mg daily) |

| | | | | |
|---|---|---|---|---|
| Nefopam | Moderate analgesic. Contraindicated in convulsive disorders. Caution in pregnancy, elderly, renal, liver disease. May cause nausea, dry mouth, sweating. | 30 mg | O or IM | 30–60 mg up to 3 times daily |
| **Opioids** | | | | |
| Codeine phosphate | Analgesic for moderate pain. Contraindicated in late pregnancy and liver disease. Avoid alcohol. May cause sedation and constipation. Reduced cough reflex. | 15 mg | O | 10–60 mg up to 6 times a day (or 30 mg IM) |
| Dextro-propoxyphene | Analgesic for moderate pain. Risk of respiratory depression in overdose, especially if taken with alcohol. May cause dependence. Occasional hepatotoxicity. No more effective as an analgesic than paracetamol/acetoaminophen or aspirin alone. | 65 mg | O | 65 mg up to 4 times a day |
| Dihydrocodeine tartrate | Analgesic for moderate pain. May cause nausea, drowsiness, constipation. Contraindicated in children, hypothyroidism, asthma renal disease. May increase postoperative dental pain. Reduce dose for elderly. Available with paracetamol as co-dydramol | 30 mg | O | 30 mg up to 4 times a day (or 50 mg IM) |
| Pentazocine | Analgesic for moderate pain. May produce dependence. May produce hallucinations. May provoke withdrawal symptoms in narcotic addicts. Contraindicated in pregnancy, children, hypertension, respiratory depression, head injuries or raised intracranial pressure. There is a low risk of dependence. | 25 mg | O | 50 mg up to 4 times a day (or 30 mg IM or IV) |
| Buprenorphine | Potent analgesic. More potent analesic than pentazocine, longer action than pentazocine, longer action than morphine, no hallucinations, may cause salivation, sweating, dizziness and vomiting. Respiratory depression in overdose. Can cause dependence. Contraindicated in children, pregnancy, MAOI, liver disease and respiratory diseases | 0.2 mg | Sublingual | 0.2–0.4 mg upto 4 times a day (or 0.3 mg IM) |

**Table 8.6** Contd.

| Analgesic | Comments | Tablet contains | Route | Adult dose |
|---|---|---|---|---|
| Fentanyl | Potent analgesic. Acts rapidly (in 1–2 min) Respiratory depression in overdose. Contraindicated in respiratory depression, head injury, alcoholism, phaeochromocytoma | | O, IM IV, patch | 50–200 µg |
| Meptazinol | Potent analgesic Claimed to have a low incidence of respiratory depression. Side effects as buprenorphine | No tablet | IM or IV | 75–100 mg up to 6 times a day |
| Phenazocine | Analgesic for severe pain. May cause nausea | 5 mg | 0 or sublingual | 5 mg up to 4 times a day |
| Pethidine | Potent analgesic. Less potent than morphine. Contraindicated in MAOI. Risk of dependence | No tablet | SC or IM | 25–100 mg up to 4 times a day |
| Morphine | Potent analgesic. Often causes nausea and vomiting. Reduces cough reflex, causes pupil constriction, risk of dependence. Contraindicated in respiratory depression, head injury, alcoholism, phaeochromocytoma. | As required | SC or IM or O or suppository | 5–10 mg |
| Diamorphine | Potent analgesic. More potent than pethidine and morphine but more euphoria and dependence. | 10 mg | SC, IM or O | 2–5 mg by injection, 5–10 mg orally |

ª There are many NSAIDs.

# Antibacterials

# Antibacterials

**Indications for the use of antibacterials** (together with appropriate surgical drainage or other measures)
- Cervical fascial space infections;
- Osteomyelitis and osteoradionecrosis;
- Odontogenic infections in ill, toxic or susceptible patients (e.g. immunocompromised);
- Acute ulcerative gingivitis;
- Specific infections such as tuberculosis, syphilis;
- Some instances of:
  - pericoronitis;
  - dental abscess;
  - dry socket;
- Prophylaxis:
  - of infective endocarditis (see Chapter 4);
  - in cerebrospinal rhinorrhoea;
  - in compound facial or skull fractures;
  - in major oral and maxillofacial surgery (e.g. osteotomies or tumour resection);
  - In surgery in immunocompromised or debilitated patients, or following radiotherapy to the jaws.

▶ Drainage is essential if there is pus: antibacterials will not remove pus;

**Choice of antibacterial** (Table 8.7)
- Odontogenic infections are typically polymicrobial.
- Anaerobes are implicated in many odontogenic infections, and these often respond to penicillins or metronidazole.
- Most bacteria causing odontogenic infections are penicillin-sensitive.
- Very high blood antimicrobial levels can be achieved with oral amoxicillin, with good patient compliance.
- Use another antimicrobial if the patient is allergic, or has had penicillin with the previous month (resistant bacteria).
- Metronidazole may be preferred as an alternative to a penicillin.
- Erythromycin is an alternative for penicillin-resistant infections where a β-lactamase producing organism is involved. However, many organisms are now resistant to erythromycin or rapidly develop resistance and its use should therefore be limited to short courses.
- Erythromycin is an alternative for infections in penicillin-allergic patients.
- Pus (as much as possible) should be sent for culture and sensitivities, but antimicrobials should be started immediately following sampling, if they are indicated.
- For prophylaxis of infective endocarditis (Chapter 4).

- Clindamycin is no more effective than penicillins against anaerobes and there may be cross-resistance with erythromycin-resistant bacteria, so it should not be used for routine treatment of odontogenic infections.

## Failure of an infection to respond to an antibacterial

If an infection fails to respond within 48 h, reconsider possible:
- inadequacy of drainage of pus;
- inappropriateness of the drug or dose;
- antimicrobial insensitivities of micro-organism (staphylococci are now frequently resistant to penicillin and some show multiple resistances—e.g. meticillin-resistant *Staphylococcus aureus* [MRSA]);
- patient non-compliance (or non-concordance, to be politically correct!);
- local factors (e.g. foreign body);
- unusual type of infection;
- impaired host defences (unusual and opportunistic infections are increasingly identified, particularly in the immunocompromised patient);
- non-infective cause for the condition!

In serious or unusual cases of infection, consult the clinical microbiologist.

## Routes of antibacterial administration

*Oral preparations* of antimicrobials are preferred in most instances.
*Topical antibacterials*, should usually be avoided, as they may produce sensitization and may cause the emergence of resistant strains.
*Parenteral administration* of antibacterials may be indicated where:
- no oral preparation is available;
- high blood levels are required rapidly (e.g. serious infections);
- the patient cannot or will not take oral medications (e.g. unconscious patient);
- the patient is to have a GA within the following 4 h.

**Table 8.7** Some antibacterials

|  | Comments | Route | Dose |
|---|---|---|---|
| _Penicillins_ | Most oral bacterial infections respond to penicillin. Oral phenoxymethyl penicillin is usually effective and is cheap. Amoxicillin is often used and is usually effective, but almost four times as expensive. |  |  |
| Amoxicillin | Orally active (absorption better than ampicillin). Broad-spectrum penicillin derivative _Staphylococcus aureus_ often resistant. Not resistant to penicillinase. Contraindicated in penicillin hypersensitivity. Rashes in infectious mononucleosis, cytomegalovirus infection lymphoid leukaemia, lymphoma, allopurinol. May cause diarrhoea. | O, IM or IV | 250–500 mg 8-hourly (see Table 4.7) about endocarditis) |
| Augmentin | Mixture of amoxicillin and potassium clavulanate (inhibits some penicillinases and therefore is active against most _Staph. aureus_; inhibits some lactamases and is therefore active against some Gram-negative and penicillin-resistant bacteria). Contraindicated in penicillin hypersensitivity. | O | 1 tablet 8-hourly |
| Ampicillin | Less oral absorption than amoxicillin Otherwise as for amoxicillin. (There are many analogues but these have few, if any, advantages). Contraindicated in penicillin hypersensitivity. | O, IM or IV | 250–500 mg 6-hourly |
| Benzylpenicillin | Not orally active. Most effective penicillin where organism sensitive. Not resistant to penicillinase. Contraindicated in penicillin hypersensitivity. Large dose may cause ↓$K^+$ and ↑$Na^+$. | IM or IV | 300–600 mg 6-hourly |
| Flucloxacillin | Orally active penicillin derivative. Effective against most but not all penicillin-resistant staphylococci (most staphylococci). Contraindicated in penicillin hypersensitivity. | O or IM | 250 mg 6-hourly |
| Phenoxymethyl penicillin (penicillin V) | Orally active. Best taken on an empty stomach. Not resistant to penicillinase. Contraindicated in penicillin hypersensitivity. | O | 250–500 mg 6-hourly |
| Procaine penicillin | Depot penicillin. Not resistant to penicillinase. Contraindicated in penicillin hypersensitivity. Rarely psychotic reaction. | IM | 300 000 units every 12 h |

**Table 8.7** Contd.

|  | Comments | Route | Dose |
|---|---|---|---|
| Triplopen (trade name) | Depot penicillin. Contains benzyl (300 mg), procaine (250 mg) and benetha-mine (475 mg) penicillins. Not resistant to penicillinase. Contraindicated in penicillin hypersensitivity. | IM | 1 vial every 2–3 days |
| *Sulphonamides* | The main indications for sulphonamides are in the prophylaxis of post-traumatic meningitis but meningococci increasingly are resistant. Contraindicated in pregnancy and in renal disease. In other patients, adequate hydration must be ensured to prevent the (rare) occurrence of cystalluria. Other adverse reactions include erythema multiforme, rashes and blood dyscrasias. |  |  |
| *Co-trimoxazole* | Combination of trimethoprim and sul-phamethoxazole. Orally active. Broad spectrum, occasional rashes or blood dyscrasis. Contraindicated in pregnancy, liver disease. May increase the effect of protein-bound drugs. Now used mainly for the treatment of *Pneumocystic carinii* pneumonia. | O or IM | 960 mg twice daily or 3–4.5 mL IM twice daily. |
| *Tetracyclines* | Tetracyclines have a broad antibacterial spectrum, but of the many preparations there is little to choose between them. However, doxycycline is useful sine a single daily dose is adequate, whilst minocycline is effective against meningo-cocci; both are safer for patients with renal failure. Most other tetracyclines are nephrotoxic. Tetracyclines discolouration of developing teeth and have absorption impaired by iron, antac-ids, milk, etc. Use of tetracyclines may predispose to candidosis, and to nausea and GI disturbance. |  |  |
| Tetracycline | Orally active. Broad spectrum. Contra-indicated in pregnancy and children up to at least 7 years (tooth discolour-ation). Reduce dose indicated in renal failure, liver disease, elderly. Frequent mild GI effects. | O | 250–500 mg 6-hourly |

**Table 8.7** Contd.

|  | Comments | Route | Dose |
|---|---|---|---|
| Doxycycline | Orally active. Single daily dose. Broad spectrum. Contraindicated in pregnancy and children up to at least 7 years (tooth discolouration. Safer than tetracyclines in renal failure (excreted in faeces). Reduce dose in liver disease and elderly. Mild gastrointestinal effects. | O | 100 mg once a day |
| Minocycline | Orally active. Broad spectrum: active against meningococci. Safer than tetracycline in renal disease (excreted in faeces). May cause dizziness and vertigo. Absorption not reduced by milk. Contraindicated in pregnancy and children up to 7 years (tooth discolouration). May rarely also cause pigmentation in adults. | O | 100 mg twice a day |
| *Beta lactams* Cephalosporins and cephamycins | Cephalosporins are broad-spectrum, expensive antibiotics with few absolute indications for their use in dentistry, although they may be effective against *Staph. aureus*. They produce false positive results for glucosuria with 'Clinitest'. Hypersensitivity is the main side-effect. Some cause a bleeding tendency. Some are nephrotoxic. Cefuroxime is less affected by penicillinases than other cephalosporins and is currently the preferred drug of the many available. |  |  |
| Cephalexin and cephradine | Orally active. Cheaper than most cephalosporins. Contraindicated if history of anaphylaxis to penicillin. | O | 250–500 mg 6-hourly |
| Cefotaxime and ceftazidine | Not orally active. Broad-spectrum activity. Contraindicated if history of anaphylaxis to penicillins. Expensive. | IM or IV | 1 g 12-hourly |
| Cefuroxime | Not orally active. Broad-spectrum activity. Contraindicated if history of anaphylaxis to penicillins. | IM or IV | 250–750 mg 8-hourly |
| *Macrolides* Erythromycin | Erythromycin has a similar antibacterial spectrum to penicillin and is therefore used in penicillin-allergic patients. Active against most staphylococci, *Mycoplasma* and *Legionella*, but not always against oral bacteroides. Do not use erythromycin estolate, which may cause liver disease. |  |  |

**Table 8.7** Contd.

|  | Comments | Route | Dose |
|---|---|---|---|
| Erythromycin stearate | Orally active. Useful in those hypersensitive to penicillin. Effective against most staphylococci and streptococci. May cause nausea, rapid development of resistance. Reduced dose indicated in liver disease. Can increase ciclosporin absorption and toxicity, enhances anticoagulants. | O | 250–500 mg 6-hourly |
| Erythromycin lactobionate | Used where parenteral erythromycin indicated. Give not as bolus but by infusion. Comments as above. | IV | 2 g daily |
| Azithromycin | Has slightly less activity than erythromycin against Gram-positive bacteria but enhanced activity against some Gram-negative organisms including *H. influenzae*. It has a long tissue half-life and once daily dosage is recommended. Cause fewer GI side-effects than erythromycin. Contraindications: liver disease | O | 500 mg once daily for 3 days |
| Clarithromycin | An erythromycin derivative with slightly greater activity than the parent compound. Tissue concentrations are higher than with erythromycin. It is given twice daily. Causes fewer GI side-effects than erythromycin. Avoid concomitant administration with pimozide or terfenadine | O | 250 mg every 12 h for 7 days |
| *Aminoglycosides* Gentamicin | Reserved for use in pregnancy and myasthenia gravis. Reduce dose in renal disease | IM or IV | Up to 5 mg/kg daily |
| Clindamycin | Clindamycin is active against Gram-positive cocci, including penicillin-resistant staphylococci and also against many anaerobes, especially *Bacteroides fragilis*. Has only a limited use because of serious side-effects, mainly antibiotic-associated colitis. It is recommended for staphylococcal joint and bone infections such as osteomyelitis. Clindamycin is used for prophylaxis of endocarditis in patients allergic to penicillin (unlicensed indication). | O, IM | 150–300 mg every 6 h |

**Table 8.7** Contd.

|  | Comments | Route | Dose |
|---|---|---|---|
| Metronidazole | Orally active. Effective against anaerobes. Use only for 7 days (or peripheral neuropathy may develop, particularly in liver patients). Avoid alcohol (disulfiram-type reaction). May increase warfarin effect. May cause tiredness IV preparation available but expensive. Suppositories are effective. Contraindicated in pregnancy. | O or IV | 200–400 mg or 250–500 mg, 8-hourly with meals |
| Rifampicin | Reserved mainly for treatment of tuberculosis. May be used in prophylaxis of meningitis after head injury as *Neisseria meningitidis* may be resistant to sulphonamides. Safe and effective but resistance rapidly occurs. Body secretions turn red. May interfere with oral contraception. Occasional rashes, jaundice or blood dyscrasias. | | |
| *Glycopeptides* | | | |
| Vancomycin | Reserved for serious infections, prophylaxis of endocarditis, and treatment of pseudomembranous colitis. Extravenous extravasation causes necrosis and phlebitis. May cause nausea, rashes, tinnitus, deafness. Rapid injection may cause red neck syndrome. Contraindicated in renal disease, deafness. Very expensive. | O or IV | 500 mg 6-hourly for pseudomembranous colitis, IV by slow injection for prophylaxis of endocarditis. |
| Teicoplanin | Similar to vancomycin but is not given by mouth and can be given IM and has significantly longer duration of action allowing once-daily administration. | IM, IV | 400 mg |

# Antifungals

- The most common oral fungal infections are associated with *Candida albicans*.
- Predisposing factors are usually local (dry mouth; antibacterial use; steroid use; wearing of appliances; smoking).
- Systemic predisposing factors include any immune defect.
- Antifungals are used to treat oral or oropharyngeal fungal infections but underlying predisposing factors should first be considered.
- In immunocompromised patients, antifungals are increasingly used for prophylaxis, and increasingly systemically, such as with the azoles (ketoconazole, fluconazole, miconazole, itraconazole, voriconazole).
- Antifungal resistance is now a significant problem to immunocompromised persons, especially those with a severe immune defect, who may show *Candida* species resistant to fluconazole and, sometimes, to other azoles.
- Antifungal resistance may sometimes be overcome by using higher drug doses, or changing the agent (Table 8.8).
- Antifungals should be continued for at least 1 week following resolution of clinical manifestations.

**Table 8.8** Antifungals

|  | Comments | Oral dose |
|---|---|---|
| Amphotericin[a] | Active topically. Negligible absorption from GI tract. Given IV for deep mycoses. | 10–100 mg, 6-hourly |
| Nystatin[a] | Active topically. Negligible absorption from GI tract. Pastilles taste better than lozenge. | 500 000 unit lozenge, 100 000 unit pastille or 100 000 unit per mL of suspension. 6-hourly. |
| Miconazole[a] | Active topically. Also has antibacterial activity. Absorption from GI tract. Theoretically the best anti-fungal to treat angular cheilitis. Interacts with terfenadine cisapride, astemizole and warfarin. Avoid in pregnancy, porphyria. | 250 mg tablet 6-hourly or 25 mg/ml gel used as 5 mL 6-hourly, for 14 days |
| Ketoconazole | Absorbed from GI tract. Useful in intractable candidosis. May cause nausea, rashes, pruritus and liver damage. Contra-indicated in pregnancy and liver disease. Interacts with terfenadine cisapride, and astemizole. | 200–400 mg once daily with meal, for 14 days |
| Fluconazole | Absorbed from GI tract. Useful in intractable candidosis. May cause nausea, diarrhoea, rash. Contraindicated in pregnancy, liver and renal disease. Interacts with terfenadine, cisapride and astemizole. | 50–100 mg daily for 14 days |
| Itraconazole | Absorbed from GI tract. Useful in intractable candidosis. May cause nausea, neuropathy, rash. Contraindicated in pregnancy, liver disease. Interacts with terfenadine, cisapride and astemizole. | 100 mg daily for 14 days |
| Voriconazole | Absorbed from GI tract. Useful broad-spectrum antifungal licensed for use in life-threatening infections, e.g. invasive fluconazole-resistant *Candida* spp. May cause nausea, neuropathy, rash. Contraindicated in pregnancy, liver disease. Interacts with terfenadine, cisapride and astemizole. | 400 mg twice daily for 14 days |

[a] Dissolve in mouth slowly.

# Antivirals

- The most common orofacial viral infections are associated with herpesviruses, human papillomaviruses, and enteroviruses.
- HIV and other viruses may also cause orofacial lesions.
- Management of viral infections is predominantly supportive, as, at present, there are few antiviral agents of proven efficacy.
- Most antivirals will achieve maximum benefit if given early in the disease.
- Immunocompromised patients with viral infections may well benefit from active antiviral therapy, as these infections may spread locally and systematically (Table 8.9).
- Systemic aciclovir should be used with caution in pregnancy and renal disease. Aciclovir may cause ↑ liver enzymes, and urea, rashes and CNS effects.
- Famciclovir should also be used with caution in pregnancy and renal disease. Famciclovir may cause headache and nausea.

**Table 8.9** Antiviral therapy of oral viral infections

| Virus | Disease | Otherwise healthy patient | Immunocompromised patient |
|-------|---------|---------------------------|---------------------------|
| Herpes simplex | Primary herpetic gingivostomatitis Recurrent herpetic ulcers | Consider oral aciclovir[a] 100–200 mg, five times daily as suspension (200 mg/5mL) or tablets. 5% aciclovir cream or penciclovir 1% cream every 2 h. | Aciclovir 250 mg/m$^2$ IV every 8 h. Consider aciclovir as above depending on risk of patient infection. |
| Herpes varicella | Chickenpox | — | Aciclovir 500 mg/m$^2$ (5 mg/kg) IV every 8 h |
| | Zoster (shingles) | 3% aciclovir ophthalmic ointment for shingles of ophthalmic division of trigeminal | As above. Or famciclovir 250 mg three times daily, or 750 mg once daily. |

[a] In neonate, treat as if immunocompromised.

# Immunosuppressive agents

**Topical immunosuppressants** (Tables 8.10 and 8.11) are useful in the management of many immunologically related oral lesions:

- Recurrent aphthous stomatitis
- Oral manifestations of Behçet's disease, Reiter's syndrome, MAGIC (Mouth and Genital Ulcers and Interstitial Chondritis) syndrome, PFAPA (Periodic Fever, Adenitis, Pharyngitis and Aphthae) syndrome, ulcerative colitis, Crohn's disease, OFG (orofacial granulomatosis), Sweet's syndrome, among others
- Dermatoses
  - Lichen planus
  - Pemphigoid
  - Pemphigus (only cases with oral lesions alone and low titres of circulating antibodies. Weekly clinical follow-up and monthly measurement of circulating antibody titres are mandatory)
  - Erythema multiforme
  - Dermatitis herpetiformis
  - Linear IgA disease

**Intralesional corticosteroids** (Table 8.12) are occasionally useful, for example in the management of intractable erosive lichen planus, keloid scars and localized granulomatous lesions (e.g. OFG).

**Intra-articular corticosteroids** (Table 8.13) are occasionally indicated, e.g. for intractable pain from a non-infective arthropathy.

**Systemic corticosteroids** (Table 8.14) are indicated in the management of anaphylaxis, adrenal crisis and pemphigus. They may also be needed in other disorders, such as giant cell arteritis and Bell's palsy, and can be used to reduce postoperative and post-traumatic oedema.
Because of their serious adverse effects (see Chapter 4), systemic steroids must always be used with caution. Patients should be given a steroid card, warned of possible adverse reactions, and informed of the need for an increase in the dose if ill or traumatized, or having an operation. The BP, glucose and bone density should be monitored.

**Other immunomodulatory agents** (Table 8.15) used increasingly for their 'steroid sparing' effect, include azathioprine, colchicine, thalidomide, dapsone, pentoxifylline, tacrolimus and pimecrolimus. Interferon is being used to control diseases such as Sjögren syndrome. Imiquimod is an immunostimulatory drug used to treat papillomavirus infections.

**Table 8.10** Examples of topical corticosteroids ranked according to potency (from higher to lower)

| Steroid | Potency |
|---|---|
| Clobetasol propionate<br>Halcinonide | Very potent |
| Betamethasone dipropionate<br>Desoximethasone<br>Fluocinonide<br>Fluticasone<br>Mometasone<br>Triamcinolone acetonide | Potent |
| Fluocinolone acetonide | Mild–moderate–potent depending on strength |
| Desoximetasone<br>Fluocortolone | Moderate |
| Hydrocortisone | Low |

**Table 8.11** Examples of topical immunosuppressants used in dentistry

| | Drugs | Concentration % | N° applications/day | Application time (mins) |
|---|---|---|---|---|
| Corticosteroids | Clobetasol propionate | 0.05 | 2–3 | 5 |
| | Fluocinonide | 0.05 | 5–10 | 5 |
| | Triamcinolone acetonide | 0.1–0.2 | 10 | 5 |
| Alternatives to topical corticosteroids (not licensed for oral use) | Tacrolimus | 0.03–0.1 | 2 | 5 |
| | Pimecrolimus | 1.0 | 2 | 5 |

These formulations can be prepared in aqueous preparations or adhesive vehicles. When a prolonged treatment is predicted (>10 days) they should be used in combination with an antifungal (e.g. 100 000 IU/mL nystatin).

**Table 8.12** Intralesional corticosteroids

| Corticosteroid | Comments | Dose |
|---|---|---|
| Prednisolone sodium phosphate | Short-acting | Up to 22 mg |
| Methylprednisolone acetate | Also available with Lignocaine/lidocaine | 4–80 mg every 1–5 weeks |
| Triancinolone acetonide | — | 2–3 mg every 1–2 weeks |
| Triamcinolone hexacetonide | — | Up to 5 mg every 3–4 weeks |

**Table 8.13** Intra-articular corticosteroids

| Corticosteroid[a] | Comments | Dose |
|---|---|---|
| Dexamethasone sodium phosphate | More expensive than hydrocortisone acetate | 0.4–5 mg at intervals of 3–21 days |
| Hydrocortisone acetate | Usual preparation used | 5–50 mg |

[a] Also used are those listed under intralesional corticosteroids.

**Table 8.14** Systemic corticosteroids

| | Comments | Dose |
|---|---|---|
| Prednisolone | In dentistry may be indicated systematically for treatment of pemphigus and Bell's palsy, and occasionally in other disorders | Initially 40–80 mg orally each day in divided doses, reducing as soon as possible to 10 mg daily. Give as enteric-coated prednisolone with meals |
| Deflazacort | In dentistry may be indicated systematically for treatment of pemphigus and Bell's palsy, and occasionally in other disorders High glucocorticoid activity; purported to have less adverse effects than above | Initially up to 120 mg orally each day in divided doses, reducing as soon as possible to 3–18 mg |
| Dexamethasone | May be useful to reduce post-surgical oedema after minor surgery | 5 mg IV with premedication then 0.5–1.0 mg each day for 5 days, orally if possible. |

**Table 8.14** Contd.

|  | Comments | Dose |
|---|---|---|
| Betamethasone | May be useful to reduce post-surgical oedema after minor surgery | 1 mg orally the night before operation. 1 mg orally with premed. 1 mg IV at operation 1 mg orally every 6 h for 2 days postoperatively |
| Methylpredisolone | May be used to reduce post-surgical oedema after major surgery | Methylprednisolone sodium succinate 1 g IV at operation then 500 mg IV on the evening of operation, followed by 125mg IV every 6 h for 22 h. The methylprednisolone acetate 80 mg every 12 h for 22h |

**Table 8.15** 'Steroid-sparing' immunosuppressants

|  | Comments | Oral dose daily |
|---|---|---|
| Azathioprine | Steroid sparing for immunosuppression. Myelosuppressive and hepatotoxic and long term may predispose to neoplasms. Contraindicated in pregnancy. | 2–2.5 mg/kg |
| Colchicine | Steroid sparing for immunosuppression. May cause nausea, rashes, GI upset blood dyscrasias or neuropathy. Contraindicated in pregnancy, elderly, cardiac, renal or hepatic disease. | 500 µg 3 times |
| Dapsone | May be useful for dermatitis herpetiformis and other mucocutaneous disorders. May cause rashes, fever, eosinophilia, headache, haemolysis, neuropathy, nausea. Contraindicated in G6PD deficiency, pregnancy, cardiorespiratory disease. | 1 mg/kg |
| Mycophenolate mofetil | Myelosuppressive, May cause nausea, rashes, GI upset. Contraindicated in pregnancy Long term may predispose to neoplasms. | 1 g twice |
| Pentoxifylline | May cause headache, GI upset, dizziness. Contraindicated in cerebrovascular haemorrhage, MI. | 400 mg twice |

# CNS-active drugs (see also page 375)

## Hypnotics (Table 8.16)

Hypnotics are used in the management of insomnia. This may be caused by pain, anxiety or depression.

In hospital, patients may temporarily need a hypnotic, but this should not be prescribed without forethought and certainly not regularly.

Hypnotics potentiate other CNS depressants (e.g. alcohol) and may impair judgement and dexterity. They may be contraindicated in people with liver or respiratory disease, and the elderly.

*Z drugs (Table 8.16)* and *benzodiazepines* (BZPs) are generally the preferred hypnotics, but are contraindicated as above and both groups are addictive, BZPs especially so. They are also anxiolytic (see below).

▶Hypnotics cause unsteadiness, some confusion, drowsiness (particularly when used together with alcohol) and impaired judgement. Patients should therefore be warned of the dangers of driving, operating machinery, or making important decisions.

▶*Barbiturates and glutethimide* should not be used; barbiturates are addictive, and both are dangerous in overdose.

## Anxiolytics (Table 8.17)

*Benzodiazepines*, which act on GABA receptors are the main anxiolytics. All may produce dependence (especially lorazepam) and there is often little to choose in terms of anxiolytic effect between the different BZPs.

*Buspirone*, which acts on serotonin receptors, is also commonly used and does not cause dependence but may take 2 weeks to have effect.

Doses of anxiolytics should be reduced for the elderly, and BZPs may have anomalous effects in children.

*Beta-blockers* (e.g. propranolol) may be more useful if anxiety is causing tremor and/or palpitations.

▶Identify and treat the cause of the patient's anxiety wherever possible.

▶Differentiate if possible between simple anxiety and agitated depression—the treatment is different.

## Tranquillizers (neuroleptics or antipsychotics) (Table 8.18)

Atypical antipsychotics (olanzapine, clozapine, risperidone) are the major tranquillizers now used. Phenothiazines are less popular as they can cause extrapyramidal disorders, postural hypotension, confusion and hypothermia and therefore should be avoided in the elderly. They should not be stopped suddenly after prolonged or high dosage, as withdrawal symptoms or acute psychoses may result.

## Antidepressants (Table 8.19)

- Depression is treated with psychotherapy and possibly drugs and occasionally physical treatments (ECT).
- Cognitive behavioural therapy (CBT) is used for depression.
- Self-help groups can be useful.
- If there is any possibility of a suicide attempt the patient must be seen by a psychiatrist *as a matter of urgency.*

- Antidepressants can be very effective but there may be an interval as long as 3–4 weeks before the antidepressant action takes place.
- Monitoring of plasma concentrations of antidepressants may be helpful in ensuring optimal dosage.
- Prescribe only limited amounts of antidepressants, as there is a danger that the patient may use them in a suicide attempt. SSRIs are safer in these cases.
- Antidepressant doses should be reduced for the elderly patient.
- Antidepressants often cause a dry mouth, but the complaint of dry mouth may also be a manifestation of depression.
- The natural history of depression is of remission after 3–12 months. Do not withdrawal antidepressants prematurely.
- SSRIs are popular antidepressants, less liable to drug interactions, adverse effects and safer in overdose than the more traditional drugs.
- SSRIs should not be used with TCAs or within 2 weeks of MAOIs.
- SSRIs are contraindicated in epilepsy, cardiac disease, diabetes, glaucoma, bleeding tendencies, liver disease, renal disease and pregnancy. Fluoxetine is epileptogenic.
- TCAs are also commonly used in the management of depression, and of chronic pain.
- Adverse effects of TCAs may include:
  - Cardiovascular (postural hypotension; cardiotoxicity; arrhythmias)
  - Neurological (seizures; dizziness; ataxia; tremor; insomnia; agitation; drowsiness)
  - Liver (jaundice)
  - Blood (leucopenia)
  - Others (dry mouth, sexual dysfunction; nausea; constipation; urinary retention; blurred vision)
  - TCAs interact with noradrenaline, but not significantly with the adrenaline (epinephrine) in dental local anaesthetic solutions.
- MAOIs are now rarely used but adverse effects include:
  - xerostomia
  - hypotension
  - anorexia, nausea and constipation
- MAOIs do not significantly interact with adrenaline (epinephrine) in dental local anaesthetic solutions, though there are multiple other interactions (see Table 8.28).

## Anticonvulsants (Table 8.20)

- Anticonvulsants and other drugs are used in the treatment of idiopathic trigeminal neuralgia, once organic causes have been excluded.
- Carbamazepine is the standard anticonvulsant used, but phenytoin may also be required if the pain is not controlled.
- As either drug may cause blood dyscrasias or hepatic dysfunction, it may be helpful to monitor full blood counts, liver function and BP.

**Table 8.16** Hypnotics

| Hypnotic | Comments | Route | Dose (at night) |
|---|---|---|---|
| Chlormethiazole | Contraindicated in liver disease; useful in elderly; may cause dependence. | O | 192 mg capsule or 250 mg/5ml syrup 500 mg |
| Diazepam | BZP. May cause dependence. Reduce dose in elderly. Useful as hypnotic only for severe insomnia. | O | 5 mg or 10 mg 5–10 mg |
| Dichloralphenazone | Derivative of chloral hydrate; contraindicated in oral anticoagulants, porphyria. Useful in elderly. | O | 650 mg 1300 mg |
| Nitrazepam | BZP. No more useful than diazepam; avoid in the elderly; may cause dependence; hangover effect. | O | 5 mg 5–10 mg |
| Temazepam | BZP. Less 'hangover' effect than nitrazepam; may cause dependence; useful in elderly. | O | 10 mg 10–20 mg |
| Clonazepam | BZP. Potential effects on neurogenic pain. | O | 0.5 mg Up to 2 mg daily |
| Zaleplon | Shorter action than benzodiazepines. Lower risk of dependence than benzodiazepines. Very short action. Contraindicated in liver disease, drug abuse, pregnancy, sleep apnoea, myasthenia gravis. Reduce dose in elderly. | O | 5 mg or 10 mg 10 mg |
| Zolpidem | Shorter action than benzodiazepines. Lower risk of dependence than benzodiazepines. Contraindicated in liver disease, drug abuse, pregnancy, sleep apnoea, myasthenia gravis. Reduce dose in elderly. | O | 5 mg or 10 mg 10 mg |
| Zoplicone | Shorter action than benzodiazepines. Lower risk of dependence than benzodiazepines. Contraindicated in liver disease, drug abuse, pregnancy, sleep apnoea, myasthenia gravis. Reduce dose in elderly. | O | 3.75 mg or 7.5 mg |

All may enhance alcohol, and impair skills including driving.

**Table 8.17** Anxiolytics

|  | Comments | Preparations contain | Route | Dose |
|---|---|---|---|---|
| Diazepam | BZP anxiolytic; reduce dose in elderly. Can cause dependence | 2 mg, 5 mg or 10mg | O | 2–30 mg a day in divided doses. |
| Lorazepam | BZP anxiolytic; reduce dose in elderly. Shorter action than diazepam. Can cause dependence | 1 mg or 2.5 mg | O | 1–4 mg a day |
| Temazepam | BZP anxiolytic; reduce dose in elderly. Shorter action than diazepam. Can cause dependence | 10 mg or 20 mg | O | 10–20 mg a day |
| Propranolol | Useful anxiolytic does not cause amnesia, but reduces tremor and palpitations; contraindicated in asthma, cardiac failure, pregnancy. | 10 mg or 40 mg | O | 80–100 mg daily |
| Buspirone | Useful anxiolytic that does not cause amnesia or dependence; contraindicated in epilepsy, liver disease, reneal disease, pregnancy. | 5 mg or 10 mg | O | 5–10 mg daily |

Benzodiazepines and buspirone may enhance alcohol, and impair skilled tasks, such as driving.

**Table 8.18** Tranquillizers

|  | Comments | Preparation contains | Route | Dose |
|---|---|---|---|---|
| Chlorpromazine | Major tranquillizer. May cause dyskinesia photosensitivity; eye defects and jaundice. Contraindicated in epilepsy. IM use causes pain and may cause postural hypotension. | 25 mg tab; 25 mg/5 mL syrup; 50 mg/2 mL injection | O or IM | 25 mg 8-hourly |
| Chlordiazepoxide | Anxiolytic; reduce dose in elderly. | 5 mg or 10 mg | O | 5-10 mg 8-hourly |
| Thioridazine | Phenothiazine with fewer adverse effects than chlorpromazine, Major tranquillizer. Rare retinopathy. | 10 or 25mg | O | 10-50 mg 8-hourly. |
| Haloperidol | Major tranquillizer; useful in the elderly; may cause dyskinesia. | 500 µg | O | 500 µg 12-hourly |

**Table 8.19** Some useful antidepressants

|  | Comments | Preparation Contains | Route | Dose |
|---|---|---|---|---|
| Amitriptyline | Tricyclic antidepressant. Effect may not or be seen until up to 30 days after start. Sedative effect also. Contraindicated after recent MI. | 25 mg 50 mg | O | 25–75 mg daily in divided doses when treatment established use single dose at night |
| Dothiepin | Tricyclic anxiolytic. Effect also useful in atypical facial pain. | 25 mg or 75 mg | O | 25 mg three times a day or 75 mg at night When treatment established, use single dose at night |
| Clomipramine | Tricyclic. Equally as effective as amitriptyline but less sedative effect. Useful in phobic or obsessional states. | 10 mg or 25 mg | O | 10–100 mg daily in divided doses |
| Fluoxetine | A selective serotonin re-uptake inhibitor (SSRI). Low sedation, antimuscarinic or cardiac effects. Causes GI side-effects. Contraindicated in epilepsy, cardiac disease, pregnancy, liver, kidney disease, allergy or mania. | 20 mg | O | 20 mg daily |
| Flupenthixol | Not a tricyclic or MAOI. Fewer side-effects. Contraindicated in cardiovascular, hepatic or renal disease, Parkinsonism, or excitable or overactive patients. | 0.5 mg or 1 mg | O | 1–3 mg daily in the morning |
| Venlafaxin | An SNRI (serotoxin and noradrenaline re-uptake inhibitor). Less sedation or dry mouth. Contraindicated in cardiovascular, mania, bleeding disorders glaucoma or renal disease. Avoid sudden withdrawal. | 37.5 mg or 75 mg | O | 37.5 mg twice daily |

**Table 8.20** Drugs for treatment of trigeminal neuralgia[a]

|  | Comments | Dose |
| --- | --- | --- |
| Carbamazepine | Prophylactic for trigeminal neuralgia—not analgesic. Occasional dizziness, diplopia, and blood dyscrasia, often with a rash and usually in the first 3 months of treatment. Potentiated by cimetidine, dextropropoxyphene and isoniazid. Potentiates lithium, interferes with contraceptive pill. Contraindicated in cardiac, renal and liver disease, glaucoma and pregnancy. | Initially 100 mg once or twice daily. Many patients need about 200 mg 8-hourly. Do not exceed 1800 mg daily |
| Gabapentin | Similar adverse effects to carbamazepine. Headache common. Contraindicated in psychiatric disease renal disease, diabetes and pregnancy. Avoid sudden withdrawal. | 300 mg up to three times daily |
| Phenytoin | Similar adverse effects to carbamazepine. Contraindicated in liver disease and pregnancy. Produces gingival swelling. | 150–300 mg daily |
| Baclofen | Common adverse effect of sedation. Contraindicated in peptic ulceration and pregnancy. Avoid abrupt withdrawal. | 5 mg three times daily |

[a] All may cause drowsiness and impair driving and skilled tasks.

# Antiemetics

The most commonly used antiemetics are listed in Table 8.21.

*Postoperative nausea and vomiting* may be prevented by cyclizine, prochlorperazine, or ondansetron ± dexamethasone (which has an antiemetic effect as well as reducing postoperative oedema).

*Cytotoxic therapy-associated nausea* may be prevented by metoclopramide or ondansetron ± dexamethasone.

**Table 8.21** Antiemetics

| Drug | | Comments | Route | Dose |
|---|---|---|---|---|
| Cyclizine | An antihistamine | May cause drowsiness and urinary retention; caution in liver disease and severe heart failure | PO/IM/IV | 50 mg, 3 times daily |
| Metoclopramide | | Contraindicated if GI bleeding, GI surgery, and breastfeeding; caution in pregnancy, children, and renal or hepatic failure; may cause extrapyramidal side-effects (especially in the young) | PO/IM/IV | 10 mg, 3 times daily |
| Ondansetron | A 5HT$_3$ antagonist | Caution in pregnancy, breast-feeding and liver failure; may cause flushing, headache, and constipation | PO/IM/ IV/PR | 8–16 mg, twice daily |
| Prochlorperazine | A phenothiazine | For adverse effects see antipsychotics (page 396) | PO | 5–10 mg, 3 times daily |

# Other drugs

### Salivary substitutes and sialogogues

Patients with dry mouth should avoid:

- dry foods;
- drugs that worsen xerostomia (see page 409);
- smoking;
- alcohol.

*Parasympathomimetics* such as pilocarpine and cevimeline are sialogogues, increasing salivation if functional salivary tissue remains. The main hazards of pilocarpine are bradycardia, arrhythmias, colic, broncho-spasm and sweating but, apart from the latter, these are uncommon. Pilocarpine is contraindicated in asthma, cardiac disease, biliary disease, glaucoma, pregnancy, peptic ulcer, liver disease and kidney disease. Patients should also be warned that pilocarpine may interfere with vision, especially at night, and that if that is the case, they should not drive.

*Salivary substitutes* may help symptomatically, but often sips of water suffice. Salivary substitutes usually contain carboxymethylcellulose (Glandosane, Luborant, Salivace, Saliveze) or mucin (Saliva Orthana). The latter contains fluoride, but may be unsuitable for use by certain religious groups, as it contains pork mucin.

### Antifibrinolytic agents

See Table 8.22.

### Retinoids

Retinoids (Table 8.23) are sometimes used to control lichen planus or leucoplakias, but are teratogenic and their effect abates once the drug is discontinued. Isotretinoin is used in the treatment of acne.

**Table 8.22** Antifibrinolytic drugs

|  | Comments | Route | Dose |
|---|---|---|---|
| Epsilon amino caproic acid | Useful in some bleeding tendencies. May cause nausea, diarrhoea, dizziness, myalgia. Contraindicated in pregnancy, history of thromboembolism, renal disease. | O | 3 g, 4–6 times daily |
| Tranexamic acid | Comments as above, but tranexamic acid is usually the preferred drug. Can be used to good effect in patients on warfarin, or in those with coagulation defects. | O | 1–1.5 g, 6-or 12-hourly |
|  |  | IV | Slow IV injection 1 g 8-hourly |

**Table 8.23** Retinoids

| Drug | Comments | Route | Dose |
|---|---|---|---|
| Etretinate | Vitamin A analogue may be used in treatment of erosive lichen planus. Effect begins after 2–3 weeks. Treat for 6–9 months, followed by a similar rest period. Most patients develop dry, cracked lips. May cause epistaxis, pruritus, alopecia. Contraindicated in pregnancy, liver disease. | O | Initially 1 mg/kg in two divided doses |
| Acitretin | Metabolite of etretinate, Contraindicated in pregnancy, Liver and renal disease. Avoid tetracyclines and methotrexate. Similar adverse effects as etretinate. | O | 25–50 mg daily |

# Immunizations

Dental and PCD students and staff before exposure to clinical work, should be immunized against hepatitis B, as well as receiving the standard immunizations (Table 8.24). HBV immunization takes up to 6 months to confer adequate protection; the duration of immunity is not known precisely, but a single booster 5 years after the primary course may be sufficient to maintain immunity for those who continue to be at risk.

Hepatitis B vaccine is used in individuals at high risk of contracting hepatitis B, including healthcare personnel (including trainees) who have direct contact with blood or blood-stained body fluids or with patients' tissues, and:

- parenteral drug abusers;
- individuals who change sexual partners frequently;
- close family contacts of a case or carrier;
- infants born to mothers who either have had hepatitis B during pregnancy, or are positive for both hepatitis B surface antigen and hepatitis B e-antigen, or are surface antigen positive without e markers (or where they have not been determined); active immunization of the infant is started immediately after delivery and hepatitis B immunoglobulin is given at the same time as the vaccine (but preferably at a different site). Infants born to mothers who are positive for hepatitis B surface antigen and for e-antigen antibody should receive the vaccine but not the immunoglobulin;
- individuals with haemophilia, those receiving regular blood transfusions or blood products, and carers responsible for the administration of such products;
- patients with chronic renal failure including those on haemodialysis. Haemodialysis patients should be monitored for antibodies annually and re-immunized if necessary. Home carers (of dialysis patients) who are negative for hepatitis B surface antigen should be vaccinated;
- occupational risk groups such as morticians and embalmers;
- staff and patients of day-care or residential accommodation for those with severe learning difficulties;
- inmates of custodial institutions;
- those travelling to areas of high prevalence who are at increased risk or who plan to remain there for lengthy periods;
- families adopting children from countries with a high prevalence of hepatitis B.

**Table 8.24** Immunization schedule

| Timing | Routine immunization | Comments |
|---|---|---|
| During first year of life | *Haemophilus influenzae* type b vaccine (Hib) combined with adsorbed diphtheria, tetanus and [whole-cell] pertussis vaccine [DTwP] Meningococcal group C conjugate vaccine Poliomyelitis vaccine, live (oral) | *Only for neonates at risk:* BCG vaccine |
| During second year of life | Measles, mumps and rubella vaccine, live (MMR) | *If not previously immunized: Haemophilus influenzae* type b vaccine (Hib) |
| Before school or nursery school entry | Adsorbed diphtheria, tetanus and pertussis (acellular component) vaccine [DTaP] Poliomyelitis vaccine, live (oral) Measles, mumps and rubella vaccine, live (MMR) | Single booster doses |
| Before leaving school or before employment or further education | Adsorbed diphtheria [low dose] and tetanus vaccine for adults and adolescents Poliomyelitis vaccine, live (Oral) | Single booster doses |
| During adult life | *High-risk groups:* Hepatitis A vaccine Influenza vaccine Pneumococcal vaccine Hepatitis B vaccine[a] | *If not previously immunized:* Adsorbed diphtheria [low dose] and Tetanus vaccine for adults and adolescents Poliomyelitis vaccine, live (oral) *For women of child-bearing age susceptible to rubella:* Measles, mumps and rubella vaccine, live (MMR) |

[a] Contains inactivated hepatitis B virus surface antigen (HBsAg) made biosynthetically using recombinant DNA technology adsorbed on aluminium hydroxide adjuvant.

# Adverse drug reactions

- Almost any drug may produce unwanted or unexpected adverse reactions.
- The true incidence of adverse drug reactions is often not known, and many adverse reactions are probably not, at present, recognized as drug related.
- Adverse drug reactions should be reported using the 'yellow card' system.
- Drugs can cause a wide range of adverse reactions affecting the mouth.
- The commonest or most important oral effects of drugs are listed on Table 8.25.
- Patients should be warned if serious adverse reactions are predictable and likely to occur (e.g. systemic corticosteroids), and provided with the appropriate warning card to carry.

**Table 8.25** Oral side-effects of drug treatment (most are rare)

**Drugs most commonly implicated in:**

Xerostomia

Alpha receptor antagonists for treatment of urinary retention

Anticholinergics

Antidepressants (tricyclics, serotonin agonists, or noradrenaline and/or serotonin re-uptake blockers)

Antipsychotics such as phenothiazines

Appetite suppressants

Atropinics

Muscarinic receptor antagonists for treatment of overactive bladder

Protease inhibitors

Salivary gland pain

Antihypertensives

Chlorhexidine

Cytotoxics

Iodides

Sialorrhoea

Anticholinesterases

Clozapine

Causing red saliva

Clofazimine

L-dopa

Rifabutin

Rifampin

Taste disturbances

Antithyroids

Aurothiomalate

Azithromycin

Aztreonam

Baclofen

Biguanides

Calcitonin

Captopril

Cilazapril

Clarithromycin

Cytotoxic drugs

Metronidazole

Penicillamine

Protease inhibitors

Terbinafine

Thiouracil

**Table 8.25** Contd.

Oral ulceration
  Cytotoxics
  Immunosuppressive agents
  NSAIDs, e.g. indometacin
Candidosis
  Broad-spectrum antimicrobials
  Corticosteroids
  Drugs causing xerostomia
  Immunosuppressives
Stomatitis
  Antibiotics
  Antiseptics
  Barbiturates
  Dentifrices
  Mouthwashes
  Phenacetin
  Sulphonamides
  Tetracyclines
Lichenoid reactions
  ACE inhibitors
  Antimalarials
  Beta-blockers
  NSAIDs
Pemphigoid-like reactions
  Furosemide
  Penicillamine
Pemphigus-like reactions
  Diclofenac
  Penicillamine
  Rifampicin
Erythema multiforme
  Allopurinol
  Barbiturates
  Carbamazepine
  NSAIDs
  Penicillin
  Phenytoin
  Sulphonamides
Cheilitis
  Etretinate
  Isotretinoin

**Table 8.25** Contd.

    Protease inhibitors
    Vitamin A
Hyperpigmentation
    Amalgam
    Minocycline
    Smoking /tobacco
Gingival swelling
    Amlodipine
    Basiliximab
    Ciclosporin
    Diltiazem
    Felodipine
    Lacidipine
    Nifedipine
    Oral contraceptives
    Phenytoin
    Verapamil
Paraesthesia or hypoaesthesia
    Acetazolamide
    Articaine
    Labetalol
    Protease inhibitors
    Vincristine
Dyskinesias
    L-dopa
    Metoclopramide
    Phenothiazines
Tooth discolouration
    Chlorhexidine
    Fluorides
    Iron
    Tetracyclines

# Drug contraindications

It is important to always take a full medical history, as the medical status may influence the choice of drugs used.

Certain drugs should be avoided in specific medical conditions (Tables 8.26 and 8.27).

**Table 8.26** Drugs to be avoided or only used in low dosage in specific conditions

| Condition | Drug that may be contraindicated[a] |
|---|---|
| Addison's disease (hypoadrenocorticism) | Any GA |
| Alcoholism | Antidepressants<br>Any GA<br>Aspirin<br>Baclofen<br>Carbamazepine<br>Cephamandole<br>Chlorpropamide<br>Metronidazole<br>Paracetamol/acetoaminophen<br>Salicylate<br>Tinidazole |
| Allergies | Aspirin<br>Penicillin |
| Anorexia nervosa | Paracetamol/acetoaminophen |
| Asthma | Aspirin<br>NSAIDs<br>Opiates |
| Bleeding disorders | Aspirin<br>Corticosteroids |
| Burns | Suxamethonium |
| Carcinoid syndrome | Opiates |
| Cardiovascular diseases | Adrenaline (epinephrine)<br>Aspirin<br>Chloral hydrate<br>Halothane<br>Itraconazole<br>Pentazocine<br>Rofecoxib<br>Thiopentone<br>Tricyclics |
| Cerebrovascular disease | Diazepam[b] |
| Children under 16 years | Aspirin<br>Tetracyclines |
| Chronic lymphocytic leukaemia | Amoxicillin<br>Ampicillin |
| Constipation | Codeine |
| Diabetes mellitus | Aspirin<br>Corticosteroids |
| Diarrhoea | Clindamycin<br>Mefenamic acid |

**Table 8.26** Contd.

| Condition | Drug that may be contraindicated[a] |
|-----------|-------------------------------------|
| Drug addiction | Pentazocine |
| Dystrophia myotonica (myotonic dystrophy) | Suxamethonium<br>Thiopentone |
| Elderly | Atropinics<br>Diazepam<br>Dihydrocodeine<br>Ketamine<br>Midazolam<br>NSAIDs<br>Tricyclics |
| Epilepsy | Enflurane<br>Flumazenil<br>Fluoxetine<br>Ketamine<br>Phenothiazines<br>Quinolones<br>Tricyclics |
| Glaucoma | Atropinics<br>Carbamazepine<br>Diazepam[b]<br>Steroids<br>Tricyclics |
| Glucose-6-phosphate dehydrogenase deficiency | Aspirin<br>Co-trimoxazole<br>Sulphonamides |
| Gout | Amoxicillin<br>Ampicillin<br>Aspirin |
| Head injury | Ketamine<br>Opiates |
| Hypertension | Adrenaline (epinephrine)<br>Aspirin<br>Corticosteroids<br>Ketamine<br>Pentazocine |
| Hyperthyroidism | Adrenaline (epinephrine)<br>Atropinics |
| Hypothyroidism | Any GA<br>Codeine<br>Diazepam<br>Dihydrocodeine<br>Midazolam<br>Opiates<br>Pethidine<br>Thiopentone |
| Infectious mononucleosis | Amoxicillin<br>Ampicillin |

**Table 8.26** Contd.

| Condition | Drug that may be contraindicated[a] |
|---|---|
| Liver disease | GA |
| | Antidepressants |
| | Aspirin |
| | Carbamazepine |
| | Carbenoxolone |
| | Chloral hydrate |
| | Clindamycin |
| | Corticosteroids |
| | Co-trimoxazole |
| | Dextropropoxyphene |
| | Diazepam |
| | Erythromycin |
| | estolate |
| | Etretinate |
| | Flumazenil |
| | Halothane |
| | Ketoconazole |
| | Midazolam |
| | Opiates or codeine |
| | Paracetamol/acetoaminophen/acetoaminophen |
| | Pentazocine |
| | Phenothiazines |
| | Phenytoin |
| | Rifampicin |
| | Suxamethonium |
| | Thiopentone |
| | Tricyclics |
| Malignant hyperpyrexia | Desflurane |
| | Enflurane |
| | Halothane |
| | Ketamine |
| | Sevoflurane |
| | Suxamethonium |
| Myasthenia gravis | Aminoglycosides |
| | Clindamycin |
| | GAs |
| | Lincomycin |
| | Quinolones |
| | Sulphonamides |
| | Tetracyclines |
| Neuromuscular diseases | Diazepam |
| | Midazolam |
| | Suxamethonium |
| | Tetracyclines |
| | Thiopentone |
| Parkinsonism | Benzodiazepines |
| Peptic ulcer | Aspirin |
| | Chloral hydrate |
| | Corticosteroids |
| | Mefenamic acid |

**Table 8.26** Contd.

| Condition | Drug that may be contraindicated[a] |
|---|---|
| Phaeochromocytoma | Barbiturates |
| | Enflurane |
| | Adrenaline |
| Porphyria | Carbamazepine |
| | Co-trimoxazole |
| | Dextropropoxythene |
| | Diazepam |
| | Erythromycin |
| | MAOI |
| | Metronidazole |
| | Midazolam |
| | Phenytoin |
| | Sulphonamides |
| | Thiopentone |
| Pregnancy[c] | Care with all drugs |
| | Aspirin |
| | Co-trimoxazole |
| | Diazepam |
| | Epsilon amino |
| | caproic acid |
| | Erythromycin |
| | Etretinate |
| | Flumazenil |
| | Mefenamic acid[c] |
| | Metronidazole |
| | Midazolam |
| | Opiates |
| | Phenytoin |
| | Sulphonamides |
| | Tetracyclines |
| Psychiatric disease | Ketamine |
| Raised intracranial pressure | Ketamine |
| | Opiates |
| Renal disease | Any GA or CNS depressant or NSAID |
| | Aciclovir (systemic) |
| | Aspirin |
| | Carbamazepine |
| | Cephaloridine |
| | Cephalothin |
| | Chloral hydrate |
| | Clindamycin |
| | Co-trimoxazole |
| | Diazepam |
| | Dihydrocodeine |
| | Erythromycin |
| | Mefenamic acid |
| | Metronidazole |
| | Midazolam |
| | Opiates |
| | Paracetamol/acetoaminophen/acetoaminophen |

**Table 8.26** Contd.

| Condition | Drug that may be contraindicated[a] |
|---|---|
| | Sulphonamides |
| | Suxamethonium |
| | Tetracyclines |
| Respiratory disease | Any GA |
| | Dextropropoxyphene |
| | Diazepam |
| | Dihydrocodeine |
| | Midazolam |
| | Opiates |
| | Thiopentone |
| Sjögren's syndrome | Co-trimoxazole |
| Suxamethonium sensitivity | Suxamethonium |
| | Local anaesthetics |
| Systemic lupus erythematosus | Tetracyclines |
| Teenagers | Metoclopramide |
| Thrombotic disease | Epsilon amino caproic acid |
| | Tranexamic acid |
| Thyroid disease | Povidone-iodine |
| Tuberculosis | Corticosteroids |
| Urinary retention (prostatic disease) | Atropinics |
| | Opiates |

[a] Contraindications are often relative, or of theoretical interest only; other drugs may also be contraindicated.
[b] Midazolam may be safer but should still be used with caution.
[c] And breast feeding.

**Table 8.27** Possible contraindications to drugs used in dentistry

| Drug | Possible contraindications | Possible reaction |
|------|---------------------------|-------------------|
| Acetoaminophen/ paracetamol | Alcoholism | Hepatotoxicity |
| | Anorexia | Hepatotoxicity |
| | Liver disease | Hepatotoxicity |
| | Renal disease | Nephrotoxicity |
| Aciclovir (systemic) | Renal disease | Urea rises |
| Adrenaline (epinephrine) | Hypertension (theoretically) | Hypertension |
| | Hyperthyroidism (theoretically) | Arrhythmias |
| | Ischaemic heart disease | Arrhythmias |
| | Phaeochromocytoma | Hypertension |
| Ampicillin (or amoxicillin) | Allergy to penicillin | Anaphylaxis |
| | Chronic lymphocytic leukaemia | Rash |
| | Gout | Rash |
| | Infectious mononucleosis | Rash |
| Antidepressants | Alcoholism | Potentiated |
| Aspirin | Allergy to aspirin including aspirin-induced asthma | Anaphylaxis |
| | Alcoholism | Gastric bleeding |
| | Bleeding disorders | Gastric bleeding |
| | Breast feeding | Reye's Syndrome |
| | Cardiac failure | Fluid retention |
| | Children under 16 years | Reye's syndrome |
| | Diabetes mellitus | Interferes with control |
| | Glucose-6-phosphate dehydrogenase deficiency | Haemolysis |
| | Gout | Gout worse |
| | Hypertension | Fluid retention |
| | Liver disease | Bleeding tendency |
| | Peptic ulcer | Gastric bleeding |
| | Pregnancy | Haemorrhage |
| | Renal disease | Fluid retention and gastric bleeding |
| Atropinics | Elderly | Confusion |
| | Glaucoma | Glaucoma exacerbated |
| | Hyperthyroidism | Tachycardias |
| | Urinary retention or prostatic hypertrophy | Urine retention |
| Carbamazepine | Alcoholism | Sedation |
| | Blood disorders | Dyscrasia |
| | Elderly | Agitation or confusion |
| | Glaucoma | Raised intraoccular pressure |
| | Liver Disease | Hepatotoxic |
| | Porphyria | Acute porphyria |
| | Pregnancy | Teratogenic |
| Carbenoxolone | Liver disease | Toxicity |

**Table 8.27** Contd.

| Drug | Possible contraindications | Possible reaction |
|---|---|---|
| Cephalosporins | Allergy to cephalosporins | Anaphylaxis |
| | Allergy to penicillins | Allergy |
| | Renal disease | Nephrotoxic |
| Chloral hydrate | Cardiovascular disease | Fluid retention |
| | Gastritis | Gastric irritation |
| | Liver disease | Coma |
| | Renal disease | CNS depression |
| Clindamycin | Diarrhoea | Aggravated |
| | Liver disease | Increased toxicity |
| | Renal disease | Increased toxicity |
| Codeine | Colonic disease | Constipation |
| | Hypothyroidism | Coma |
| | Liver disease | Respiratory depression |
| Corticosteroids | Diabetes mellitus | Diabetes worsened |
| | Glaucoma | Glaucoma exacerbated |
| | Hypertension | Increased hypertension |
| | Liver disease | Increased side-effects |
| | Peptic ulcer | Perforation |
| | Tuberculosis | Possible dissemination |
| Co-trimoxazole | Elderly | Agranulocytosis |
| | Glucose-6-phosphate-dehydrogenase deficiency | Haemolysis |
| | Liver disease | Enhanced toxicity |
| | Porphyria | Acute porphyria |
| | Pregnancy | Folate deficiency |
| | Renal disease | Increased toxicity |
| | Sjögren's syndrome | Aseptic meningitis |
| Dextropropoxyphene | Liver disease | Potentiated paralysis |
| | Porphyria | |
| | Pregnancy | Fetal depression |
| | Respiratory disease | Respiratory depression |
| Desflurane | Malignant hyperpyrexia | Pyrexia |
| Diazepam | (see Midazolam) | |
| Dihydrocodeine | Elderly | Increased toxicity |
| | Hypothyroidism | Coma |
| | Renal disease | Increased toxicity |
| | Respiratory disease | Respiratory depression |

**Table 8.27** Contd.

| Drug | Possible contraindications | Possible reaction |
|------|---------------------------|-------------------|
| Enflurane | Epilepsy<br>Halothane hepatitis<br>Malignant hyperpyrexia<br>Phaeochromocytoma | Epileptogenic<br>Hepatitis<br>Pyrexia<br>Hypertension |
| Epsilon amino caproic acid | Haematuria<br>Pregnancy<br>Thrombotic disease | Renal tract obstruction<br>Thrombosis<br>Thrombosis |
| Erythromycin | Breast feeding<br>Liver disease<br>Porphyria<br>Pregnancy<br>Renal disease | Enters milk<br>Hepatotoxic<br>Paralysis<br>?teratogenic<br>Toxicity |
| Etomidate | Adrenal disease | Adrenal suppression |
| Etretinate | Liver disease<br>Pregnancy | Hepatotoxic<br>Teratogenic |
| Fluconazole | Cardiac failure<br>Liver disease<br>Porphyria<br>Pregnancy<br>Renal disease | Cardiac failure<br>Hepatotoxic<br>Crisis<br>Teratogenic<br>Toxicity |
| Flumazenil | Allergy<br>Epilepsy<br>Liver disease<br>Pregnancy | Allergy<br>Epileptogenic<br>Delayed excretion<br>Teratogenic |
| Fluoxetine | Epilepsy | Epileptogenic |
| Halothane | Cardiac arrhythmias<br>Halothane hepatitis<br>Malignant hyperpyrexia<br>Recent anaesthesia with Halothane | Increased arrhythmias<br>Hepatitis<br>Pyrexia<br>Hepatitis |
| Isoflurane | Malignant hyperpyrexia | Pyrexia |
| Itraconazole (see also Fluconazole) | Heart failure | Heart failure |
| Ketamine | Elderly<br>Epilepsy<br>Hallucinations<br>Hypertension<br>Malignant hyperpyrexia<br>Psychiatric disease<br>Raised intracranial pressure | Hallucinations<br>Fits<br>Hallucinations<br>Hypertension<br>Pyrexia<br>Psychotic reactions<br>Increased intracranial pressure |
| Ketoconazole (see also Fluconazole) | Liver disease | Hepatotoxic |

**Table 8.27** Contd.

| Drug | Possible contraindications | Possible reaction |
|------|----------------------------|-------------------|
| Lincomycin (as for Clindamycin) | | |
| Local anaesthetics | Suxamethonium sensitivity | Respiratory depression |
| Mefenamic acid | Asthma | Bronchospasm |
| | Diarrhoea | Diarrhoea worse |
| | Peptic ulcer | Bleeding |
| | Pregnancy and lactation | ?Teratogenic |
| | Renal disease | Renal damage |
| Metoclopramide | Teenagers | Dystonic reactions |
| Metronidazole | Alcoholism | Headache |
| | Blood dyscrasias | Leucopenia |
| | Breast feeding | In milk |
| | CNS disease | Neuropathy |
| | Epilepsy | Epileptogenic |
| | Liver disease | Toxicity |
| | Porphyria | Acute porphyria |
| | Pregnancy | ?Teratogenic |
| | Renal disease | Increased drug effect |
| Miconazole (see Fluconazole) | | |
| Midazolam | Cerebrovascular disease | Cerebral ischaemia |
| | Chronic obstructive airways disease | Respiratory depression |
| | Elderly | Cerebral ischaemia |
| | Glaucoma | Increased intraocular |
| | Hypothyroidism | Coma |
| | Neuromuscular disorders | Condition deteriorates |
| | Porphyria | Acute porphyria |
| | Pregnancy | Fetal hypoxia/dependence |
| | Severe renal disease | Increased midazolam effect |
| | Severe liver disease | Increased midazolam effect |
| NSAIDs | Asthma | Bronchospasm |
| | Elderly | Toxicity |
| | Liver disease | Hepatotoxicity |
| | Peptic ulcer | Gastric bleeding |
| | Pregnancy | Patent ductus arteriosus |
| | Renal disease | Nephrotoxic |

**Table 8.27** Contd.

| Drug | Possible contraindications | Possible reaction |
|------|---------------------------|-------------------|
| Opiates | Asthma | Bronchospasm |
| | Carcinoid syndrome | Increased toxicity |
| | Chronic obstructive airways disease | Respiratory depression |
| | Head injury | Confuse 'eye signs' |
| | Hypothyroidism | Coma |
| | Liver disease | Increased respiratory depression |
| | Pregnancy | Fetal depression |
| | Renal disease | Increased respiratory depression |
| | Urinary retention or prostatic enlargement | Urinary retention |
| Penicillins | Allergy to penicillin | Anaphylaxis |
| | Renal disease | Hyperkalaemia with IM benzyl penicillin |
| Pentazocine | Hypertension | Hypertension |
| | Liver disease | Enhanced activity |
| | MI (recent) | Cardiac arrest |
| | Narcotic addict | Withdrawal syndrome |
| | Pregnancy | Fetal depression |
| Pethidine | Hypothyroidism | Coma |
| Povidone-iodine | Lactation | Toxicity |
| | Pregnancy | Toxicity |
| | Thyroid disease | Toxicity |
| Promethazine | Liver disease | Coma |
| Propofol | Children under 17 years | May cause convulsions |
| Quinolones | Epilepsy | Epileptogenic |
| | Myasthenia gravis | Muscle weakness |
| Rifampicin | Liver disease | Hepatotoxic |
| Rofecoxib | Cardiac disease | Risk of infarction |
| Sevoflurane | Malignant hyperpyrexia | Pyrexia |
| Sulphonamides | Glucose-6-phosphate dehydrogenase deficiency | Haemolysis |
| | Liver disease | Toxicity |
| | Porphyria | Acute porphyria |
| | Pregnancy | Fetal haemolysis |
| | Renal disease | Crystalluria |
| Suxamethonium | Burns | Arrhythmias |
| | Dystrophia myotonica | Increased muscle weakness |
| | Liver disease | Apnoea |
| | Malignant hyperpyrexia | Pyrexia |
| | Myasthenia gravis | Increased muscle weakness |
| | Renal disease | Apnoea |
| | Suxamethonium sensitivity | Apnoea |

**Table 8.27** Contd.

| Drug | Possible contraindications | Possible reaction |
|------|---------------------------|-------------------|
| Tetracyclines | After gastrointestinal surgery | Enterocolitis |
| | Children | Tooth staining |
| | Myasthenia gravis | Increased muscle weakness |
| | Pregnancy | Tooth staining (fetus) |
| | Renal disease | Nephrotoxicity |
| | Systemic lupus erythematosus | Photosensitivity |
| Thiopentone | Addison's disease | Coma |
| | Barbiturate sensitivity | Anaphylaxis |
| | Cardiovascular disease | Cardiovascular depression |
| | Dystrophia myotonica | Increased weakness |
| | Hypothyroidism | Coma |
| | Liver disease | Increased anaesthesia |
| | Myasthenia gravis | Increased weakness |
| | Porphyria | Acute porphyria |
| | Postnatal drip | Laryngeal spasm |
| | Respiratory disease | Respiratory depression |
| Tranexamic acid | Haematuria | Renal tract obstruction |
| | Pregnancy | Thromboses |
| Triclofos | Thromboembolic disease | Thromboses |
| Tricyclics | Cardiovascular disease | Postural hypotension |
| | | Arrhythmias |
| | Elderly | Hypotension |
| | Epilepsy | Increased fits |
| | Glaucoma | Glaucoma exacerbated |
| | Liver disease | Increased drug effect |
| Trimethoprim | Sjögren's syndrome | Trimethoprim-induced aseptic meningitis |
| Voriconazole (see Fluconazole) | | |

Many of these reactions are likely to be of more theoretical interest than clinical significance, so reference should also be made to the appropriate chapters for particular diseases.

# Drug interactions

- The number of new drugs is always increasing, as is their complexity
- Increasingly large numbers of people are treated with multiple drugs
- Keeping up-to-date with drug indications, adverse effects, contraindications and interactions is becoming increasingly difficult.
- Apart from hard copy sources of information such as the British National Formulary and the Physicians Desk Reference, electronic sources are now available, such as Epocrates.
- It is generally good practice to:
  - Never use any drug unless there are good indications.
  - Avoid polypharmacy, and use only drugs with which you are familiar.
  - Check before use, adverse effects, contraindications and interactions.

Possible interactions with drugs used in dentistry are listed on Tables 8.28 and 8.29.

**Table 8.28** Possible drug interactions in dentistry

| Drug used in dentistry | Interaction with | Possible effects |
| --- | --- | --- |
| Acetoaminophen/ paracetamol | Alcohol | Hepatotoxicity |
| | Anticonvulsants | Hepatotoxicity |
| | Carbamazepine | Hepatotoxicity |
| | Cholestyramine | Reduced absorption of paracetamol/acetoaminophen |
| | Domperidone | Increased absorption of paracetamol/acetoaminophen |
| | Isonicotinic hydrazide | Enhanced (INAH) hepatotoxicity |
| | Metoclopramide | Potentiation |
| | Oral anticoagulants | Increased bleeding tendency |
| | Zidovudine | Increased myelosuppression |
| Aciclovir | Zidovudine | Lethargy |
| Adrenaline (epinephrine) | Halothane | Arrhythmias |
| | Tricyclics | Pressor response in overdose |
| Amphotericin | Aminoglycosides | Enhanced nephrotoxicity |
| | Cyclosporin | Enhanced nephrotoxicity |
| Anaesthetics (general) | Antihypertensives | Hypotension |
| | MAOI | Enhanced hypotension; anaesthetics potentiated |
| Antibiotics | Oral anticoagulants | Enhanced anticoagulant effect |
| | Oral contraceptives | Reduced contraceptive effect |
| Aspirin | Acetoaminophen (doses >4 g/day) | Enhanced hepatotoxicity |
| | Alcohol | Increased risk of gastric bleeding |
| | Antacids | Reduced aspirin absorption |
| | Corticosteroids | Peptic ulceration |
| | Lithium | Lithium toxicity |
| | Methotrexate | Enhanced methotrexate activity |
| | Metoclopramide | Potentiation of aspirin absorption |
| | NSAIDs | Potentiation |
| | Oral anticoagulants | Enhanced anticoagulant effect |
| | Oral hypoglycaemics | Enhanced hypoglycaemic effect |

**Table 8.28** Contd.

| Drug used in dentistry | Interaction with | Possible effects |
|---|---|---|
| | Phenylbutazone | Increased liability of peptic Ulceration |
| | Phenytoin | Phenytoin toxicity |
| | Probenecid | Uricosuric action reduced |
| | Sodium valproate | Bleeding tendency |
| | Sulphinpyrazone | Uricosuric action reduced |
| | Zafirlukast | Enhanced leukotriene |
| Atropine | Metoclopramide | Antagonism |
| Azathioprine | Allopurinol | Toxicity |
| | Rifampicin | ?Transplant rejection |
| Azithromycin | Pimozide | Arrhythmias |
| | Terfenadine | Arrhythmias |
| Baclofen | ACE inhibitors | Enhanced hypotension |
| | Alcohol | Sedation |
| | NSAIDs | Toxicity |
| Barbiturates | Alcohol | May be increased sedation or resistance |
| | Antihistamines | Enhanced sedation |
| | Antihypertensives | Hypotension |
| | Corticosteroids | May precipitate hypotensive crises |
| | Ciclosporin | Reduced effect of ciclosporin |
| | MAOI | Enhanced sedation |
| | Oral anticoagulants | Reduced anticoagulant activity |
| | Phenothiazines | Tremor |
| | Phenytoin | Reduced phenytoin effect |
| | Tricyclics | Cardiac arrest |
| Carbamazepine | Calcium channel blockers | Carbamazepine toxicity |
| | Ciclosporin | Reduced effect of ciclosporin |
| | Cimetidine | Carbamazepine toxicity |
| | Clarithromycin | Carbamazepine toxicity |
| | Danazol | Carbamazepine toxicity |
| | Dextropropoxyphene | Carbamazepine enhanced |
| | Doxycycline | Reduced doxycycline effect |
| | Erythromycin | Carbamazepine toxicity |
| | Fluoxetine | Confusion |
| | Lithium | Lithium toxicity |
| | MAOI | Possible hypertension |
| | Oral anticoagulants | Reduced anticoagulant effect |
| | Oral contraceptive | Reduced contraceptive effect |
| | Paracetamol/ acetoaminophen | Liver damage |
| | Phenytoin | Reduced phenytoin effect |
| | Protease inhibitors | Interferes |
| | Sodium valproate | Reduced effect of valproate |

**Table 8.28** Contd.

| Drug used in dentistry | Interaction with | Possible effects |
|---|---|---|
| Cephalosporins | Diuretics | Increased nephrotoxicity |
| | Oral anticoagulants | Increased bleeding tendency |
| Cephamandole | Alcohol | Disulfiram-type reaction |
| | Oral anticoagulants | Increased bleeding tendency |
| Ciclosporin | ACE inhibitors | Hyperkalaemia |
| | Allopurinol | Nephrotoxicity |
| | Colchicine | Nephrotoxicity and myotoxicity |
| | Erythromycin | Ciclosporin toxicity |
| Clarithromycin | Pimozide | Arrhythmias |
| | Terfenadine | Arrhythmias |
| Codeine | MAOI | Coma |
| Colchicine | Ciclosporin | Nephrotoxicity and myotoxicity |
| Corticosteroids | ACE inhibitors | Reduced hypotensive effect |
| | Aminoglycosides | Reduced steroid effects |
| | Aspirin/NSAIDs | Increased liability of peptic ulceration |
| | Oral anticoagulants | Gastric bleeding |
| | Oral antidiabetics | Reduced effect |
| Co-trimoxazole | Methotrexate | Possible folate deficiency |
| | Oral anticoagulants | Increased bleeding |
| | Oral contraceptive | Reduced contraceptive effect |
| | Oral hypoglycaemic | Enhanced hypoglycaemia |
| | Phenytoin | Phenytoin toxicity |
| Danazol | Oral anticoagulants | Potentiated anticoagulation |
| Dextropropoxyphene | Alcohol | Central nervous system depression |
| | Carbamazepine | Carbamazepine enhanced |
| | Oral anticoagulants | Enhanced anticoagulant effect |
| | Orphenadrine | Tremor, anxiety and confusion |
| Ephedrine | MAOI | Hypertension |
| | Tricyclics | Hypertension |
| Erythromycin | Amprenavir | Erythromycin toxicity |
| | Artemether | Erythromycin toxicity |
| | Bromocriptine | Toxicity |
| | Cabergoline | Toxicity |
| | Carbamazepine | Carbamazepine toxicity |
| | Ciclosporin | Increased ciclosporin absorption |
| | Cimetidine | Erythromycin toxicity |
| | Clozapine | Convulsions |
| | Digoxin | Digoxin toxicity |

**Table 8.28** Contd.

| Drug used in dentistry | Interaction with | Possible effects |
|---|---|---|
| | Efavirenz | Erythromycin toxicity |
| | Eletriptan | Eletriptan toxicity |
| | Ergotamine | Ergotism |
| | Midazolam | Toxicity |
| | Oral anticoagulants | Increased bleeding |
| | Pimozide | Arrhythmias |
| | Rifabutin | Uveitis |
| | Ritonavir | Erythromycin toxicity |
| | Statins | Myopathy increased |
| | Tacrolimus | Tacrolimus toxicity |
| | Terfenadine | Arrhythmias |
| | Theophyllines | Toxicity |
| | Valproate | Toxicity |
| Fluconazole | Anticonvulsants | Anticonvulsant enhanced |
| | Calcium channel blockers | Cardiac failure |
| | Celecoxib | Celecoxib enhanced |
| | Ciclosporin | Ciclosporin enhanced |
| | Digoxin | Digoxin enhanced |
| | Midazolam | Midazolam enhanced |
| | Mizolastine | Mizolastine enhanced |
| | Oral anticoagulants | Enhanced anticoagulant effect |
| | Oral antidiabetics | Enhanced antidiabetic effect |
| | Oral contraceptive | May impair contraception |
| | Parecoxib | Parecoxib enhanced |
| | Pimozide | Arrhythmias |
| | Protease inhibitors (PIs) | PIs enhanced |
| | Quinidine | Arrhythmias |
| | Rifampicin | Fluconazole effect reduced |
| | Sirolimus | Sirolimus enhanced |
| | Statins | Increased myopathy |
| | Terfenadine | Arrhythmias |
| | Vincristine | Vincristine enhanced |
| | Zidovudine | Myelotoxicity |
| Flumazenil | Tricyclics | Sedation |
| Fluoxetine | Alcohol | Enhanced alcohol effect |
| | Antiepileptics | Antagonized |
| | Carbamazepine | Confusion |
| | MAOI | CNS effects |
| | Warfarin | Enhanced anticoagulant effect |
| Ganciclovir | Zidovudine | Marrow suppression |
| Gentamicin | Furosemide | Toxicity and nephrotoxicity |

**Table 8.28** Contd.

| Drug used in dentistry | Interaction with | Possible effects |
|---|---|---|
| Halothane | Aminophylline | Arrhythmias |
| | Anticonvulsants | Phenytoin toxicity |
| | Antihypertensives | Hypotension |
| | Diazepam | Enhanced activity of halothane |
| | Fenfluramine | Arrhythmias |
| | Isoprenaline | Arrhythmias |
| | L-dopa | Arrhythmias |
| | Lithium | Arrhythmias |
| | Opiates | Respiratory depression |
| | Phenothiazines | Respiratory depression; hypotension |
| Indometacin | Haloperidol | Drowsiness |
| Itraconazole (as for Fluconazole) | | |
| Ketamine | CNS depressants | Increased sedation |
| Ketoconazole (see Fluconazole) | Ciclosporin | Nephrotoxicity |
| | Simvastatin | Risk of myopathy |
| Mefenamic acid | Oral anticoagulants | Enhanced anticoagulant effect |
| | Oral hypoglycaemics | Enhanced hypoglycaemia |
| Metronidazole | Alcohol | Headache and Hypotension |
| | Anticonvulsants | Phenytoin toxicity |
| | Cimetidine | Metronidazole toxicity |
| | Fluorouracil | Fluorouracil toxicity |
| | Lithium | Lithium toxicity |
| | Oral anticoagulants | Increased bleeding tendency |
| Miconazole (as for Fluconazole) | | |
| Midazolam and other sedatives | Anticonvulsants | Midazolam potentiated |
| | Antihistamines | Enhanced sedation |
| | Azole | Midazolam potentiated |
| | Baclofen | Enhanced sedation |
| | Calcium channel blockers | Midazolam potentiated |
| | Cimetidine | Enhanced sedation |
| | Clarithromycin | Midazolam potentiated |
| | Disulfiram | Midazolam potentiated? |
| | Esomeprazole | Midazolam potentiated? |
| | Erythromycin | Midazolam potentiated |
| | Fluvoxamine | Midazolam potentiated |
| | GA | Anaesthesia enhanced |
| | L-dopa | Antagonism |
| | Lithium | Hypothermia |
| | Omeprazole | Midazolam potentiated? |
| | Opiates | Respiratory depression |
| | Oral anticoagulants | Increased bleeding tendency |
| | Pentazocine | Respiratory depression |

**Table 8.28** Contd.

| Drug used in dentistry | Interaction with | Possible effects |
|---|---|---|
| | Phenytoin | Phenytoin toxicity |
| | Protease inhibitors | Midazolam potentiated |
| | Quinupristin | Midazolam potentiated |
| | Rifampicin | Midazolam effect reduced |
| | Suxamethonium | Activity of suxamethonium reduced |
| | Telithromycin | Midazolam potentiated |
| | Tizanidine | Enhanced sedation |
| | Tricyclics | Enhanced sedation |
| Monoamine oxidase inhibitors (MAOI) | Antihypertensives | Reduced or increased hypotensive effect |
| | Codeine | Hypertension |
| | GA | Hypertension |
| | L-dopa | Hypertensive crisis |
| | Opiates | Respiratory depression |
| | Oral anticoagulants | Enhanced anticoagulant effect |
| | Oral hypoglycaemics | Enhanced hypoglycaemia |
| | Pethidine | Hypertensive crisis |
| | Propranolol | Hypertensive crisis |
| | Tricyclics | Excitation and other interactions |
| | Tyramine-containing foods | Hypertensive crisis |
| Noradrenaline (norepinephrine) | Tricyclics | Hypertension |
| NSAIDs | Acetoaminophen (>4 g/day) | Hepatotoxicity |
| | Alcohol | Gastric irritation |
| | Anticonvulsants | Phenytoin toxicity |
| | Antihypertensives | Hypotension Hyperkalaemia |
| | Baclofen | Toxicity |
| | Ciclosporin | Nephrotoxicity |
| | Corticosteroids | Gastric irrritation |
| | Cytotoxics | Toxicity |
| | Diuretics | Nephrotoxicity |
| | Lithium | Lithium toxicity |
| | Moclobemide | NSAID enhanced |
| | Oral anticoagulants | Increased bleeding tendency |
| | Oral antidiabetics | Enhanced antidiabetic activity |
| | Pentoxifylline | Increased bleeding |
| | Quinolones | Convulsions |
| | Tacrolimus | Nephrotoxicity |
| | Warfarin | Increased bleeding |
| | Zidovudine | Blood dyscrasia |
| Opiates | Diazepam | Respiratory depression |
| | Halothane | Respiratory depression |
| | MAOI | Respiratory depression or coma |
| | Thiopentone | Respiratory depression |

**Table 8.28** Contd.

| Drug used in dentistry | Interaction with | Possible effects |
|---|---|---|
| Pentazocine | Diazepam | Respiratory depression |
| Pethidine | MAOI | Hypertensive crisis |
| | Phenothiazines | Respiratory depression |
| Phenothiazines | Alcohol | May be increased sedation |
| | Antihistamines | Enhanced sedation |
| | Antihypertensives | Hypotension |
| | Diazepam | Respiratory depression |
| | Barbiturates | Tremor |
| | Opiates | Respiratory depression |
| | Oral anticoagulants | Enhanced anticoagulant effect |
| | Pethidine | Respiratory depression |
| | Tricyclics | Convulsions |
| Phenylbutazone | Aspirin | Increased liability of peptic ulceration |
| Phenytoin | Aspirin | Phenytoin toxicity |
| | Azoles | Phenytoin toxicity |
| | Baclofen | Phenytoin toxicity |
| | Carbamazepine | Reduced carbamazepine effect |
| | Cimetidine | Phenytoin toxicity |
| | Clarithromycin | Phenytoin toxicity |
| | Disulfiram | Disulfiram potentiated |
| | Isonicotinic acid hydride (INAH) | INAH potentiated |
| | Midazolam | Toxicity |
| | NSAIDs | Phenytoin toxicity |
| | Phenylbutazone | Phenylbutazone potentiated |
| Promethazine | Thiopentone | Respiratory depression |
| Quinolones | Antacids | Reduced absorption |
| | Anticoagulants | Bleeding increased |
| | Antidiabetics | Antidiabetic enhanced |
| | Anticonvulsants | Phenytoin enhanced |
| | Artemether | Toxicity |
| | Ciclosporin | Nephrotoxicity |
| | Iron | Reduced absorption |
| | Theophylline | Convulsions |
| | Zolmitriptan | Increased effect of zolmitriptan |
| Rifampicin | Antacids | Reduced rifampicin absorption |
| | Antifungals | Increased metabolism of antifungals |
| | Ciclosporin | Reduced effect of ciclosporin |
| | Oral anticoagulant | Reduced bleeding tendency |
| | Oral contraceptive | Reduced contraceptive effect |
| SSRIs | Lithium | Serotonin syndrome |
| Sulphonamides | Methotrexate | Increased methotrexate toxicity |
| | Oral anticoagulants | Enhanced anticoagulant effect |
| | Oral hypoglycaemics | Enhanced hypoglycaemia |
| | Phenytoin | Phenytoin toxicity |

**Table 8.28** Contd.

| Drug used in dentistry | Interaction with | Possible effects |
|---|---|---|
| Suxamethonium | Cytotoxic drugs | Prolonged muscle paralysis |
| | Diazepam | Activity of suxamethonium reduced |
| | Diethylstilboestrol | Prolonged muscle paralysis |
| | Digitalis | Digitalis toxicity enhanced |
| | Ecothiopate | Prolonged muscle paralysis |
| | Lithium | Onset of suxamethonium delayed; action prolonged |
| | Spironolactone | Plasma potassium rises; potential arrhythmias |
| Tetracyclines | ACE inhibitors | Reduced absorption of tetracyclines |
| | Antacids | Lower serum levels of tetracyclines |
| | Barbiturates | Reduced doxycycline blood levels |
| | Cimetidine | Reduced serum tetracycline levels |
| | Iron | Reduced serum tetracycline levels |
| | Lithium | Lithium toxicity |
| | Methoxyflurane | Renal damage |
| | Milk | Reduced tetracycline absorption |
| | Oral anticoagulants | Bleeding tendency |
| | Oral contraceptive | Reduced contraceptive effect |
| Thiopentone | Alcohol | Increased sedation |
| | Antihypertensives | Hypotension |
| | MAOI | Coma |
| | Opiates | Respiratory depression |
| | Phenothiazines | Respiratory depression |
| | Sulphonamides | Barbiturate potentiated |
| Tricyclics | Adrenaline (epinephrine) | Hypertensive response in overdose |
| | Alcohol | Enhanced central nervous system |
| | Antihypertensives | Impaired BP control |
| | Atropinics | Enhanced atropinic effect |
| | Carbamazepine | Confusion |
| | Cimetidine | Tricyclic enhanced |
| | Contraceptive pill | Tricyclic effect reduced |
| | Diazepam | Enhanced sedation |
| | GA | Cardiac arrest |
| | MAOI | Excitation and other interactions |
| | Oral anticoagulants | Enhanced anticoagulant effect |
| | Phenothiazines | Convulsions |
| Voriconazole (see Fluconazole) | | |

Many of these drug interactions are of little more than theoretical importance in dentistry, or are the result of overdose of one or both agents. However, there can be a wide range of individual variations in response to drugs, especially sedating agents.

**Table 8.29** More common drug interactions of significance in oral health care

| Drug group | Specific drugs used in dentistry | Interacting drug | Possible outcomes |
|---|---|---|---|
| Analgesics | Acetoaminophen/ paracetamol | Alcohol | Liver toxicity |
| | Aspirin | Alcohol | Risk of GI bleeding |
| | | Hypoglycaemics | Enhanced hypoglycaemia |
| | | Warfarin | Risk of GI bleeding |
| | NSAIDs | Antihypertensives | Reduced antihypertensive effect |
| | | Lithium | Lithium toxicity |
| | | Methotrexate | Methotrexate toxicity |
| | | Warfarin | Risk of GI bleeding |
| Antibacterials | Ampicillin, amoxicillin | Beta-blockers | Antihypertensive levels reduced. Increased severity of anaphylactic reactions |
| | Any | Oral contraceptives | Failed contraception |
| | Erythromycin | Benzodiazepines | High benzodiazepine levels |
| | | Carbamazepine | Carbamazepine toxicity |
| | | Ciclosporin | Ciclosporin toxicity |
| | | Digoxin | Digitalis toxicity |
| | | Statins | Muscle damage |
| | | Terfenadine | Arrhythmias |
| | | Theophylline | Theophylline toxicity |
| | | Warfarin | Bleeding tendency increased |
| | Metronidazole | Ethanol (alcohol) | Disulfiram-type reaction |
| | | Lithium | Lithium toxicity |
| | | Warfarin | Bleeding tendency |
| | Tetracyclines | Antacids | Reduced tetracycline absorption |
| | | Digoxin | Digitalis toxicity |
| Antifungals | Fluconazole | Statins | Muscle damage |
| | | Warfarin | Bleeding |
| | Miconazole | Statins | Muscle damage |
| | | Warfarin | Bleeding |

**Table 8.29** Contd.

| Drug group | Specific drugs used in dentistry | Interacting drug | Possible outcomes |
|---|---|---|---|
| Adrenaline-containing local anaesthetics | | Beta-blockers (non-selective) | Hypertension and bradycardia |
| | | Cocaine | Arrhythmias |
| | | COMT (Catechol O methyl transferase) inhibitors (tolcapone, entacapone) | Hypertension, tachy-cardias, arrhythmias |
| | | Halothane | Arrhythmias |
| | | Tricyclics | Hypertension, tachy-cardias, arrhythmias |
| Sedatives | Benzodiazepines | Alcohol | Benzodiazepine toxicity |
| | | Cimetidine | Benzodiazepine toxicity |
| | | Digoxin | Digitalis toxicity |
| | | Fluoxetine | Benzodiazepine toxicity |
| | | Isoniazid | Benzodiazepine toxicity |
| | | Oral contraceptives | Benzodiazepine toxicity |
| | | Phenytoin | Phenytoin toxicity |
| | | Protease inhibitors | Benzodiazepine toxicity |
| | | Theophylline | Theophylline toxicity |

# Alternative therapies

- Alternative therapies include, but are not limited to the following disciplines: folk medicine, herbal medicine, diet fads, homeopathy, faith healing, new age healing, chiropractic, acupuncture, naturopathy, massage, and music therapy.
- Natural (herbal) medicines are commonly used but 'natural' does not necessarily mean 'safe'. Serious adverse events, such as severe renal disease after taking Chinese herbs, and hepatotoxicity from Kava-kava (*Piper methysticum*) have been recorded and some herbal products may impair platelet aggregation prolonging bleeding (Table 8.30).

**Table 8.30** Herbal products that may interfere with haemostasis

| Herb | Substance |
|------|-----------|
| Bilberry | *Vaccinium myrtillus* |
| Bromelain | *Anas comosus* |
| Cat's claw | *Uncaria tomentosa* |
| Devil's claw | *Harpagophytum procumbens* |
| Dong Quai | *Angelica sinensis* |
| Evening primrose | *Oenothera biennis* |
| Feverfew | *Tanacetum parthenium* |
| Garlic | *Allium savitum* |
| Ginger | *Zingiber officinale* |
| Ginkgo biloba | — |
| Ginseng | *Panax ginseng* |
| Grape seed | *Vitis vinifera* |
| Green tea | *Camellia sinensis* |
| Horse chestnut | *Aesculus hippocastanum* |
| Turmeric | *Curcuma longa* |

- At present there is little evidence base for the efficacy or otherwise of most herbal medicines, but reliable published data tend to support a potential medicinal role for a few (Table 8.31).

**Table 8.31** Herbal preparations and supplements of proven efficacy

| Herbal preparation | Effective for treating | Potential adverse effects |
| --- | --- | --- |
| Saw palmetto | Benign prostatic hyperplasia | Minimal |
| Melatonin | Jet lag | — |
| St John's wort | Mild to moderate depression | Dry mouth, dizziness, GI symptoms, sunlight sensitivity, and fatigue |

USEFUL WEBSITES

http://www.fda.gov/fdac/features/1998/dietchrt.html
http://www.publications.parliament.uk/pa/ld199900/ldselect/ldsctech/123/12301.htm
http://bnf.org/bnf/bnf/
http://www.drugdigest.org/DD/Interaction/ChooseDrugs
http://vm.cfsan.fda.gov/~lrd/fdinter.html
www.mhra.gov.uk

# Analgesia, sedation and anaesthesia

# Choice of technique

### Assessing the patient's fitness for dental treatment and analgesia

Before deciding whether any dental treatment is appropriate and the technique to be used for pain control, the patient's physical status (health) should be determined. An arbitrary guideline is the classification of Physical Status of the American Society of Anesthesiology (ASA) (Table 9.1).

According to current guidelines, dental treatment must be significantly modified if the patient has an ASA score of III or above. A relatively high percentage of patients aged 65 or over do have an ASA score of III or IV.

**Table 9.1** ASA classification

| ASA | Definition |
| --- | --- |
| I | Normal, healthy patient. |
| II | A patient with mild systemic disease, e.g. well controlled diabetes, asthma, hypertension or epilepsy; pregnancy; anxiety. |
| III | A patient with severe systemic disease limiting activity but not incapacitating, e.g. epilepsy with frequent seizures, uncontrolled hypertension, recent MI, uncontrolled diabetes, severe asthma, stroke. |
| IV | A patient with incapacitating disease that is a constant threat to life, e.g. cancer, unstable angina or recent MI, arrhythmia or recent CVA. |
| V | Moribund patient not expected to live more than 24 h with or without treatment. |

### Choice of analgesic technique

- Most dental patients can be satisfactorily treated using LA alone.
- However, in some cases, conscious sedation or GA are preferable or necessary (see Tables 9.2 and 9.3).
- Non-pharmacological techniques includes
  - distraction
  - behavioural therapy/desensitization
  - hypnosis
  - acupuncture.

**Table 9.2** Indication and contraindications for sedation and GA

**Main indications for conscious sedation or GA**

Individuals who are unable to co-operate with LA

Dental phobics

Nervous children undergoing emergency treatment

Extensive oral and maxillofacial surgery

**Main contraindications for conscious sedation or GA**

Necessary equipment unavailable

Necessary staff unavailable or untrained

Patient unescorted

Patient has taken anything except plain water by mouth in the previous 6 h

Patient has a *medical contraindication* (see also Chapter 4) such as:

- Respiratory disease (e.g. respiratory tract infection) or potential airways obstruction
  - Ludwig's angina (may necessitate prior tracheostomy under LA)
  - Allergic or hereditary angioedema
  - Asthma
- Severe cardiovascular disease
  - Ischaemic heart disease, including MI in previous 6 months
  - Severe hypertension
- Bleeding tendency (e.g. haemophilia)
- Severe anaemia (e.g. sickle cell anaemia)
- Metabolic or endocrine disorders, including
  - Liver disease
  - Renal disease
  - Severe diabetes, especially if poorly controlled
  - Thyrotoxicosis
  - Hypothyroidism
  - Addison's disease or adrenocortical suppression
- Specific contraindications to anaesthetic drugs
  - Halothane sensitivity or recent anaesthesia with halothane
  - Porphyria
  - Suxamethonium sensitivity
  - History of malignant pyrexia (adverse reaction to general anaesthetics)
- Drug usage, particularly
  - corticosteroids
  - anticoagulants
  - alcohol or narcotics
  - antidepressants
- Cervical spine pathology (e.g. trauma, Down syndrome, rheumatoid arthritis)
- Pregnancy (see Chapter 5)
- Myopathies
- Disseminated sclerosis
- ▶ None of the above are absolute contraindications.

**Table 9.3** Choice between LA, sedation or GA

|  | May be indicated | May be contraindicated |
|---|---|---|
| LA | Minor surgery or procedure | Uncooperative patient |
|  | Poor risk patient for CS or GA | Very young children |
|  |  | Needle phobics |
|  | No CS or GA available | Sepsis in field |
|  | Inadequate facilities for CS or GA | Haemangioma in field |
|  |  | LA 'Allergy' very rare for amide type LAs |
|  | After a recent meal | Major surgery |
|  |  | Bleeding tendency |
|  |  | Pseudocholinesterase deficiency |
|  |  | Patients on beta-blockers if very large doses are given, |
|  |  | Patients with sensory loss in the trigeminal region |
|  |  | Liver disease |
| LA with lidocaine | Most patients | Porphyria |
|  | Pregnancy | Patients on suxamethonium (apnoea prolonged) |
| LA with prilocaine | In some patients with cardiovascular disease | G6PD deficiency (greater risk of methaemoglobinaemia) |
|  |  | Porphyria |
|  |  | Patients taking antimalarials (greater risk of methaemo-globinaemia) |
|  |  | Patients taking sulphonamides (greater risk of methaemo-globinaemia) |
| LA with articaine | Patients on beta-blockers | Porphyria |
| LA using bupivacaine | When unusually prolonged analgesia is required | Cardiac disease |
|  |  | Pregnancy (may cause maternal cardiac effects and fetal hypoxia) |
| LA containing adrenaline (epinephrine) | For maximally effective anaesthesia | After radiotherapy to the area Patients with a liability to dry socket |
|  |  | Asthmatic patients who can be sensitive to sulphites |
|  |  | Cardiac patients with cardiac bypass grafts or on digoxin (may precipitate dysrhythmias) |

**Table 9.3** Contd.

|  | May be indicated | May be contraindicated |
|---|---|---|
|  |  | Patients on beta-blockers (hypertensive crises may result) |
|  |  | Persons who have used drugs of abuse, especially cannabis, ephedrine, clenbuterol or cocaine in the previous 24 h (additive sympathomimetic effects may develop) |
|  |  | Untreated hyperthyroidism |
|  |  | Phaeochromocytoma |
| LA containing felypressin | For better anaesthesia than with prilocaine alone | Some cardiac patients |
|  |  | Patients with a liability to dry socket |
|  |  | Theoretically in pregnant patients |
| Conscious sedation | Patient too anxious to accept treatment under LA | Psychotic personalities |
|  | Many prolonged operations such as removal of third molars or preparation for multiple implants for which GA would otherwise be needed | Disablingly severe cardiac disease |
|  |  | Respiratory infections |
|  |  | Airways obstruction |
|  |  | Fascial space infections |
|  |  | Chronic obstructive pulmonary disease |
|  | Patients who faint with LA | Unescorted patient |
|  | Tendency to retch | Pregnancy |
|  | Uncooperation (e.g. learning disability) |  |
|  | Involuntary movements (e.g. chorea, Parkinsonism) |  |
|  | Where stress may induce attacks of angina |  |
|  | Where stress may induce attacks of hypertension |  |
|  | Where stress may induce attacks of epilepsy |  |
|  | Where stress may induce attacks of asthma |  |

**Table 9.3** Contd.

|  | May be indicated | May be contraindicated |
|---|---|---|
| Inhalational sedation | Children | Claustrophobia (mask phobia) |
|  | Drug-users | Pregnancy first trimester |
|  | Myasthenia gravis | Psychoses |
|  | Asthma |  |
|  | Needle phobics |  |
|  | Patients with tendency to retch |  |
|  | Epileptics |  |
| IV sedation | Upper airways obstruction | Younger children |
|  | Claustrophobic patients | Needle phobics |
|  |  | Liver disease |
|  |  | Myasthenia gravis |
|  |  | Glaucoma |
|  |  | Pregnancy |
|  |  | Unescorted patients |
| GA | Major surgery | Severe cardiac disease |
|  | Acute local infections (but not Ludwig's angina) | Severe respiratory disease |
|  | Injection phobia | Severe infections in floor of mouth |
|  | Patients unable to co-operate | Severe anaemia (especially sickle cell anaemia) |
|  | Learning disability | Severe renal disease |
|  | Ineffective LA | Severe hepatic disease |
|  | Allergy to LA | Pregnancy |
|  |  | Meal within 6 h |
|  |  | Unescorted patients |

# Local analgesia (LA)

Owing to the potentially serious risks involved both in conscious sedation (CS) and particularly GA, the preferred method of pain control during dental surgical procedures is LA, which is very safe and is adequate for most procedures. It is also used in most cases where conscious sedation and some where GA are employed.

Table 9.4 lists the local anaesthetics most commonly used in dentistry.

**Table 9.4** Injectable local anaesthetic agents

| Agent | Comments | Maximum safe dose for fit adults |
|---|---|---|
| Articaine 2% plus adrenaline 1 in 100 000[a] | Effective analgesia >90 min Occasional neurotoxicity | 7 mg/kg |
| Bupivacaine 0.25% or 0.5% | Useful where long-acting LA is required (up to 8 h) | 2 mg/kg |
| Bupivacaine 0.25% or 0.5% plus 1 in 200 000 adrenaline | Useful where long-acting LA is required (up to 8 h) | 2 mg/kg |
| Lignocaine/lidocaine 2% plain | Poor and brief analgesia (15–45 min) | 200 mg (5 × 2 mL cartridges) |
| Lignocaine/lidocaine 2% plus adrenaline 1 in 80 000 | Effective analgesia >90 min | 500 mg (12 × 2 mL cartridges) |
| Prilocaine 4% plain | Poor and brief analgesia (about 30 min). Occasional neurotoxicity Methaemoglobinaemia in excess | 400 mg (6 × 2 mL cartridges) |
| Prilocaine 3% plus felypressin 0.03/iu/mL | Effective analgesia for 90 min | 600 mg (10 × 2 mL cartridges) |
|  | Methaemoglobinaemia in excess | |
|  | May be preferred for patients on tricyclic antidepressants. Occasional neurotoxicity | |

[a]The total dose of adrenaline must never exceed 500 μg, i.e. not more than 40 mL of a 1 in 80 000 solution.

# Conscious sedation

*Definition* The use of a drug to produce a state of depression of the central nervous system enabling treatment to be carried out, *but during which verbal contact with the patient is maintained throughout* the period of sedation.

▶The drugs and techniques used should carry a margin of safety wide enough to render unintended loss of consciousness unlikely.

The level of sedation must be such that the patient:
• remains conscious,
• retains protective reflexes, and
• is able to respond to verbal commands.
*Sedation beyond this level of consciousness must be considered to be GA.*
It is helpful to use a sedation scoring system e.g. AVPU or verbal response from GCS (Chapter 11).

## Assessment and selection of patients for sedation

It is important to determine:
• The reason sedation is indicated.
• Specific fears (e.g. needles); past experiences (e.g. gagging problems).
• Any contraindications to sedation.
• Any special precautions indicated.
• Whether the patient can bring a responsible escort.
• Whether the patient's responsibilities (e.g. their job, night duty, driving, caring for young children) will permit them to receive sedation.
• The patient's expectations.
• Dental treatment required.

Dental examination may need to be carried out in a 'non-dental' chair with a pen torch and mouth mirror. Some patients will find intra-oral radiographs difficult to tolerate, so extra-oral radiographs may be more appropriate on the first visit.

▶Only patients who fall into the ASA categories I and II are suitable for treatment under conscious sedation outside a hospital department.

## Selection of sedation technique

Available techniques include:

*Oral sedation*—using a benzodiazepine such as diazepam or temazepam. This is convenient but involves a delay while waiting for the drug to take effect, and the level of sedation cannot be controlled.

*IV sedation*—using a benzodiazepine, usually midazolam. Although this is convenient both for operator and patient, and the level of sedation can be controlled, the drug cannot easily be withdrawn.

*Inhalational sedation (relative analgesia)*—using nitrous oxide and oxygen. Inhalational sedation is preferred as it is more convenient both for operator and patient, the level of sedation can be controlled, and the drug can easily be withdrawn.

### Personnel requirements for sedation

Where IV or inhalational sedation techniques are to be employed, a suitably experienced practitioner may assume the responsibility of sedation of the patient, as well as operating, *provided that, as a minimum requirement, a second appropriate person is present throughout.*

Such an 'appropriate person' might be a suitably trained dental surgery assistant or nurse, or ancillary dental worker, whose experience and training enables them to be an efficient member of the dental team and makes them capable of monitoring the clinical condition of the patient. Should the occasion arise, he or she must also be capable of assisting the dentist in case of emergency.

It is extremely important that the second person involved conforms to the definition of a second appropriate person and that emergency procedures are revised with that person at regular and frequent intervals.

The second 'appropriate person' must be present throughout the treatment and must not leave the surgery at any time. Therefore, when patients are being sedated, a third person must also be present and available to fetch, carry out administrative duties and answer the telephone.

Resuscitation training must be undertaken by the whole team at regular intervals (at least annually).

**Consent to sedation** must be informed. This means that the patient must be given an explanation of the procedure, and the nature, purpose, effects, and balance of risks. Explain fully exactly what is to be done at each visit. Get a consent form signed, giving permission for a sedation technique to be used together with LA, as well as consent for the operative procedure.

**Written instructions** with preoperative and postoperative advice must always be given (see page 471).

**Requirements before using conscious sedation** (see also www.doh.gov.uk/sdac)
- Written medical history.
- Previous dental history.
- Written instructions have been provided pre- and postoperatively.
- The presence of an accompanying adult.
- The patient has complied with pre-treatment instructions.
- The medical history has been checked and acted on.
- Records of drugs employed, dosages and times given including site and method of administration.
- Previous conscious sedation/GA history.
- Pre-sedation assessment.
- Any individual specific patient requirements.
- Suitable supervision has been arranged.
- There is written documentation of consent for sedation (consent form).
- Records of monitoring techniques.
- Full details of dental treatment provided.
- Post-sedation assessment.

# Oral sedation

### Advantages
- Easy to administer
- Helpful for the moderately apprehensive patient
- Relatively safe, as protective reflexes are maintained.

### Disadvantages
- Variability in absorption time (the patient may become sedated too soon, possibly endangering themselves en route to the surgery [risk minimized by administering drug on arrival], or may become sedated too late, then delaying treatment).
- Level of sedation is unpredictable and uncontrollable.
- Unpredictable effect of benzodiazepines in certain patients.
  - Some children become hyperexcitable.
  - Some children are rather resistant.
  - Elderly patients may be very sensitive.

### Agents used
Diazepam and temazepam are the main drugs used for oral sedation (Table 9.5).

#### Diazepam
Diazepam can either be taken as a single dose (5–15 mg for an adult) 1 h before treatment, or in divided doses (e.g. 5 mg the night before treatment, a further 5 mg on waking and another 5 mg 1 h before treatment. Diazepam has a long half-life and is used infrequently for outpatient sedation.

#### Temazepam
Temazepam has the advantage of a more rapid-onset and shorter action with less hangover than diazepam. A dose of 30 mg temazepam may be taken 1 h preoperatively to provide a level of sedation almost the same as that seen with IV diazepam in lipid emulsion (Diazemuls).

**Table 9.5** Oral sedation for outpatients

|  |  | Time | Route | Dose |
|---|---|---|---|---|
| Adult |  |  |  |  |
|  | Temazepam | 0.5–1 h preoperatively | O | 10–30 mg |
|  | Diazepam | 0.5–1 h preoperatively | O or IM | 5–15 mg |
| Child |  |  |  |  |
|  | Diazepam | 1.5 h preoperatively | O or IM or rectal | 2 mg (or more according to age) |
|  | Midazolam | 45 min preoperatively |  | 500 micrograms/kg (max 15 mg) |
|  | Temazepam | 45 min preoperatively |  | 1 mg/kg (max 30 mg) |

# Inhalational sedation (relative analgesia: RA)

## Indications
- Anxiety
- Marked gagging (retching)
- Some casual patients

## Contraindications
- Psychological.
- Fear or non-acceptance of the nasal mask.
- Inability to communicate with the patient.
- Severe psychiatric disease, where co-operation is not possible.
- Nature of procedure warrants GA.
- Medical contraindications such as:
  - Temporary (e.g. heavy cold) or permanent (e.g. deviated nasal septum) nasal obstruction;
  - Cyanosis at rest due to chronic cardiac (e.g. congenital cardiac disease) or respiratory disease (e.g. chronic bronchitis or emphysema)—these patients are theoretically dependent on low $O_2$ levels for their respiratory drive;
  - First trimester of pregnancy;
  - Some neuromuscular disease.

## Advantages
- Patient remains conscious and co-operative.
- Non-invasive.
- No strict fasting is required beforehand.
- Level of sedation is easily controlled.
- Protective reflexes are minimally impaired.
- The drug can be easily and rapidly ↑, ↓, or discontinued.
- The drug is administered and excreted through the lungs, and virtually total recovery takes place within the first 15 min of cessation of administration. The patient may, therefore, attend and leave surgery or hospital unaccompanied.
- Provides a degree of analgesia (although LA is often still required).
- Provides some degree of amnesia.
- No significant hypotension or respiratory depression.

## Disadvantages
- The level of sedation is largely dependent on psychological reassurance/back up.
- The nitrous oxide must be administered continuously while required.
- Amnesia or a distortion of time may occur, but this may be advantageous.
- Nitrous oxide pollution of the surgery atmosphere. This can be reduced by:
  - scavenging equipment;

- venting the suction machine outside the building;
- minimizing conversation from the patient;
- testing the equipment weekly for leakage;
- keeping the equipment well maintained with 6-monthly servicing;
- ventilating the surgeries with fresh air (e.g. open window and door fan, and open window air conditioning);
- monitoring the air (e.g. Barnsley $N_2O$ monitor).

## Essential advice to the patient

- On the day of treatment:
  - Do eat as normal before treatment.
  - Do take your routine medicines at the usual times.
  - DO NOT drink any alcohol.
- After treatment:
  - The effects of the sedative gas normally wear off very quickly and you will be fit to go back to work or travel home.

▶ Although recovery is very rapid and patients may be safely discharged without an escort, they should be discouraged from driving, particularly two-wheeled vehicles, immediately after treatment, or taking alcohol or other drugs.

# Procedure for RA

- *Check* that the RA machine is ready and working, that extra $N_2O$ and $O_2$ are available and that you are completely familiar with the machine. Use a scavenging system.
- *Lie the patient* comfortably supine in the chair with legs uncrossed, and the equipment as unobtrusive as possible.
- *Explain* the procedure to the patient.
- *Allow $O_2$ to flow* (e.g. 5 L/min for a small adult, 7 L/min for a large adult).
- *Close the air entrainment port* if present on the nasal mask.
- Ask the patient to *place the facemask* on his or her nose. Adjust the mask and tubing to give a good fit.
- *Warn* the patient that the $O_2$ will feel cold.
- *Check the $O_2$ flow volume is adequate* by:
  - asking the patient if he/she is receiving the right amount of air (do not directly suggest too much or too little);
  - watching whether the patient is mouth-breathing to supplement the flow;
  - watching the reservoir bag to see if it is under or over inflating, in which case the flow is wrong.
- *Adjust the rate of $O_2$ flow* until a comfortable minute volume is achieved. The correct volume for each patient must be found at each visit.
- *Turn $N_2O$ flow to 10%* (90% $O_2$), informing the patient that he/she may feel changes, such as a feeling of warmth, heaviness/light-headedness, tingling of hands and feet, a feeling of remoteness, and a change in visual and auditory acuity.
- *The signs of inhalation sedation are positive and pleasant:*
  - relaxation;
  - warmth;
  - tingling or numbness;
  - visual or auditory changes;
  - slurring of speech;
  - slowed responses (e.g. reduced frequency of blinking, delayed response to verbal instructions or questioning).
- *Maintain 10% $N_2O$ for 1 min;* continue the verbal reassurance at all times.
- *Increase the $N_2O$ flow to 20%* and maintain that for 1 further minute.
- *Proceed in minute-long increments of 5% $N_2O$* until the patient appears and feels quite relaxed, reiterating suggested sensation changes all the time.

*Machine output flows of between 20% and 35% $N_2O$ in $O_2$* commonly allow for a state of detached sedation and analgesia, without any loss of consciousness or danger of obtunded reflexes. At these levels, patients are aware of operative procedures and are co-operative without being fearful. Never exceed 50% of $N_2O$.

*If the normal patient cannot maintain an open mouth* then he/she is too deeply sedated. A possible exception may be in the case of a handicapped patient, unable to maintain an open mouth even without sedation. If a prop is then used, extra careful observation of the depth of sedation is essential.

*If after a period of relaxation, the patient becomes restless or apprehensive*, this usually means the level of $N_2O$ is too high and the percentage should be ↓ to a more comfortable level. The patient can then be maintained at an appropriate level until the operative procedure (or that part of it which the patient does not normally tolerate) is complete.

- *Give the LA* injection.
- *Monitor the patient* throughout by checking the pulse and respiratory rate at frequent intervals. The patient should be conscious and able to respond when directed. Dozing is safe, but snoring indicates partial airways obstruction and must be corrected immediately. Both operator and assistant should carefully monitor the patient.
- *When the sedation is to be terminated*, the $N_2O$ flow is hit off, so that *100% $O_2$ is given for 2 min* to counteract possible diffusion hypoxia.
- *Remove the facemask.*
- Slowly bring the patient upright over the next few minutes.
- The patient will usually be *fit to leave after 15 min*. Check that he/she is totally alert and well before leaving the clinic.

# IV sedation

### Advantages
- Adequate level of sedation is attained pharmacologically rather than with psychological back up.
- Amnesia removes unpleasant memories.
- The patient may take a light meal up to 2 h before treatment.

### Disadvantages
- Benzodiazepines produce no added analgesia—therefore adequate LA is needed.
- Once administered, the drug cannot be 'discontinued' or 'switched off' (compared with RA).
- There is a short period after injection when laryngeal reflexes may be impaired and therefore a mouth-sponge/gauze or rubber dam must be used to protect against accidental inhalation of water or debris.
- Patient must be accompanied home from surgery and may not drive or work machinery (including domestic appliances), make important decisions, or drink alcohol for 24 h.
- Risk of over-sedation.

### Contraindications
- Psychological: frightened of needles and injections.
- Social: responsibilities (e.g. caring for young children, shift work), inability to bring an escort.
- Medical, such as:
  - previous reactions to IV agents or any benzodiazepine;
  - pregnancy (also caution during breast feeding);
  - severe psychiatric disease;
  - liver or kidney disease;
  - glaucoma (benzodiazepines contraindicated);
  - alcohol or narcotic dependency (may render usual doses ineffective).
- Children: there is a considerable variability in reaction to diazepam. RA is the method of choice in most cases.

### Potential drug interactions (see also tables 8.28 and 8.29)
- Cimetidine (for gastric ulceration).
- Disulfiram (for treatment of alcoholism).
- Drugs for Parkinsonism, e.g. levodopa.
- Drugs that decrease cardiovascular and respiratory function, e.g. antihypertensive drugs, antihistamines, narcotic analgesics, hypnotics, sedatives and anti-epileptics.

It should be noted that these drug interactions are not necessarily absolute contraindications to the careful use of IV or oral benzodiazepines.

### Perioperative care
The procedure of IV sedation is described on page 460. The pre- and postoperative advice given to patients and routine checks and procedures before and after IV sedation are similar to those for day-case (out-patient) GA (see Chapter 10)—an important difference is that the fasting period prior to surgery with IV sedation is only 2 h.

# Drugs used for IV sedation

The benzodiazepines used for IV sedation are diazepam or midazolam (Table 9.6).

IV administration of a benzodiazepine produces:

- acute detachment for 20–30 min;
- a state of relaxation for a further hour or so;
- some anterograde amnesia for about the same period;
- minimal cardiovascular depression (a small degree of hypotension and bradycardia may simply be a relief of the hypertension and tachycardia caused by anxiety).

**Diazepam** is a non-water soluble benzodiazepine and IV administration may cause pain and/or thrombophlebitis (to overcome this, it is usually administered as Diazemuls [see Table 9.6]). It is presented in a 2 mL ampoule in a concentration of 5 mg/mL for IV or IM injections. It undergoes an enterohepatic circulation and metabolites may be sedating; so action may be unpredictably prolonged or recurring.

**Midazolam** is a water-soluble benzodiazepine available in a 2 mL ampoule in a concentration of 5 mg/mL or in a 5 mL ampoule in a concentration of 2 mg/mL. Note that both presentations contain the same amount of drug, 10 mg midazolam, in one ampoule.

Midazolam is preferred to diazepam because it:

- is non-irritant in aqueous solution (↓ risk of venous thrombosis);
- has a much shorter half life (in the region of 1–2 h);
- has no significant metabolites, so that recovery is both quicker and smoother;
- has more predictable amnesic properties.

Midazolam is now the most commonly used drug for IV sedation. The dental practitioner using midazolam must be aware of the drug's possible:

- *Adverse reactions* (hiccough; cough; oversedation; pain at the injection site; nausea and vomiting; headache; blurred vision; fluctuations in vital signs; hypotension; respiratory depression; respiratory arrest)
- *Contraindications* (hypersensitivity to midazolam; erythromycin use [potentiates midazolam]; concomitant use of barbiturates, alcohol, narcotics, or other CNS depressants; glaucoma; depressed vital signs; shock or coma)

**Table 9.6** Agents for conscious IV sedation

| Drug | Proprietary names | Adult dose | Comments |
|------|-------------------|------------|----------|
| Diazepam | Valium | Up to 20 mg | Acts via the GABA (gamma amino butyric acid) receptor. |
| | | | Disadvantages: may cause pain or thrombophlebitis; drowsiness returns transiently 4–6 h postoperatively due to metabolism to desmethyldiazepam, triazolam and oxazepam and entero-hepatic recirculation. |
| | | | May cause mild hypotension and respiratory depression. |
| | Diazemuls | Up to 20 mg | Advantages over Valium: most of the actions above, but less thrombophlebi-tis and therefore can be given into veins on dorsum of hand. |
| | | | Disadvantage: expensive. |
| Midazolam | Hypnovel | 0.07 mg/kg (up to 7.5 mg total dose) | Acts via the GABA receptor. |
| | | | Advantages over diazepam: onset of action quicker (30 s); amnesia more profound, starting 2–5 min after administration and lasting up to 40 min (with no retrograde amnesia); recovery more rapid; virtually completely eliminated within 5 h, without any recurrence of drowsiness; less incidence of venous thrombosis; at least twice as potent. |
| | | | Flumazenil is the antidote. |
| | | | Disadvantages: signs of sedation less pre-dictable; very slow injection required. |
| | | | Occasional deaths in elderly. |
| Propofol | Propofol, Diprivan | 2 mg/kg | Acts via the GABA receptor at a site different than that of the benzodi-azepines. |
| | | | Advantages: IV injection produces hypnosis rapidly with minimal excita-tion, usually within 40 s and recovery is also rapid; safe to use in porphyria and malignant hyperthermia. |
| | | | Disadvantages: may cause pain on injection and occasional fits or anaphy-laxis; after induction with propofol, apnoea may occur; there is no antidote. |
| | | | Contraindicated in patients taking anticonvulsants. |
| | | | There have been several cases of sepsis 2° to contaminated ampoules. |

# Procedure for IV sedation

*Select a suitable site for venepuncture* in the antecubital fossa or dorsum of the hand. A 21G (green) needle is usually used, but an indwelling needle of the butterfly type can be used so that a patent vein can be maintained throughout the procedure. The arm should be kept straight with a board if the antecubital fossa is used.

*Occlude the venous return* above the elbow with a tourniquet, or ask an assistant to squeeze the arm. Alternatively, place the tourniquet above the wrist and use the back of the hand.

*Cleanse the skin* with a suitable antiseptic (e.g. isopropanol 70% or chlorhexidine 0.5%).

*Select the most readily palpable vein* that is remote from the brachial artery.

*Tap the vein* gently, until it becomes reflexly dilated, and tense the skin with one hand distal to the chosen puncture site.

*Place the needle* at a 30° angle to the skin, bevel upwards, without obstruction from the needle hub or syringe barrel and press downwards. Once through the skin, which is the most painful part of the procedure, the needle can be manipulated so that the technique of entering the vein from the side can be used. At this point, the needle should be almost parallel to the skin. Advance the needle until 2/3 of its length is within the vein. The appearance of blood within the tubing on aspiration confirms correct positioning.

*Secure the needle* with non-allergenic tape.

*Give a small IV flush* (2 mL normal saline) to ensure that the needle is in a vein and that there is no adverse reaction (Table 9.7). If for any reason the end of the needle is no longer into the vein, injection can be painful and may create a small lump under the skin.

*Slowly inject the prepared drug*, warning the patient of a possible cold sensation at the needle site or as the drug tracks up the arm. Provided one is sure that the needle is correctly positioned, the patient should be reassured that this sensation will pass within a short period of time. Stop injecting if pain is felt locally (indicating injection into the subcutaneous tissue) or radiating down the forearm (indicating entry into an artery).

*Inject 3 mg midazolam over 30 s*, then pause for a further 90 s.

*Give further increments of 1 mg midazolam* every 30 s, until sedation is judged to be adequate. Watch for any adverse responses and particularly any respiratory impairment.

*The correct dose* has been given when there is slurring of speech and the patient is relaxed. Ptosis is *not* a reliable end point; adequate sedation with midazolam may occur before ptosis is evident.

*Monitor injection site* for extravasation, local reaction, phlebitis .

*Give LA.*

*Protect the airways*, especially in conservation procedures, i.e. use rubber dam, butterfly sponges, etc. The airways must be protected because laryngeal reflexes are impaired after the administration of benzodiazepines.

*Protect the patient's eyes* during operation.

*Operative procedures may be started* in the usual way, when adequacy of LA has been confirmed. Approximately 30 min of sedation time is available for the operator. As there may be considerable muscle relaxation, a prop may be needed to maintain the mouth open. A barrier to prevent accidental inhalation of debris must be used, and this may be a rubber dam, butterfly sponge or gauze square. Some advocate the use of a small dose of either hyoscine or atropine in addition to benzodiazepines to reduce the risks arising from excessive salivation or bronchial secretion, but the advantages gained are outweighed by the discomfort of a very dry mouth and the potential dangers of using atropinics.

*Monitor the patient* frequently by means of the pulse, respiratory rate and the patient's colour. The patient should remain conscious and able to respond when directed.

*At the end of the procedure*, slowly bring the patient upright over 5 min. The patient should recover over at least another 15 min under the direct supervision of a member of the dental team or his escort. The patient must not be discharged until at least 1 h has elapsed since the drug was given.

*The patient should be discharged into the care of the escort* and instructed to rest quietly at home for the remainder of the day and refrain from driving or operating machinery or making important decisions for 24 h. Postoperative instructions, together with any pertaining to the dentistry performed, should be given on a written sheet for the patient to refer to later, as he/she may still be under the effects of the amnesic properties of the drug.

**Table 9.7** Possible complications of IV injections

| Complication | Cause | Treatment |
|---|---|---|
| Haematoma | Leakage of blood, because of inadequate pressure on vein after needle removed. Mainly occurs from dorsum of hand veins. | Avoid by using antecubital veins and applying firm pressure after needle removal. |
| Extraneous injection | Needle moves during injection. Mainly causes problems with thiopentone and diazepam. | Inject normal saline (or plain lignocaine/lidocaine 2% at site. |
| Intra-arterial injection | Ensure that the blood vessel is not pulsating before injecting. Main problem is with thiopentone. | Inject plain lignocaine(5mL). Call for medical assistance. |
| Venous thrombosis | Viscous or irritant solutions injected into small veins. Main problems are with thiopentone, and diazepam | Icthammol in glycerine application. Analgesics. Rest. Plus antibiotics if not resolved in 7 days. |

Any of these may be a cause of pain.

# Benzodiazepine reversal agent

**Flumazenil** is a specific benzodiazepine antagonist which allows rapid reversal of conscious sedation with benzodiazepines, by specific competitive inhibition for benzodiazepine receptors.

Flumazenil has a short duration of action (half life approx. 40 min); therefore, repeated doses may be required until all possible central effects of the benzodiazepine have subsided. If drowsiness recurs, an infusion of 100–400 micrograms/h may be employed.

Flumazenil is available as 5 mL ampoules containing 500 micrograms. The initial dose is 200 micrograms (2 mL) over 15 s. If the desired level of consciousness is not obtained within 60 s, give 100 micrograms at 60-s intervals, up to a maximum of 1 mg. Usual dose required: 300–600 micrograms.

## Contraindications

- Hypersensitivity to benzodiazepines or flumazenil
- Pregnancy
- Epilepsy
- Impaired liver function (metabolized in liver)
- Psychotropic drugs (e.g. tricyclics)

## Adverse effects (rare)

- Flushing
- Nausea/vomiting
- Anxiety/palpitations/fear
- Seizures
- Transient rise in BP and pulse rate

▶Patients given flumazenil require longer post-operative observation before discharge (2h following the last dose of flumazenil is suggested).

▶Patients given flumazenil following IV sedation procedures must still follow the normal instructions given after sedation (i.e. no driving, operating machinery, etc.).

# General anaesthetics

Agents used as GA may be divided into those that are inhaled (Table 9.8) and those given intravenously (Table 9.9).

**Table 9.8** Gaseous (inhalational) anaesthetic agents[a]

| Drug | Proprietary names (UK) | Comments |
|------|-----------------------|----------|
| Desflurane | Suprane | Less potent than isoflurane. May cause apnoea or coughing. |
| | | Contraindicated in children and in malignant hyperthermia. |
| Enflurane | Ethrane Alyrane | Less potent anaesthetic than halothane but less likely to induce dysrhythmias or affect liver. Powerful cardiorespiratory depressant. Non-explosive. |
| | | Contraindicated in malignant hyperthermia. |
| Halothane | Fluothane | The most widely used GA agent worldwide. Non-explosive. Anaesthetic but weak analgesic. Causes fall in BP, cardiac dysrhythmias and bradycardia. Hepatotoxic on repeated administration[b]. Postanaesthetic shivering is common, vomiting rare. |
| | | Contraindicated in malignant hyperthermia. |
| Isoflurane | Forane Aerrane | Isomer of enflurane. It causes less cardiac but more respiratory depression than halothane. Induction is slower than with halothane. Recovery is quicker |
| | | Contraindicated in malignant hyperthermia. |
| Sevoflurane | Sevoflurane | Rapid action and recovery. May cause agitation in children. |
| | | Contraindicated in malignant hyperthermia. |
| Nitrous oxide[c] | | Analgesic, but weak anaesthetic. Non-explosive. No cardiorespiratory effects. Mainly used as a vehicle for other anaesthetic agents, or for sedation. |
| | | Safe in malignant hyperthermia. |

[a] Gas scavenging should be used.
[b] Do not give halothane if patient has had halothane within the previous 12 weeks or has previously had an adverse reaction to halothane, or unexplained postoperative fever or jaundice.
[c] Abuse may lead to disturbed vitamin $B_{12}$ metabolism, megaloblastosis, and neurological sequelae.

**Table 9.9** IV anaesthetic agents

| Drug | Proprietary names (UK) | Adult dose | Comments |
|---|---|---|---|
| Etomidate | Hypnomidate | 0.2 mg/kg | Pain on injection: use large vein and give fentanyl 200 μg first. After operation give naloxone 0.1–0.2 mg and oxygen. Little cardiovascular effect. Often involuntary movements, cough and hiccup, nausea and vomiting. Hepatic metabolism. Avoid in repeated doses in traumatized patient—may suppress adrenal steroid production. |
| Ketamine | Ketalar | 0.5–2 mg/kg | Rise in BP, cardiac rate, intraocular pressure. Little respiratory depression. Often hallucinations. Rarely used in dentistry.<br><br>Contraindicated in hypertension, psychiatric, cerebrovascular or ocular disorders. |
| Propofol | Diprivan | 2 mg/kg | See Table 9.5. Commonly used for induction of anaesthesia. |
| Thiopentone | Intraval | 4 mg/kg (2.5% solution) | Ultra short-acting barbiturate. No analgesia. Danger of laryngospasm. Rapid injection may cause apnoea. Irritant if injected into artery or extravascularly. Useful in epileptics. |

# Muscle relaxants

Muscle relaxants (neuromuscular blocking drugs) are used during the induction of GA (to allow laryngeal relaxation), in order to permit intubation, and also to relax the jaw and other muscles.
►Assisted ventilation is necessary while the drug is active.

## Depolarizing muscle relaxants

*Suxamethonium* is ideal for the brief muscle relaxation needed during the induction of GA. Effect appears rapidly and persists for ~5 min. Respiration must be assisted, as the patient is paralysed and unable to breathe. Recovery is rapid and spontaneous; drug reversal is not feasible.

Adverse effects include postoperative muscle pain, hypersalivation (↓ if atropine is given), arrhythmias, prolonged respiratory depression, hyperthermia and hypertension.

Suxamethonium is contraindicated in suxamethonium sensitivity (pseudocholinesterase deficiency), personal or family history of malignant hyperthermia, fascial space infections, major trauma, recent burns, muscular dystrophy and neurological disorders with muscle wasting.

## Non-depolarizing (competitive) muscle relaxants

Non-depolarizing muscle relaxants have a more prolonged action than suxamethonium, and are therefore useful in situations where prolonged mechanical ventilation is required (e.g. in intensive care). Paralysis may be reversed by anticholinesterases (e.g. neostigmine).

*Atracurium* has an effect that appears within 3 min and persists for 15 to 35 min. It undergoes non-enzymatic metabolism and is therefore safe in long-term use, even when liver and/or renal function is impaired. Side-effects of atracurium include hypotension, facial flushing and bronchospasm because of histamine release.

*Cisatracurium, rocuronium, and vecuronium* are newer non-depolarizing muscle relaxants, which produce less histamine release and are therefore more popular. Choice depends primarily on the timing of action onset and duration.

## Other considerations

Drugs that may complicate, or be complicated by, conscious sedation or GA are listed on Table 9.10 along with suggested actions.

Other aspects of preoperative, intraoperative and postoperative management of patients undergoing GA are discussed on Chapters 10 and 11.

**Table 9.10** Preoperative modification of regularly used medications before operation under sedation or GA[a] (see also Table 10.3)

| Medication | Conscious sedation | GA |
|---|---|---|
| ACE inhibitors | Continue | Continue |
| Analgesics | Continue | Continue (but see Table 10.3) |
| Antiarrhythmics | Continue | Continue |
| Anticoagulants | Consult haematologist | Consult haematologist |
| Anticonvulsants | Continue | Continue |
| Antidepressants | Continue | Withdraw monoamine oxidase inhibitors slowly 2 weeks before major surgery. Others can be continued |
| Beta-blockers | Continue | Continue |
| Contraceptive pill | Continue | Continue unless major surgery, in which case stop 4 weeks before (use alternative contraception) |
| Corticosteroids | Continue and raise dose | Continue and raise dose |
| Digoxin | Continue | Continue |
| Diuretics (potassium-sparing) | Continue | Omit on morning of operation |
| Diuretics (thiazides or loop) | Continue | Continue |
| Insulin or antidiabetics | Consult diabetologist | Consult diabetologist |
| Lithium | Continue | Stop 1–3 days before major surgery |

[a] Always discuss with the physician responsible for the patient

USEFUL WEBSITES

www.doh.gov.uk/sdac
http://omni.ac.uk/browse/mesh/C0079159L0079159.html

# Perioperative management

# Day-stay surgery: preparations

### Advance arrangements

- Most procedures concerning booking a patient for day-stay surgery depend on local protocols, set by the hospital administration, responsible consultant, secretary and senior departmental nurse.
- The patient is booked on the appropriate operating list, and a letter of information is sent to the patient confirming details of the agreed plan.
- Patients should be clearly instructed of
  - preoperative instructions
  - the time they should arrive
  - what they should bring
  - what to do about medication they take (see Tables 10.3 and 10.4)
  - the anticipated duration of stay
  - postoperative instructions

*Written informed consent* must be obtained from all patients having an operation. The possible benefits of treatment must be weighed against risks and always discussed by the person carrying out the procedure, or, if for some good reason this is not possible, a delegated person with the appropriate expertise to do so.

'Informed' consent means that the patient must be fully aware of the procedure, its intended benefits, its possible risks and the level of these and of the risks and benefits of not having the procedure. In particular, patients must be warned carefully and comprehensibly:

- about preoperative preparation;
- of possible adverse effects or outcomes (e.g. deformity);
- about postoperative sequelae (e.g. pain, swelling, bruising);
- where they will be during their recovery (e.g. ITU);
- of the possibility of IV infusions, catheters, nasogastric tubes, etc.

*The warnings must be properly recorded in the case notes and signed by operator and patient.*

*Certain investigations* (e.g. radiographs, blood tests, etc.) may be indicated, depending on the actual operation needed and the general health of the patient (see Chapter 3, and below).

*A pre-admission appointment* in the week prior to the operation is a good opportunity to complete the medical history, obtain informed consent, finalize investigations, and give advance instructions and advice.

## Advance instructions

Essential advice to patients having out-patient GA or IV sedation should be in the form of verbal and written instructions along the following lines Table 10.1.

---

**Table 10.1** Instructions for patients planned for day-stay surgery

---

Some drugs that you will be given before and during the operation may affect you for the rest of the day and possibly longer; therefore:

- You must NOT eat or drink anything for 6 h before operation[a]
- You must bring a responsible adult escort, who should accompany you home and stay with you until the next morning.
- You must NOT, for the 24 h after the procedure:
  - drink alcohol or take recreational drugs,
  - ride a bicycle, or drive any vehicle,
  - operate machinery,
  - go to work,
  - do housework or cooking,
  - undertake any responsible business matters,
  - sign important documents.

---

[a] or, better, give an exact time to stop (e.g. after 3am)

Certain information about the surgical procedure and its implications should also be given. An example is given in Table 10.2.

---

**Table 10.2** Removal of wisdom teeth

---

Dear Patient,

As you know we feel that your wisdom teeth should be removed. Here is some information, which we hope will answer some of your questions.

Wisdom teeth removal is often necessary because of infection (which causes pain and swelling), decay, serious gum disease, the development of a cyst or because teeth are overcrowded. Wisdom teeth are removed under local anaesthetic (injection in the mouth), sedation or general anaesthetic in hospital, depending on your preference, the number of teeth to be removed and the difficulty of removal.

It is often necessary to make a small incision in the gum, which is stitched afterwards. After removal of the teeth, your mouth will be sore and swollen and mouth movements will usually be stiff. Slight bleeding is also very common. These symptoms are quite normal, but can be expected to improve rapidly during the first week. It is quite normal for some stiffness and slight soreness to persist for two to three weeks. Pain and discomfort can be controlled with ordinary painkillers, such as paracetamol/acetoaminophen, and you might be prescribed antibiotic tablets. A dentist will be available to see you afterwards if you are worried, and will want to check that healing is satisfactory.

Complications are rare, but occasionally wisdom tooth sockets become infected, when pain, swelling and stiffness will last longer than normal. Occasional patients suffer from tingling or numbness of the lower lip or tongue after lower wisdom teeth removal. This is because nerves to these areas pass very close to the wisdom teeth and are occasionally bruised or damaged. The numbness nearly always disappears after about one month, but very occasionally lasts for a year or more.

Please let us know if we can give you any more information.

---

# Day-stay surgery: procedures

### Routine checks before the procedure

ALWAYS CHECK:

- Patient's full name, date of birth, address and hospital number.
- Nature, side and site of operation.
- That any teeth marked for extraction agree with those entered in the:
  - consent form;
  - patient's notes;
  - referring practitioner's notes.
- Medical history, particularly of cardiorespiratory disease or bleeding tendency. Ensure that any relevant medical history is drawn to the anaesthetist's attention.
- Availability of suitable social support on discharge.
- Consent has been obtained in writing from the patient or, in a person under 16 years of age, from a parent or guardian, and that the patient adequately understands the nature of the operation and sequelae. Ensure that the consent form has been signed by the patient or guardian and relevant clinician (member of staff).
- Necessary investigations are available. If permanent teeth are to be removed, check radiographs showing complete roots are available.
- Patient has had nothing by mouth for at least the previous 6 h.
- Patient has emptied bladder.
- Patient has removed any contact lenses.
- Patient's dentures or other removable appliances are removed and bridges, crowns and loose or damaged teeth have been noted by the anaesthetist.
- Necessary premedication and, where indicated, regular medication (e.g. the contraceptive pill, anticonvulsants) have been given (Tables 10.3 and 10.4).
- Equipment and suction apparatus are working satisfactorily, correct drugs are available and drug expiry date has not passed.
- Emergency kit is available and drug expiry date has not passed.
- A responsible assistant is present.
- Patient will be escorted by a responsible adult.
- Patient has been warned not to drive, operate machinery, drink alcohol or make important decisions for 24 h postoperatively.

**Table 10.3** Therapies that may need to be modified before maxillo-facial surgery (always consult physician and anaesthetist)(see also Table 9.10). Restart normal medication once the patient is again eating.

| Medication | Comments |
| --- | --- |
| Anticoagulants | Decision to discontinue anticoagulants should balance risk of increased perioperative bleeding against hazard of thromboembolism. |
|   Aspirin | Usually stop at least 1 week before surgery. |
|   Clopidogrel | Usually stop at least 1 week before surgery. |
|   Ticlopidine | Usually stop 10–14 days before surgery. |
|   Warfarin | Before *major* surgery usually stop at least 4–5 days, substituting warfarin with low molecular weight heparin (LMWH). |
| Corticosteroids | Continue and raise dose. See Chapter 4 |
| Diabetic medications<br>  Insulin | See Chapter 4 |
|   Oral antidiabetic agents | If procedure is short and can be performed early in the morning, and the patient is expected to eat shortly after the procedure, then the usual diabetic regimen can just be shifted to a few hours later in the day. Otherwise, discontinue most drugs the day before surgery. Discontinue biguanides (metformin) on the day of surgery because renal function changes arising intraopera-tively may potentiate the risk of lactic acidosis. Sulfonylureas are withheld on the operative day. |
| Diuretics; furosemide, bumetanide, chlorthalidone, metolazone, spironolactone | Usually withhold morning dose to avoid dehydra-tion and hypovolaemia as well as inconvenience of diuresis to patients. |
| Herbal medicines | Best discontinued a few days before surgery. |
| Lithium | Lithium should be discontinued 1–3 days before major surgery and resumed when renal function and electrolyte levels are stable. Levels may need to be monitored. |

**Table 10.3** Contd.

| Medication | Comments |
| --- | --- |
| Monoamine oxidase inhibitors (MAOIs); phenelzine, tranylcypromine | May need to be stopped slowly 2 weeks before surgery. Decisions should be made in consultation with the patient's physician, anaesthetist or psychiatrist. |
| NSAIDs | |
| Non-selective NSAIDs; aspirin, ibuprofen, naproxen, indo-metacin, ketorolac, ketoprofen | Usually stop at least 1 week prior to surgery. Can usually substitute alternative analgesic, e.g. paracetamol/acetaminophen ± narcotic. |
| Selective COX-2 inhibitors; celecoxib, valdecoxib | Little effect on platelet function, but may be prudent to stop 1 week before *major* surgery. |
| Potassium supplements | Stop day before operation and consider checking potassium level. |

**Table 10.4** Therapies usually NOT to be modified before maxillofacial surgery (always consult physician). The following should almost always be continued up to and including the day of surgery[a].

| Drugs | Comments |
| --- | --- |
| Antibiotics and antiretrovirals | — |
| Antireflux medication; ranitidine, omeprazole | — |
| Cardiovascular drugs | |
| Antihypertensives | ACE inhibitors and angiotensin II receptor blockers are occasionally withheld, especially in patients undergoing cardiopulmonary bypass. Diuretics are usually *withheld on the day* of surgery (see *above*) |
| Antianginals; beta-blockers, calcium antagonists, nitrates | — |
| Antiarrhythmics | Continue if used to treat serious arrhythmias |
| Beta-blockers | Beta-blockers provide the single best therapy for prevention of ischaemia perioperatively. Abrupt withdrawal may adversely affect the heart rate and blood pressure and may precipitate MI |
| Digoxin | — |
| Hormones and drugs for endocrine problems | |
| Oral contraceptives | Risk of venous thromboembolism must be balanced against risk of pregnancy. Continue unless major surgery, in which case stop 4 weeks before (use alternative contraception) |
| Antithyroid medications; propylthiouracil, methimazole | — |

**Table 10.4** Contd.

| Drugs | Comments |
|---|---|
| Corticosteroids | Steroid cover may be indicated |
| Thyroxine | Start thyroxine postoperatively as soon as the patient is on oral liquids. The long half-life (7 days) means that it can be stopped for a few days without problems. |
| Lipid-lowering drugs; gemfibrozil, atorvastatin, lovastatin, niacin, cholestyramine | Controversial. May be associated with postoperative rhabdomyolysis. But, recent *evidence* suggests that discontinuation of statins increases risk of cardiac events. |
| Neurological or psychological medications | |
| Antiepileptics | Phenytoin and phenobarbital should be continued with parenteral formulations. Carbamazepine and valproic acid are not available in parenteral form and the patient must be changed to phenytoin until they resume eating. |
| Antiparkinson medication | Patients who take dopamine must stay on their usual medication perioperatively because no parenteral form of Sinemet is available and withholding drug can cause parkinsonian crisis. Anticholinergics may be given IM perioperatively without serious cardiovascular risk. L-dopa should be resumed postoperatively as soon as possible, and the patient monitored for hypotension. |
| Antidepressants tricyclic antidepressants, serotonin reuptake inhibitors | *Exception:* monoamine oxidase inhibitors (usually need to stop these 2 weeks before surgery) |
| Antipsychotics | Given the complications associated with untreated psychoses, continued treatment with antipsychotic drugs is warranted perioperatively unless there is cardiac disease. |
| Benzodiazepines and opioids | Patients who have been on these for a long time develop tolerance and have an increased risk of serious withdrawal problems. |
| Drugs for myasthenia gravis; pyridostigmine, neostigmine | — |
| Respiratory drugs | |
| Beta agonists | — |
| Theophylline | — |
| Inhaled medications; steroids salbutamol, ipratropium bromide | Ask patients to bring their inhalers to the hospital. |

[a] Fasting reduces the risk for aspiration of stomach contents when the patient has GA. However, liquids are cleared from the stomach within 2 h of ingestion, and no differences in the volume or pH of gastric contents is noted in those patients taking clear fluids 2 h before surgery compared with those taking clear fluids 9 h before surgery. Therefore, patients can be given their routine medications with sips of water up to 2 h before GA. Where medications are to be continued throughout the perioperative period, a change of formulation or substitution may be needed.

## The procedure

Theatre procedures during day-stay surgery do not differ from those relevant to in-patients (discussed below), except for the fact that the operation should be completed by early afternoon, to allow adequate recovery time before dicharge. The procedures involved in IV sedation have been discussed on Chapter 9.

## After operation

- Complete immediately the case notes and daybook (must be dated and signed by the responsible member of clinical staff).
- Consider whether analgesics and/or antibiotics need to be prescribed.
- Return any dentures, etc.
- Check patient, particularly for complete consciousness and clear airways (and speak to accompanying responsible adult) before discharge.
- Check the patient understands postoperative instructions.
- Check the patient knows where and how to obtain advice in the event of emergency/complication.
- Give an advice sheet to complement the one given preoperatively. This should once again outline the main instructions regarding drug effects (see Tables 10.3 and 10.4), and possible adverse effects and complications. In particular, instructions regarding postoperative bleeding should now be given in more detail, as in Table 10.5.

**Table 10.5** Instructions following tooth extraction

After a tooth has been extracted, the socket will usually bleed for a short time, but then the bleeding stops because of a healthy clot of blood in the tooth socket. These clots are easily disturbed and, if this happens, more bleeding will occur. To avoid disturbing the clot:

DO NOT

- rinse your mouth out for 24 h,
- disturb the clot with your tongue or fingers, or anything else
- take food which requires chewing (for the rest of the day),
- chew on the affected side for at least 3 days (if both sides of your mouth are involved, you should have a soft diet for 3 days)
- take hot drinks, hot baths, alcohol, exercise,
- talk too much or get excited or too hot.

If the tooth socket continues to bleed after you have left the clinic or hospital, do not be alarmed; much of the liquid that appears to be blood, will be saliva. Make a small pad from a clean handkerchief or cotton wool, or use a tea bag, and place it directly over the socket and close the teeth firmly on it. Keep up the pressure for 15–30 min.

If the bleeding still does not stop, seek advice from us, or the hospital or clinic resident dental surgeon.

# Indications for in-patient care

## Indications for urgent hospital admission of the dental patient

### Trauma

- Loss of consciousness.
- Patients in shock.
- Head injury (see Chapter 11).
- Cervical spine injury.
- Other serious injuries.
- Laryngeal trauma.
- Fractured jaws
  - Middle facial third;
  - Mandibular—unless simple or undisplaced;
  - Zygomatic—where there is danger of eye damage.

### Inflammatory lesions and infections

- Cervical/facial fascial space infections.
- Oral infections if patient is 'toxic' or severely immunocompromised.
- Necrotizing fasciitis.
- Tuberculosis (some).
- Deep mycoses (some).
- Severe viral infections, especially in severely immunocompromised.
- Severe vesiculo-bullous disorders (pemphigus and Stevens–Johnson syndrome).

### Blood loss

- Severe or persistent haemorrhage (particularly if bleeding tendency).
- Less severe bleeding but in a highly anxious patient.

### Other reasons

- Collapse of uncertain cause.
- Airways obstruction.
- Vulnerable patients who have no social care or support.
- Disturbed, severely depressed or some other psychiatric patients.
- Children or others who are being, or might be, abused.
- Diabetics out of control because of oral pain or infection.

▶In many of the indications mentioned above (including head injury, uncontrolled diabetes, etc.), you, as a dental surgeon, may have a significant role to play in patient management, but often the full care may be beyond your scope of practice. Always discuss the case with the senior or delegated responsible member of staff. It could be more appropriate for the patient to be admitted by another hospital speciality service, at least in the first instance, or under 'shared care'.

## Indications for routine admission for in-patient care

### Major operations

- Cancer surgery.
- Craniofacial surgery.
- Orthognathic surgery.

- Cleft surgery.
- Surgery involving vascular lesions.
- Some trauma surgery.
- Some orthodontic surgery.
- Some preprosthetic surgery.
- Multiple or complicated extractions.

*Serious systemic disease, where this may significantly influence*
- anaesthesia (e.g. cardiorespiratory disease, sickle cell anaemia, drug abuse);
- disease control (e.g. unstable diabetes or epilepsy);
- surgery (e.g. bleeding disorder);
- dental treatment indirectly (e.g. occasionally where treatment might otherwise necessitate multiple antibiotic courses for infective endocarditis prophylaxis);
- immunity (e.g. HIV/AIDS, immunosuppressive therapy);
- behaviour (e.g. some mental health disorders, some drug abusers).

*Other reasons*
- Complicated investigations required.
- Social reasons, e.g. some patients:
  - living alone, with irresponsible carers, or far from medical care;
  - having difficulty eating;
  - subject to abuse;
  - with disabilities.

## Exceptions to admission for routine in-patient care

Patients with a communicable infection, or a recent history of contact with one, should only be admitted if there is a good indication—when the occupational health department should be informed and involved in management.

# The day of a routine hospital admission

Patients are best admitted on the day of operation unless there are special preoperative preparations or treatment to be carried out. Patients should, however, be admitted early enough for the consultant to see them on the ward round before operation.

*Points to remember*
- No admission is 'routine' to the patient, partner or family.
- Patients need reassurance and, if they are admitted the night before the operation, may well benefit from a hypnotic (Chapter 8 and page 494).
- Reassure patients (and partner or family) about the various preoperative and postoperative procedures, particularly if the patient is to recover with deformity, bruising or swelling, in a strange ward (e.g. intensive care), or if nasogastric tubes, IV infusions, catheters, etc. will be used.
- Check the patient has given informed consent to the operation. Record in writing whether warnings about possible complications have been given and are appreciated and understood.
- Inform the anaesthetist of the medical history and courteously enquire if he/she wants any special measures or requires any investigations.
- Check that any necessary investigations have been performed, the results are available, and checked. If unsure, contact someone senior and enquire whether any further investigations are needed. For example, if there is more than 50:50 chance of severe haemorrhage, such as in major surgery or patients with a bleeding tendency, take blood for autologous transfusion and for grouping and cross-matching.
- Carry out necessary preoperative dental procedures (e.g. impressions), and ensure necessary dental items are in theatre at operation.
- Warn:
  - the radiographers if radiographs will be required—fill out the necessary request forms before operation;
  - the pathologists if frozen sections will be required;
  - the photographers if they will be required.
- Check the patient has appropriate social support for discharge.
- Tell the patient and relatives when the operation will take place, and roughly how long recovery will take.
- Clerk in the patient (see following section).

## Dealing with patients, partners and relatives
*Patients' reactions to hospitalization and illness*
Many people who have been waiting to come in to hospital know that, in the next few days, they have before them discomfort and perhaps danger. At the very least, their routine has been upset; they have left the security and privacy of their own homes and comfort of partners or relatives for an alien world, which they may often regard with fear. Any operation is a forbidding and usually new prospect to most patients. They feel vulnerable and at a disadvantage. Patients admitted as emergencies may be acutely ill and often also disturbed by trauma and an ambulance journey.
The most normal and self-sufficient individual will find these circumstances daunting: the vulnerable, old, and very young may well be overwhelmed

and become distressed. Patients of different cultural and ethnic backgrounds also vary in their emotional response to separation from their family, and to illness, pain, operation or hospitalization.

This situation may have become routine to you, but for the patient it may well be one of the most important and stressful experiences of their life. Try to be understanding and show your empathy to the patient and family in every way you can. Everything you say or do at this stage, including body language, they may well remember for a long time. Even if you have no further role to play in the patient's management, being the first person they deal with, you probably have the greatest effect on whether this experience is going to be a pleasant or haunting one! Be patient, gentle, calm and confident, and try not to hurt or upset the patient in any way. Give the patient and family as much information as they want, within your scope of knowledge, and reassure them that you will try to find out what you do not know. The idea that the patients are happier if they do not know what is planned for them is nonsense: they are entitled to be told what is going to happen to them, and in a language they can understand.

The difficulty about talking to patients is how to explain things without frightening or confusing them. However, it is probably better to risk this than to have an apprehensive patient complaining about apparent secrecy. Most patients are not interested in technical details, but require a simple explanation, and reassurance.

### Relatives and partners

- Relatives and partners are usually interested and concerned, although occasionally intrusive or abusive.
- Allow the patient time with their friends and relatives—this is usually important in helping them to cope.
- Do not forget the question of confidentiality (see Chapter 13) but, with this in mind, the date and time of the operation and discharge may well be needed by caring relatives or partners.
- Speak personally to the relatives and partners at a pre-arranged visit by them, *provided the patient consents*. Ask a senior member of staff whether they would prefer to do this themselves.
- Phone calls from relatives and partners should be handled by nursing staff in the first instance. Try to avoid being bleeped (or paged) by relatives and partners. Be careful and tactful in what you say and *never give personal or medical details by phone or email, or on an answer-phone*.

# Clerking in the patient

Patients must be clerked on the day of admission. Do not allow unclerked patients to be on the ward for more than a very short time (an hour or so, at the most).

## Admitting

*Urgent admissions:* Ensure everyone is informed about the admission. The responsible specialist, or their deputy, must always be informed if a patient is admitted under their care. The appropriate arrangements for a bed must be made, usually via the surgical bleep-holder (a senior hospital nurse), and the relevant ward sister must be told.

An example of urgent admission clerking is shown in Table 10.6.

*Non-urgent (planned) admissions:* Ensure everyone is informed about the admission as above.

An example of planned admission clerking is shown in Table 10.7.

## History taking (see also Chapter 1)

A detailed history of the presenting complaint, as well as all relevant medical history, must be taken from all patients, especially those admitted for major operations or expected to stay in hospital.

## Examination (see also Chapter 2)

Patients with a proven diagnosis admitted for operation, should be re-examined specifically to confirm:

- oral findings;
- their fitness for a GA;
- their ability to withstand the operative procedures planned.

## Investigations (see also Chapter 3)

- All patients admitted for a GA should have estimations of:
  - weight and body mass index (BMI);
  - temperature, pulse, BP, and respiratory rate (Fig. 10.1);
  - urinalysis;
  - haemoglobin.
- Patients of over 50 years of age and any patient with a history of severe cardiac or respiratory disease should have an ECG read, and a CXR.
- Patients with a possible high alcohol intake should have LFTs.
- Patients from some ethnic groups may need special investigations (e.g. SickleDex, for sickle-cell anaemia) (see Chapter 3).
- Investigations relevant to the oral procedure may also be indicated.

**Summarize** your findings and write down a consequent plan.

**Table 10.6** Clerking example of an urgent admission

01/01/05    Urgent admission on X ward (via A & E) (under care of Mr A.Bloggs)
(03:00 am)                                                              John Smith
                                                               21 y.o. college student

PC
• Swelling and pain left side of face
• Inability to close mouth

HPC
• Alleged assault 2 h ago, outside a nightclub (police involved)
• Has had 5 pints of lager prior to incident
• Punched once on the chin
• °LOC, °Vomiting, °Headache
• Feels his bite is different and has difficulty swallowing
• Has had analgesia (diclofenac IM) in A & E

RMH
• No significant medical history (°RF, °Asthma, °bleeding-tendency, °DM)
• No previous hospitalizations
• No previous operations

Drugs
• Nil
• °Known allergies

RDH
• Registered with a dentist back home
• Has yearly check-ups (no significant dental problems)

SE
• °CVS symptoms
• °RS symptoms (except for occasional dry cough)
• °GI symptoms
• °NS symptoms

FH
• Parents and siblings fit & well
• No diseases running in the family

SH
• Lives in a flat, which he shares with 3 other students
• Smokes 15 cigarettes/day
• Drinks ~25 units of alcohol/week

OE
• Alert & orientated GCS: 15/15
• No signs of intoxication
• T: 36.5°C    BP: 114/72
• Pulse: 72 bpm, regular, good volume and character
• RR: 12 rpm O₂ Sat: 99% (on air)
• Trachea: central Apex: 5th LICS, MCL
• HS: I + II + 0 (°murmurs)
• Chest: symmetrical, no deformities, good air entry (L = R)
• PN: resonant    BS: vesicular (°added sounds)
• Abdomen: soft, °tenderness, °masses
• Liver, spleen, and kidneys cannot be palpated

Face
• Swelling ++ over left angle of mandible
• Hypoaesthesia lower left lip and left chin

**Table 10.6** Contd.

*Mouth*
- *Bleeding from LL8 area*
- *Ecchymosis left retromolar region and left buccal sulcus*
- *Premature contact LL8*
- *Occlusion: deranged*

*OPTG and PA mandible*
- *Displaced fracture of left mandibular angle along partially erupted LL8*

☐  *Diagnosis explained to patient and treatment options discussed*

☐  *2nd on call informed*

☐  *Blood taken for FBC, U & Es, LFTs (considering alcohol intake)*

☐  *Case discussed with anaesthetist*

☐  *Booked on Theatre emergency list*

☐  *Patient consented*


*Plan*
- *Regular and PRN analgesia*
- *IV antibiotics*
- *IV fluids*
- *Chlorhexidine mouthrinses*
- *NBM*
- *Check blood results*
- *ORIF of fractured left mandibular angle—tomorrow*
- *Give advice re: alcohol intake before discharge*

°: nil; PN: percussion note; BS: breathing sounds; LL: lower left; NBM: nil by mouth.

**Table 10.7** Clerking example of a planned admission

*10/01/05    Planned admission on X ward (under the care of Mr A. Bloggs)*
*(6 pm)*                                                                *Mary Jones*
                                                      *72 y.o. retired school teacher*

*RA*
- Tracheostomy
- Resection of SCC right floor of mouth and marginal mandibular resection
- Radical right neck dissection and selective left neck dissection
- Reconstruction with left free forearm flap

*HPC*
- First noticed soreness right tongue/throat, 5/52 ago
- Saw GP who referred pt to GDP, as ill fitting dentures were suspected of causing ulcer noted on right floor of mouth
- GDP eased sharp edge of denture, 4/52 ago
- At RV 1 week later ulcer still present and felt indurated
- Urgent referral was sent to OMFS unit
- Biopsy taken in O/P dept. 2/52 ago: reported as SCC
- Small neck lump was noted (FNA: suggestive of 2° SCC)
- Diagnosis was discussed with pt who opted for surgical Rx
- Soreness has been increasing (managed with Difflam mouthwash and codeine phosphate)
- Pt eating less (some dysphagia), has lost ~3 kg of weight

*RMH*
- Hypertension (generally well controlled with medication)
- ? Angina (no attacks for >5 years)
- Osteoarthritis (primarily affecting knees)
- Previous hospitalizations: pneumonia '72
- Operations: hysterectomy '83
- °DM, °RF, °MI, °CVA, °DVT, °TB, °bleeding tendency, °anaemia, °liver disease

*Drugs*
- propranolol 50 mg od
- bendrofluazide 2.5 mg od
- GTN spray PRN
- paracetamol/acetaminophen 1 gr (2–4 times a day depending on knee pain)
- codeine phosphate 30 mg qds (started last week)
- °HO steroids

*Allergies*
- Penicillin (rash)

*RDH*
- Has been edentulous for ~10 years
- Dentures 'not fitting perfectly anymore, but used to them'

*SE*
- General: feeling rather nervous, not sleeping very well last few nights, not eating very well, has lost 3 kg
- CVS: chest pain (last ~6 years ago), swollen ankles occasionally, °SOB, °orthopnoea, °PND, °palpitations, °claudication, °dizziness or black-outs, can walk >500 yards on the flat before stopping (from knee discomfort)
- RS: cough usually in the morning (very occasionally productive), sputum (occasionally as above, but clear), °dyspnoea, °chest pain, °wheeze
- GI: Dysphagia (see HPC), constipation (only last few days—on codeine), °indigestion, °nausea or vomiting, °abdo pain, °jaundice, °significant bowel habit changes

**Table 10.7** Contd.

- GU: moderate frequency and nocturia, °dysuria, °haematuria, °incontinence
- NS: °headaches, °faints or funny turns, °fits, °visual or auditory problems, °weakness, °numbness, °paraesthesiae
- MSS: pain and stiffness of knees (particularly after use), but only occasional swelling
- °Endocrine symptoms

*FH*
- Father died of heart attack, age 56
- Mother died of old age
- Has a 69 y.o. sister who is well
- Has 2 sons who are well

*SH*
- Lives in a bungalow, with her 76 y.o. husband (both independent)
- Does most of the housework herself, but gets some help with shopping from one of her sons who lives near by
- Smokes 10 cigarettes/day for the last 50 years (25 packet-years)
- Drinks ~12 units of alcohol/week (mainly wine)

*OE*
- Well presented, rather thin lady. Arrived with her husband.
- Appears comfortable at rest and well hydrated
- Hands: nicotine stains, °cyanosis, °finger clubbing, °nail or joint abnormalities
- T: 36.1°C   BP: 148/96 (admits to having been a bit stressed)
- Pulse: 84 bpm, regular, good volume and character
- °Radial-radial or radial femoral delay
- Peripheral pulses present
- JVP not raised
- No signs of anaemia, jaundice or cyanosis on the face
- RR: 12 rpm %O Sat: 99% (on air)
- Trachea: central Apex: 5th LICS, MCL
- °Precordial heave or thrill
- HS: I + II + 0 (°murmurs)
- °Sacral or ankle oedema
- Chest: symmetrical, no deformities, good air entry (L = R)
- PN: resonant   BS: vesicular (°added sounds)
- Abdomen: soft, °tenderness, °masses
- PEG in place (inserted 4/7 ago)
- Liver palpated ~1 cm below right costal margin
- Spleen and kidneys cannot be palpated
- Bowel sounds: normal
- Cranial nerves: all intact (including XI)
- PNS: not examined
- MSE: appears normal
- Gait appears normal. Arms, legs and spine not properly assessed

*Mouth/neck*
- Right ventral tongue/floor of mouth ulcer ~1.5 cm in diameter, indurated, with associated white plaque extending to right alveolar process
- Edentulous with some ill-fitting dentures, but still fair amount of alveolar process preserved
- The rest of mucosa appears healthy (no signs of candidosis)
- Hard, fixed, non-tender, upper superficial anterior cervical LN ~2 cm

**Table 10.7** Contd.

- *Parotid glands and thyroid: normal*
- *Facial artery palpable*

*Sp: Inv:*
- *Bx: moderately differentiated SCC*
- *FNA (right neck lump): suggestive of metastatic SCC*
- *OPTG: no bony invasion seen (but suspected clinically)*
- *Endoscopy (upper airways): NAD*
- *ECG: normal*
- *CXR: normal*
- *FBC: normal (Hb 13.1, WBC 8, Plt 310)*
- *U & Es: normal*
- *LFTs: normal*
- *Glucose: 6.7 (random)*
- *Urinalysis: NAD*
- *Coagulation screen: normal*
- *Cross-matching: 6 units available for operation*

*Sum: Reasonably healthy 72 y.o. lady, for major Head & Neck surgery tomorrow morning*

☐ *Pt appears to have good insight of the disease and understands treatment planned*

☐ *Drug chart written up*

☐ *Seen by Dr B.M.F. (anaesthetist) who has written up pre-meds*

☐ *Have confirmed arrangements with Theatre and ITU*

☐ *Pt has given consent*

*Plan*
- *NBM after midnight, but*
- *Should have normal antihypertensives at 6 am with some water*
- *Check BP in the morning*
- *Pre-op RV 8 am at consultant WR*

RA: reason for admission; MSE: mental state examination; NAD: Nothing abnormal detected; WR: ward-round; °: nil; PN: percussion note; BS: breathing sounds; NBM: nil by mouth.

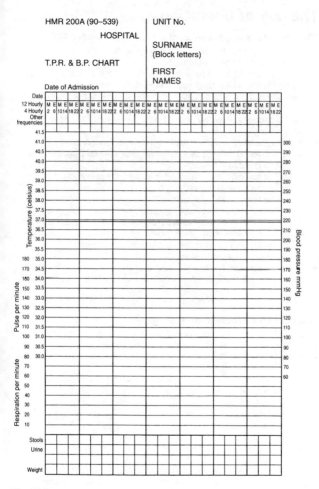

**Fig. 10.1** Temperature, pulse, respiration and blood pressure chart

# The day of operation

## Checks before in-patient dental treatment under GA

- Patient's full name, date of birth and hospital number.
- Nature, side, and site of operation.
- Medical problems, particularly of cardiorespiratory disease or bleeding tendency, should be highlighted and known by everyone involved.
- Consent has been obtained in writing from the patient or, in a person under 16 years of age (18 in Australia), from a parent/guardian, and that the patient adequately understands the nature of the operation and sequelae.
- Theatre is booked, and any special equipment needed, is prepared.
- Necessary dental items such as splints, radiographs, and models are available in the correct theatre.
- Patient has had nothing by mouth for at least the previous 6 h.
- Patient has an empty bladder.
- Patient has removed any contact lenses.
- Dentures and other removable appliances have been removed, and bridges, crowns, and loose teeth have been noted by the anaesthetist.
- Necessary premedication (see following section) and, where indicated, regular medication (such as the contraceptive pill, anticonvulsants or antidepressants) has been given.
- Make sure that for patients with special requirements (e.g. those on steroid therapy, those at risk of infective endocarditis, and diabetics) appropriate arrangements have been made.
- Necessary investigations (blood, etc.), if needed, have been completed.

## Checks before maxillofacial surgery

In addition to the checks needed before in-patient dental treatment under GA, the following are required preoperatively:

- Ensure that the patient, partner and relatives are made aware that the patient may awake postoperatively:
  - with deformity, swelling and possible bruising;
  - in the intensive care unit;
  - with nasal tubes;
  - with intravenous cannulae;
  - with facial sutures;
  - with a tracheostomy;
  - with intermaxillary fixation;
  - with hair shaved;
- Ensure that a bed is booked in intensive care (if indicated).
- Blood (if indicated). Autologous blood for transfusion should be collected 3 weeks preoperatively. Otherwise group and crossmatch blood.
- A CXR; the anaesthetic is likely to be prolonged and this is useful as a baseline, if there are postoperative complications.
- ECG (if indicated).
- Haemoglobin level.
- Urea and electrolytes, and urinalysis.

- Investigations relevant to the surgical procedure:
  - Radiographs (and tracings);
  - Photographs;
  - Models and templates.
- Discuss the case with the anaesthetist.
- Ensure that nurses are conversant with the postoperative management.

Give the necessary information to all involved in the patient's care. Ensure that the ward, consultant, theatre, anaesthetist, partner and relatives are informed if the patient is returning to a different ward (also inform the new ward of the patient's details and management).

### Other preparations in major cases
You may be expected to put up an IV infusion line, so that there is ready access to a vein before GA. Enquire about specific size of cannula, especially if blood transfusion may be needed.

# Surgical operations: safeguards

## Operating on the wrong patient

### Causes
- Tiredness or lack of care.
- Notes attached to the wrong patient following emergency admission.
- Rearrangement of beds in the ward on day of operation.
- Last minute changes in theatre lists.
- Patients with the same or similar name on the ward.

### Prevention
- Care.
- Patients should have one hospital number, which should always be quoted on every paper.
- All patients should be labelled.
- The label should bear the patients surname, forenames, date of birth and accident or in-patient number.
- Labelling the patient should be the responsibility of the sister or her deputy, or, at night, by the nurse in charge or her deputy.
- All unconscious patients admitted through the accident department should be labelled before being taken to the ward.
- The surgeon or accident officer should see that unconscious patients are escorted by a nurse to the ward or theatre.
- The dental surgeon who is to operate should check the patient before operation in the theatre suite, check that the medical or dental record relates to the patient and ask the patient their name and the operation they are to have.
- The anaesthetist should check that the medical record relates to the patient.
- The operations list should carry the patient's surname in full, forenames, hospital number, date of birth and the operation planned.
- The operations list should be displayed in the surgery or theatre, in the anaesthetic room, and in every ward that has a patient on the list or is to receive a patient from the list.
- When sending from theatre for a patient, the theatre porter should bring a slip bearing the surname, forenames, and number of the patient.
- The ward sister or her deputy should be responsible for seeing that:
  - the correct patient is sent to theatre;
  - the patient has signed a consent form;
  - the patient has received the prescribed premedications;
  - where appropriate, the side of the operation has been marked;
  - the correct records and radiographs accompany the patient
- In theatre, the theatre superintendent or deputy should be responsible for sending for patients.
- Day patients for minor operations and out-patients for any operation under GA should be labelled in the same way as in-patients.

## Operating on the wrong side or area

### Causes
- Tiredness or lack of care.
- Wrong information on case papers.

- Illegible case papers.
- Abbreviation of the words 'right' and 'left'.
- Mistakes in dental charting.
- Failure to check the entry on the operating lists against the notes in theatre, together with the wrong case papers or the preparation of the wrong side or area.
- Wrong radiographs.
- No routine procedure for marking operation side.

*Prevention*
- It is the responsibility of the surgeon who explains the operation to the patient, to witness the patient signing the correct consent form.
- The surgeon should mark the side area with an indelible skin pencil before the patient is sent to theatre.
- Sisters should inform the operating surgeon if they find that a patient due to be sent to theatre has not been so marked, but they should not undertake the marking themselves.
- The words LEFT and RIGHT should always be written in full and in block letters, at least on theatre lists.
- When extracting teeth, especially for orthodontic reasons (where the teeth may not be carious), count the teeth carefully, and double-check/confirm with a colleague, if present at operation. As silly as you think this may appear, it may be what saves the patient from losing a tooth unnecessarily (and you from a medico-legal nightmare!).

# Premedication

The objects of premedication (Tables 10.8a, b and c) are to:
- allay anxiety;
- reduce cardiac excitability;
- reduce bronchial secretion;
- reduce GI complications ($\downarrow$ stomach acid);
- provide some analgesia;
- aid the induction of anaesthesia;
- provide some amnesia.

*Note:*
- Premedication (premed) details should be arranged with the anaesthetist and ward sister.
- Problems of cardiac rhythm irregularities are most common in infants and young children, and thus occasionally children < age of 12 years require premedication before in-patient GA (Table 10.8a and b).
- The anaesthetist usually accepts responsibility for premedication and often has his/her own regimen. Establish the protocol that the anaesthetist wishes you to follow.
- Not every patient needs premedication—every drug has potential problems including adverse effects, hypersensitivity, prolonged sedation, drug interactions, etc.

## *Timing of premedication*
- Premedication is effective for about 4 h; therefore, do not give it too early.
- Do not give premedication too late; if there is not 30–60 min available before the operation, leave the anaesthetist to give suitable drugs intravenously before induction. Atropine IM takes effect within 30 min; morphine takes about 1 h.
- If the operation is delayed for >3 h, repeat only the dose of atropine.

## Contraindications and adverse reactions (see also Chapter 8)
- Atropine is contraindicated in glaucoma.
- Hyoscine may cause confusion and should be avoided in the elderly.
- Atropine and hyoscine may cause drowsiness, blurred vision, urine retention and dry mouth.
- Morphine is contraindicated in patients who have a head injury or respiratory disorders.
- Benzodiazepines are contraindicated in glaucoma and respiratory disorders.

**Table 10.8a** Inpatient child preoperative medication (see also Chapter 8)

| Drugs | Time before operation | Route | Dose |
|---|---|---|---|
| Midazolam | 30 mins | O | 500 micrograms/kg (max 15mg) |
| Atropine | 30 mins | O/IM | 40 mg/kg (or 20 mg/kg IM) |
| Paracetomol/ acetaminophen | 1 hr | O | 10 mg/kg |
| Diclofenac | 1 hr | O | 1 mg/kg |
| Temazepam | 1 hr | O | 500 micrograms/kg |
| Diazepam | 1 hr | O | 250 micrograms/kg (max 10 mg) |
| Trimeprazine | 1.5 hr | O | 2 mg/kg |

**Table 10.8b** Alternative agents for child premedication[a]

| Drugs | Time before operation | Route | Dose |
|---|---|---|---|
| Morphine | 30 mins | SC | 100 micrograms/kg |
| Cycllizine | 30 mins | SC | 1 mg/kg |

[a]If a sub-cutaneous cannula is *in situ*.

**Table 10.8c** In-patient adult perioperative medication (see also Chapter 8)

| Drugs | Time before operation | Route | Dose |
|---|---|---|---|
| *Anxiolysis* | | | |
| Lorazepam | 2 hrs | O | 1–2 mg |
| Temazepam | 1 hr | O | 10–20 mg |
| *Analgesia* | | | |
| Morhine (opiod) | 30 mins | IM/sc | 10 mg |
| Pethine (opiod) | 30 mins | IM | 50 mg |
| Diclofenac | 1.2 hrs | O/PR | 50–100 mg |
| Paracetamol/ acetaminophen | 1 hr | O/PR | 1 g |
| *Antisialogogue* | | | |
| Glycopyrollate | 30 mins | IM | 200 micrograms |
| *Antiemetic* | | | |
| Cyclizine | 1 hr | IM/IV | 50 mg |
| Prochlorperizine | 1 hr | IM | 12.5 mg |
| Metaclopramide | 1 hr | IM/IV/O | 10 mg |
| Ondansetron | 1 hr | O | 10 mg |
| *Antacid* | | | |
| Ranitidine | 2 hr | O | 150 mg |
| Lansoprazole | 2 hr | O | 30 mg |
| Rabeprazole | 2 hr | O | 20 mg |

# Theatre lists

## Regular theatre operating list
- The operating list should not be made too long.
- Time must be allowed for each operation for induction of anaesthesia (usually about 15 min per patient), any over-running and breaks.
- Arranging the patient sequence for operation is decided on the basis of:
    - diabetic, highly anxious patients, or those unable to cooperate, should be done early in the list;
    - 'day' cases should be completed before 15.00 h;
    - 'dirty' cases (e.g. opening an abscess) should be done at the end;
    - patients with blood-borne infections (e.g. hepatitis or HIV/AIDS) should be done last of all;
    - the surgeon's preference.
- The list should note the:
    - patient's full name, hospital number, date of birth, ward, operation, side/site of operation (in block capitals) and type of anaesthetic;
    - name of the operator, responsible consultant surgeon and anaesthetist;
    - start time;
    - theatre venue.
- The list should be sent to the theatre, ward, anaesthetist, surgeon and house officer on duty.
- If the order of the list changes, all must be informed—including the patient, partner and relatives.

## Emergency theatre list

Emergency lists usually run 24 h/day but, at night, will only usually operate for *real* emergencies (see box below). It is the duty of the house officer to book an emergency case in theatre as soon as they know what the planned management is, and after the senior surgeon in charge and the anaesthetist have been consulted, and a ward bed arranged.

It is good practice to see what the emergency/trauma list situation is like, and communicate with on-call doctors of other specialties, and the anaesthetist, regarding the prioritization of cases. It is rare that maxillo-facial operations need to be done early for life-saving reasons but, when one of your cases needs to be treated as a priority, you will usually find all parties concerned will be understanding and cooperative as long as relations are not broken! So do not argue with, or try to bully, colleagues.

---

### CEPOD classification of emergencies

| | |
|---|---|
| *Elective* | Operation time to suit patient and surgeon. |
| *Scheduled* | An early operation, but not immediately life-saving (usually within 3 weeks). |
| *Urgent* | Operation asap after resuscitation (within 24h). |
| *Emergency* | Immediately life-saving operation (resuscitation simultaneous with surgery). |

---

# In theatre

Ensure that last minute jobs have been done, such as checking that everything for theatre is ready, and that all necessary phone calls are made. Ensure someone can answer necessary calls on your page/bleep, or mobile telephone. Then scrub and gown.

## Scrubbing up and gowning

- Lather the hands and forearms with soap or a special solution (Table 10.9).
- Scrub with a brush for 1 min, especially the nails and hands. Vigorous scrubbing is open to the criticism that bacteria may be brought out of skin pores and increase rather than reduce skin bacterial counts.
- Lather and rinse hands and forearms vigorously for a further 5 min— turn taps on with elbows.
- Rinse off soap, holding your hands at a higher level than the elbows.
- Dry with a sterile towel. It is important to prevent the towel touching unsterile skin at the elbow and then wiping the opposite hand with it.
- The sterile gown is unfolded and the arms pushed into the armholes; then the arms are held up. A nurse should then pull down the shoulders and body of the gown and tie it behind. It is inadvisable to pull the sleeves up yourself because of the risk of inadvertently touching the mask or collar.
- Gloves are donned (know your glove size), care being taken not to touch the outside with the skin of the opposite hand. This is probably the most important stage, and possibly the one hardest to explain; ask a senior colleague or a theatre nurse to show you on your first day in theatre, if you do not feel perfectly comfortable with your technique.
- Thereafter, observe a 'no touch' technique, keeping your hands near your abdomen or chest while waiting or moving around in theatre.

Surgical personnel have traditionally been required to scrub their hands for 10 min preoperatively, but studies have found that scrubbing for 5 min reduces bacterial counts as effectively and may help prevent skin damage associated with such lengthy hand-washing. Surgical hand-washing protocols also have required surgical staff to scrub hands with a brush, which can also damage skin and result in increased shedding of bacteria from the hands; some studies have indicated that scrubbing with a disposable sponge or combination sponge-brush is as effective, while other studies have indicated that neither a brush or sponge is necessary to reduce bacterial counts on the hands of surgical staff to acceptable levels. A two-stage surgical scrub using an antiseptic detergent, followed by application of an alcohol-containing preparation has been demonstrated to be effective.

Surgical hand scrubs with 60–95% alcohol alone or 50–95% when combined with limited amounts of a quaternary ammonium compound, or chlorhexidine gluconate, more effectively lower bacterial counts on the skin immediately post-scrub than other agents. The next most active agents, in order of decreasing activity, are: chlorhexidine gluconate, iodophors, triclosan and plain soap (http://www.cdc.gov/handhygiene/).

## Preparing the patient

### Painting up

- The eyelids should be carefully closed by the anaesthetist and covered with gauze pads, smeared with a little Vaseline, and secured with tape, micropore or strapping prior to antiseptic preparation of the face. Some centres also use plastic or other eye guards.
- The operation site and several centimetres around in all directions should be painted with an antiseptic, dried with a sterile swab and then painted with a bactericidal agent.
- Cetrimide solution or povidone iodine solution (provided there is no iodine sensitivity) are most suitable for preparing the face. It is not essential to paint inside the lips and mouth prior to oral and maxillofacial surgery, although some do.
- Spirit solutions must not be used to prepare the skin around the eyes.

### Towelling

- The anaesthetist will disconnect the airline and lift up the head.
- Two towels are passed under head and pulled down behind the neck.
- The top towel is folded over the patient's forehead or face if only the neck needs to be exposed, and secured with a towel clip. It is important to cover all areas that do not need to be exposed during the operation, as this seals off potential sources of microorganisms.
- The lower towel is then drawn down over the shoulder on both sides, and the chest covered by another towel.
- Keep the towel edge, which will be next to the exposed skin, in view at all times by holding it between the two hands, allowing the rest of the towel to trail.

## Diathermy

*Monopolar diathermy* is frequently used for cutting through muscles and coagulating blood vessels. The diathermy point carries a positive electric charge, which runs to earth through the patient. Unless the patient is earthed by means of a large electrode bandaged to the thigh the tissue may become overheated by the electric current passing through it, leading to a severe burn. It is essential that no other part of the patient is in contact with a conductor, as the current will often flow through and burn the skin at this point.

▶Before towelling, therefore, all theatre staff must ensure that no part of the patient is touching metal fittings or the metal tabletop.

*Bipolar diathermy* does not need earthing, and may also be used for coagulation of small blood vessels. Although less effective, it is less destructive and is preferred in operations of the face.

▶Diathermy is absolutely contraindicated if any explosive anaesthetic agents are used, or if the patient has a cardiac pacemaker.
▶Biopsy material obtained by diathermy will be distorted and difficult for the histologist to interpret.

**Table 10.9** Characteristics of main hand hygiene and surgical antisepsis products

| Product | Constituents | Mechanisms of antimicrobial activity | Comments |
|---|---|---|---|
| Plain soaps | Detergent-based and contain esterified fatty acids and sodium or potassium hydroxide | Detergent | Minimal antimicrobial activity. Fail to remove pathogens. Contaminated soap may lead to colonization of hands with Gram-negative bacilli. |
| Alcohols | Contain either isopropanol, ethanol, n-propanol, or a combination | Microbial denaturation | Solutions containing 60–95% alcohol are most effective. Excellent activity against Gram-positive and Gram-negative vegetative bacteria, including multidrug-resistant pathogens (e.g. MRSA and VRE), *Mycobacterium tuberculosis*, various fungi, viruses (e.g. herpes simplex virus, HIV, influenza virus, respiratory syncytial virus, vaccinia virus, hepatitis B virus and hepatitis C virus. |
| | | | Very poor activity against bacterial spores, protozoan oocysts, and nonenveloped viruses (e.g. rotavirus, adenovirus, and enteroviruses). |
| | | | Activity is not substantially affected by organic matter. Alcohols are flammable. Contamination of alcohol-based solutions seldom reported. |
| Chlorhexidine | Cationic bisbiguanide | Attachment to, and subsequent disruption of, microbial cytoplasmic membranes | FIRST CHOICE. Active against Gram-positive bacteria, but less against Gram-negative bacteria, fungi and enveloped viruses (e.g. herpes simplex virus, HIV, cytomegalovirus, influenza, and RSV). |
| | | | Low activity against tubercle bacilli, spores and nonenveloped viruses. |
| | | | Activity not substantially affected by organic matter. Potentially ototoxic. Has occasionally become bacterially contaminated. |

| | Composition | Mechanism | Comments |
|---|---|---|---|
| Hexachlorophene | | Inactivates essential microbial enzyme systems | Only modest efficacy after a single handwash. Potential neurotoxic effects on infants. |
| Iodine and Iodophors | Composed of elemental iodine, iodide or tri-iodide, and a polymer carrier | Complexes with microbial amino acids and unsaturated fatty acids | AVOID IN PATIENTS WITH THYROID DISEASE OR ON LITHIUM. Bactericidal against Gram-positive, Gram-negative, mycobacteria, viruses, and fungi but not spores. Activity substantially reduced in presence of organic substances. Iodophors cause less skin irritation and fewer allergic reactions than iodine, but more irritant contact dermatitis than other antiseptics, and have occasionally become bacterially contaminated. |
| Quaternary ammonium compounds | Benzethonium chloride, cetrimide, and cetyl-pyridium chloride | Causes leakage of low molecular weight microbial cytoplasmic constituents | Active more against Gram-positive bacteria than against Gram-negative or viruses. Weak activity against mycobacteria and fungi. Activity substantially reduced by organic substances. |
| Triclosan | 2,4,4'-trichloro-2'-hydroxy-diphenyl ether | Binds to microbial enoylacyl carrier protein reductase, and affects cytoplasmic membranes and synthesis of RNA, fatty acids, and proteins | Active more against Gram-positive bacteria than against Gram-negative or viruses. Reasonable activity against mycobacterial and Candida spp. Has occasionally become bacterially contaminated. Activity not substantially affected by organic matter. |

# Assisting at operations

### General points

- To assist well requires an informed knowledge of the steps in the operation, concentration, stamina and tact.
- Try not to talk unless so encouraged.
- If swabbing, take care not to re-introduce into the mouth (and hence the larynx!) any roots, teeth, etc. that may have been placed on the swab with the intention of disposing of them.

### Handling instruments

- Many surgical instruments, for example artery forceps and some suture holders, have a ratchet device to keep them closed. The assistant must be adept at opening and closing these with either hand.
- Scissors can be most accurately controlled if the thumb and ring finger are placed in the rings and the tip of the index finger placed along the shaft.
- Ligatures or sutures should be cut with the ends of the blades; scissors seldom need to be opened more than 1 cm at the tip and the blades should be held at right angles to the skin.
- Scissors inexpertly wielded can be a danger both to the patient and the surgeon.

### Biopsy specimens (see also Chapter 3)

- If a frozen section biopsy is to be taken at operation, the houseman/intern should warn pathology before the day, write out the request form before scrubbing up, and check with the laboratory by telephone to ensure that they will be ready to process the specimen.
- Ensure that the necessary specimens are collected. For example, if immunological tests are required (direct immunofluorescence), the tissue must be snap frozen, while if tuberculosis is suspected, some of the tissue should be sent unfixed, for culture.
- The houseman/intern is responsible for sending or taking the biopsy, with the correct form duly filled in, to the laboratory.

### Operation records

- In ink (red ink has traditionally been favoured for this purpose, but it copies poorly; so check local preference), record in the case notes:
  - the name of the operator and assistant;
  - the name of the anaesthetist;
  - the name of the nurse;
  - the date, time and place of operation;
  - the overall description of the operation and, especially, any deviations from routine or any complications;
  - any blood loss;
  - postoperative instructions.
- Sign and date the entry.

▶Remember possible medico-legal implications.

# Early postoperative care

## Immediate postoperative care

- The early postoperative period is one of the most dangerous times for the patient who is recovering from a GA or conscious sedation, and who has impaired reflexes. *The airway must be protected.*
- It is imperative to ensure that the airway is protected until the patient fully recovers reflexes. The patient should be kept in the tonsillar or head injury (recovery) position (see Chapter 11) with an airway in place and constantly attended by a trained person, until the cough reflex has fully recovered.
- The anaesthetist should be, and remain, present.

*If the patient is slow to regain consciousness*
- The following checks should be carried out:
  - airways and respiration;
  - pulse and BP;
  - pupil diameter and reactivity.
- Consider whether there has been a drug reaction/overdose, or an MI or other medical complication.

## When reflexes have returned

- Remember to give any medication the patient should normally receive daily (e.g. anticonvulsants).
- Monitor the temperature, pulse, respiration and BP (see Fig 10.1, page 489).
- About 50% of patients have transient and self-resolving drowsiness, hangover, nausea, sore throat (after intubation and/or packing), and aches and pains (from suxamethonium). Prescribe, for use as required, appropriate analgesics and anti-emetics.

## Leaving theatre

Even after reflexes have recovered, the patient normally needs to spend some time (usually at least an hour) in the recovery area to ensure that the anaesthetist and surgeon have quick access to the patient, if need be. Airways compromise (e.g. airways obstruction due to aspiration of large blood clots), or rapidly progressing swellings (e.g. haematoma due to arterial bleed under a surgical flap) need urgent attention by the anaesthetist and the surgeon; so make sure that theatre staff know where you are (ideally remain in the vicinity of the theatre area)—and that you know where your senior colleague in charge is.

# Local postoperative complications

### Wound pain

- Postoperative wound pain is usually present for the 24 h or so after operation; at first constant, but eventually present only on moving or touching the area.
- For the first 48 h postoperatively, wound pain should be controlled with analgesics (see Chapter 8) given regularly.
- If pain persists longer than 48 h, or increases, it is likely that there is some pathological process, such as wound infection, present (e.g. dry socket). The patient should be encouraged to seek advice.
- Severe pain may need to be controlled by morphine or papaveretum given subcutaneously every 4–6 h. The dosage and drug used will depend on the weight and the age of the patient. For a small adult, 5–10 mg morphine will usually suffice. For the heavier adult, 15 mg of morphine may be needed.

### Wound infection

- The diagnosis of wound infection is usually obvious as, at about 3–7 days after operation, the wound appears inflamed, swollen and tender, and there may be discharge of pus and pyrexia.
- If pus is draining, there may be no need to give antibiotics, as the infection may settle spontaneously within a few days. However, pus or a swab should be taken to identify the organism and test sensitivity to antibiotics.
- If the wound is not draining but is fluctuant, one or more sutures should be removed from the most inflamed area, sinus forceps inserted and gently opened to allow drainage of pus.
- If the wound infection is only trivial, with no obvious suppuration, antibiotics may alone suffice.
- Infection under neck flaps is particularly dangerous as the carotid artery may be eroded.

### Dry socket

*Diagnosis* is usually obvious from the history of increasing and sometimes severe pain 2–4 days after extraction, often with halitosis and an unpleasant taste. The socket is empty of clot, but may contain debris. The affected area is very tender to palpation. Radiography is usually needed to exclude retained roots, foreign body, jaw fracture or other pathology. If there are other additional features such as pyrexia, intense pain or neurological changes (e.g. labial anaesthesia), the possibility of a fracture or acute osteomyelitis must be considered.

*Management* is primarily by gentle irrigation of the extraction socket with warm (50°C) sterile normal saline or aqueous 0.2% chlorhexidine. Gently dress the socket to permit granulation. A number of different concoctions may be used, suggesting that there is little significant difference in efficacy between them. Give analgesics as required.

## Oedema

The amount of oedema that occurs postoperatively depends largely on the extent of trauma, but varies between individual patients, and can be reduced by:

- minimizing the duration of operation;
- minimizing the trauma, in terms of lifting of the periosteum and removal of cortical bone;
- use of corticosteroids (e.g. 4–8 mg dexamethasone IV), ice packs or other methods that help reduce oedema;
- nursing patient in head-up position.

## Trismus

- Trismus can be reduced by minimizing the same factors as for oedema, and also by minimizing the stripping of muscle off the bone.

## Antral complications

*Loss of tooth or root into the antrum*

- Radiograph the area (periapical, occlusal ± OM) to locate the object.
- If it is extra-mucosal, remove with a sucker or other instrument and use primary closure.
- If not, further operation will be required. Meantime, give antimicrobial and nasal decongestant, and advise patient to avoid blowing their nose.

*Oro-antral fistula (OAF)*

- Patients should not blow their nose.
- Give antimicrobial and nasal decongestant.
- Primary closure may be possible if this is detected early.
- Other OAFs may close spontaneously, or may need flap closure.

## Other, rarer complications

*Seroma* is the accumulation of serous fluid under large surgical flaps, particularly in the neck. This appears as a large fluctuant swelling that is neither warm nor tender. Seromas may have to be drained several times using large syringes and needles or cannulae. Moderate pressure dressings should be applied to prevent quick re-filling of the surgical space.

*Sialocele* is a swelling occasionally appearing over the area of the parotid following partial parotidectomy. It is due to leakage of saliva produced by the remaining gland into the subcutaneous tissue. Sialoceles usually settle with time, but may need to be managed in a manner similar to seromas.

# Systemic postoperative complications

The most important systemic postoperative complications are summarized in Tables 10.10 [p.510], 10.11 [p.511] and 10.12 [p.512].

## Deep vein thrombosis (DVT)

### Predisposing factors

- Major operation with immobility of legs
- Elderly
- Obese
- Pregnancy or the contraceptive pill
- Inherited tendency to thrombosis
- Malignancy.

### Prophylaxis

*May be indicated in:*

- long major operations;
- patients likely to be immobilized after operation;
- the elderly;
- the obese;
- pregnancy;
- patients with a history of DVT;
- patients with an inherited tendency to thrombosis;

*Consists of:*

- avoiding oestrogens (e.g. contraceptive pill);
- using graduated compression stockings for intermittent pressure;
- giving low dose subcutaneous heparin (5000 units 2 h preoperatively and then 8–12 hourly for 5 days postoperatively), or low molecular weight heparin (Clexane 20 mg).

### Diagnosis

- Leg tender, warm and oedematous
- Investigations
  - Venography
  - Doppler ultrasound
  - Radio-iodine fibrinogen uptake

### Possible consequences

- Local pain and swelling (of the calf usually)
- Pulmonary embolism (may be lethal)
- Late development of varicose veins

### Management

- Anticoagulation (IV heparin for 4–10 days depending on severity of DVT; then warfarin for at least 3 months)
- Gradually mobilize as pain and oedema resolve
- Leg exercises
- Leg bandaging.

*If pulmonary embolism is suspected* (*dyspnoea; chest pain*)
• Give 100% oxygen
• Consult the physicians immediately
• Give IV normal saline (monitor pulse and BP) and IV morphine or diamorphine 5 mg.

## Postoperative jaundice

May be due to:
• Liver disease
  - Halothane hepatitis—may occur if there are repeated administrations.
  - Gilbert's syndrome—a benign enzyme defect in which jaundice may follow anaesthesia, ingestion of alcohol, or starvation.
  - Viral hepatitis (uncommon)—may follow blood transfusion.
• Other reasons
  - Sepsis.
  - Hepatotoxic drugs (e.g. erythromycin estolate).
  - Haemolysis (haemolytic anaemias or incompatible transfusion).
  - Resorption of blood from haematoma (rare).
  - Incidental hepatobiliary disease (e.g. gallstone disease).

## Problems with eating

Apart from nausea and dysphagia and possibly transient anorexia, some patients, especially those with intermaxillary fixation, may need a special soft or liquidized diet. Consult the dietician.

Special diets may also be required for other reasons including:
• religious or cultural grounds;
• ethical grounds (vegetarians and vegans);
• diabetes mellitus;
• those on MAOI;
• severe renal disease;
• severe liver disease;
• food fads.

Patients with difficulty eating should be weighed daily, and nutrition may need to be give:
• by nasogastric (NG) or orogastric tube, or better through percutaneous endoscopic gastostomy (PEG). Continuous infusion of a liquid feed is now preferred, as intermittent feeding may cause diarrhoea;
• parenterally, i.e. via an IV catheter in the subclavian or jugular veins (total parenteral nutrition; TPN). This is best avoided but, if it is necessary, regularly monitor the fluid balance, blood glucose, urea and electrolytes, and liver function.

**Table 10.10** Immediate postoperative complications

| System | Complication | Comments | Postoperative observations required |
|---|---|---|---|
| Cardiovascular | Haemorrhage Hypotension | See Chapter 4 Usually caused by autonomic suppression from GA. Treat by placing patient head down and giving vasopressor IV (ephedrine 5–15 mg or metaraminol 0.5–5 mg). | Haemoglobin, BP, pulse rate |
| | Cardiac arrest | See Chapter 6 | Conscious level BP, pulse rate |
| Respiratory | Obstruction | Place patient in 'tonsillar' position postoperatively. Snoring or stridor suggest obstruction. Treat by extending head, using pharyngeal airways (e.g. Guedel airway) and aspirating with sucker. CXR to exclude aspirated foreign body if recovery impaired. (See Chapter 6) | Respiratory rate |
| | Depression | Often caused by drugs. Suggested by shallow or slow breathing and cyanosis. Treat by ventilating with oxygen and giving naloxone 0.4 mg or doxapram 2 mg IM or IV. Maintain airways. | |
| GI | Nausea, vomiting | May be caused by drugs or swallowed blood. Protect airway and give metoclopramide 5 mg IM or 10 mg orally; or domperidone orally for teenagers, or ranitidine (or see antiemetics in Table 8.21, p.402). If there is inhalation of any vomit, suck out the pharynx and larynx. Give hydrocortisone 200 mg IV and call the physician, to avoid possible bronchospasm, ulmonary oedema and circulatory collapse (Mendelson's syndrome). Aminophylline and antimicrobials may be indicated. | |

**Table 10.11** Postoperative complications appearing usually within first 24 h

| System | Complications | Comments |
| --- | --- | --- |
| Pharynx | Sore throat | Endotracheal intubation or throat pack may be responsible. Gargle with soluble aspirin. |
| Neuromuscular | Muscle pains | Suxamethonium frequently causes pain in the back and shoulders. |
| | Nerve damage | Pressure, or extravasation of drugs may be responsible. |
| Respiratory[a] | Infection, atelectasis | Atelectasis and infection are predominantly problems in smokers or those with pre-existent respiratory disease. Exclude aspiration of foreign body. Consider antimicrobials and physiotherapy. |
| Cardiovascular | Superficial venous thrombosis | Superficial vein thrombosis may be caused by diazepam, dextrose, or thiopentone. |
| Renal | Urinary retention | Usually functional. Sit patient up. Give analgesia if abdominal pain. Give warm bath. If all else fails, catheterize or give carbachol. |
| CNS | Confusion or collapse | May be due to one of several factors (See Chapter 4): Over-sedation or drug reaction Pain Respiratory failure or infection MI Urinary retention or infection Dehydration Metabolic disturbance (e.g. diabetes) Septicaemia Stroke or other CNS disorder |

[a]May take up to 72 h to appear.

**Table 10.12** Postoperative pyrexia

| Usual time of appearance (days) | Causes | Prevention | Management |
|---|---|---|---|
| 0–3 | Septicaemia | Aseptic techniques especially with IV infusions | Antimicrobials |
| | Transfusion reaction | (See page 532) | Stop transfusion, ±chlorpheniramine 4 mg orally 4 times daily. |
| | Drug reaction, e.g. to halothane | Avoid repeated exposure | Obtain medical advice[a] |
| 1–3 | Respiratory complications | Stop patient smoking | Drainage (physiotherapy) |
| | Infection Bronchopulmonary segmental collapse | Physiotherapy Antimicrobials Avoid respiratory depressants | Antimicrobials ± oxygen Aspiration of obstruction |
| 3–5 | Localized infection | Aseptic technique Minimal trauma Antimicrobials | Drainage Antimicrobials |
| 6–10 | Deep vein thrombosis/ pulmonary embolism (See Chapter 4 and page 510) | Avoid pressure on calf Low dose heparin 5000 units SC 2 h before and every 8–12 h after surgery | Rest Bandage Anticoagulants (heparin/warfarin) |

[a]This may be malignant hyperpyrexia.

# Shock

Shock (see also Chapter 6) may follow a major operation, because of severe haemorrhage, infection, allergy or other reason (see below).

**Shock is defined as** the failure of the circulation to oxygenate the body tissues. It is recognised by:

- hypotension;
- acidosis;
- oliguria (urine output <0.5 mL/kg/h for the average adult).

**Causes** include:

- hypovolaemia (loss of blood or body fluids);
- septicaemia;
- acute respiratory obstruction;
- vascular obstruction;
- cardiac failure;
- adrenocortical insufficiency;
- neurogenic;
- allergic.

**If untreated**, shock may lead to cerebral hypoxia, acute renal failure and death.

**Management**

- Lay patient flat with legs raised.
- Maintain airways; give oxygen (10–15 L/min).
- Monitor pulse and BP.
- Consult a physician.
- Set up an IV infusion.
- Catheterize (12F gauge Foley catheter) to monitor urine output hourly.
- Consider central venous pressure (CVP) line (see below).
- Treat manifestations (Table 10.13).
- Establish and, where possible, treat the cause.

## CVP measurement

- assesses pressure in the region of the right atrium of the heart;
- is a useful guide to fluid replacement in shocked, ill and hypovolaemic patients.

**Setting up a CVP line** is a procedure requiring skill and is associated with potential dangers outside the scope of normal activities of junior dental surgeons. The causes of change in CVP include those listed in Table 10.14.

### Plasma volume expanders (Table 10.15)

- Plasma volume expanders are useful for temporarily replacing volume lost in acute haemorrhage, while blood is grouped and cross-matched.
- Gelatins, dextrans, or hydroxyethyl starch (hetastarch or pentastarch) should be used.
- Plasma protein fraction can be used, but carries the risk that it may transmit viral infections.
- Substantially salt free freeze-dried albumins are available, which can be reconstituted with sterile water to the required protein concentration.
- Albumin solutions are available.
- Care should be taken to avoid fluid overload and allergies.

▶Crystalloids (e.g. saline) are not satisfactory for this purpose as they do not remain intravascularly.

**Table 10.13** Treatment of shock

| Manifestation | Management |
|---|---|
| Hypotension | IV infusion. Monitor CVP |
| Acidosis | IV sodium bicarbonate 8.4% (about 200 Meq/24 h) |
| Oliguria | IV infusions as above. Plus diuretic, e.g. IV 100 mL of 25% mannitol solution |
| Hypoxia | Give oxygen |
| Capillary sludging | Give low molecular weight dextran IV (dextran 40 in glucose 5%) |

**Table 10.14** Changes in central venous pressure

| Falling | Rising |
|---|---|
| Loss of blood volume | Circulatory overload |
|   Bleeding | Over-transfusion |
|   Dehydration | Cardiac failure |
| Impaired venous return | Raised intrathoracic pressure |
| Increased cardiac efficiency | Haemothorax |
| | Pneumothorax |
| | Pleural effusion |
| | Cardiac tamponade |

**Table 10.15** Plasma volume replacement[a]

| Product | Used in | Comments |
|---|---|---|
| Gelatins | Severe acute haemorrhage (before blood available) | Lack of osmotic diuresis of dextrans, but have their other disadvantages. Give IV infusions (Gelofusine or Haemacel). |
| Dextrans | Severe acute haemorrhage (before blood available) | Take blood for grouping and cross-matching before starting dextrans as they interfere with these procedures. They only replace volume, not oxygen carrying capacity. May be dangerous in congestive cardiac failure and coagulopathies. Dextran 70 is the only dextran really suitable. Others are either large (110, 150) and cause red cell aggregation or small (40) and do not remain in the circulation. |
| Etherified starches | Severe acute haemorrhage | May interfere with blood clotting (Hexastarch; Hydroxyethyl starch; Pentastarch). |

[a]Must be used with caution in patients with cardiac or renal disease. Close monitoring of haematocrit, fluid and electrolytes, urine output, and for hypersensitivity reactions is indicated.

# Fluid balance

There is normally a fine balance of water and salt intake and loss (Table 10.16), with variations in oral intake reflected in proportionate changes in urine output. However, the excessive loading or loss of fluid may overwhelm compensatory mechanisms, especially in the compromised postoperative patient.

Postoperatively, patients are more prone to dehydration and electrolyte imbalances than to iatrogenic fluid overload. Fluid can be lost by several different routes and, depending on the quantity and the particular fluid lost (Table 10.17), this can lead to circulatory failure.

▶Children, in particular, are prone to dehydration as their body surface area is proportionally large.

A wide range of fluids is available to be given IV to avoid this (Table 10.18).

*Causes of postoperative fluid and electrolyte disturbances*
- Losses of blood, or other body fluids (e.g. vomiting, sweating).
- Inadequate fluid intake orally.
- Retention of sodium and loss of potassium as a reaction to trauma (this response persists for at least 24 h).

*Assessment of sodium and water balance* is based on:
- History
- Clinical examination; skin turgor may be reduced.
- Daily fluid balance chart (fluid intake and loss, including urine output).
- Daily body weight.
- Plasma urea and electrolyte levels (hyponatraemia is commonly due to water excess, rather than sodium depletion).
- Haemoglobin level and PCV.

*Fluid replacement therapy* is based on:
- Supplying the normal intake of fluids and electrolytes (water 30 mL/kg/24 h; $Na^+$ 1.4 mmol/kg/24 h; $K^+$ 1.0 mmol/kg/24 h, for adults).
- Replacing additional losses depending on the specific clinical situation.
- Modifying the above requirements where renal function is impaired.

Postoperative fluid balance in an adult can usually be maintained by infusing ~2.5 L of crystalloid solution per day, provided there are no losses of body fluids (e.g. through vomiting). However, fluid balance should always be assessed carefully (see Table 10.16).

The following IV crystalloid solutions are roughly isotonic and are used specifically to supply:
*Water*: use 5% dextrose (glucose)
*Sodium*: use 0.9% sodium chloride (150 mmol/L)
*Sodium and bicarbonate*: use 1.4% sodium bicarbonate (150 mmol/L).
*Potassium*: must always be given with great caution, as it can interfere with cardiac function. Potassium (usually as potassium chloride) can be added to the above solutions, or given as solutions to which potassium in different concentrations has already been added (the latter is considered safer). The maximum concentration of potassium to be given in infused fluid is 40 mmol/L. The maximum rate of infusion = 13 mmol (1 g)/2 h. Potassium may also be given orally (SandoK).

**Table 10.16** Average water and salt balance in healthy adults per 24 h

|  |  | Water (mL) |  | Sodium (mmol) |
|---|---|---|---|---|
| Intake[a] | Moist food and drink | 2000 | Food, drink, seasoning | 170 |
|  | Dry food and oxidation | 500 |  |  |
| Pool | Plasma | 3000 | Plasma | 450 |
|  | Tissue fluid | 12 000 | Rest of body | 3500 |
|  | Cell fluid | 30 000 |  |  |
| Output | Insensible loss | 1000 | Insensible loss | — |
|  | Urine | 1300 | Urine | 150 |
|  | Faeces | 200 | Faeces | 20 |
|  | Sweat | Variable | Sweat | Variable |

[a]Minimum requirement: water 1500 mL; 50 mmol sodium. Normal intake of potassium is 80 mmol/24 h. Ideally calculate fluid requirement by the formula (especially applicable to children and small adults): 4 mL/kg/h for the first 10 kg of body weight + 2 mL/kg/h for next 10 kg + 1 mL/kg/h for the rest of the body weight.

**Table 10.17** Average water and salt balance in healthy adults per 24 h

| Body fluid | Electrolyte concentrations (mmol/L) | | | Fluid lost mainly in |
|---|---|---|---|---|
|  | $Na^+$ | $K^+$ | $Cl^-$ |  |
| Serum | 135–140 | 3.5–5.0 | 98–106 | Burns Peritonitis |
| Gastric | 60 | 9.5 | 100 | Vomiting |
| Biliary | 145 | 5.5 | 100 | Vomiting |
| Pancreatic | 140 | 5.0 | 75 | Diarrhoea |
| Small intestinal | 120 | 5.0 | 100 | Fistulae |

**Table 10.18** Approximate ionic contents of IV fluids

| One bottle replacement | $Na^+$ | $K^+$ | $Cl^-$ | $HCO_3^-$ or equivalent | $H^+$ or equivalent | Calories/L |
|---|---|---|---|---|---|---|
| Sodium chloride (150 mmol/L isotonic saline) | 150 | 0 | 150 | 0 | 0 | 0 |
| Glucose 5% (dextrose) | 0 | 0 | 0 | 0 | 0 | 200 |
| Sodium chloride 30 mmol/L with 4.3% glucose | 30 | 0 | 30 | 0 | 0 | 170 |
| Sodium lactate 160 mmol/L | 160 | 0 | 0 | 160 | 0 | 0 |
| Sodium bicarbonate 150 mmol/L | 160 | 0 | 0 | 160 | 0 | 0 |

# IV cannulation

IV cannulation is commonly needed in hospital in-patients to allow re-peated or continuous administration of fluids or to:
- replace blood volume.
- give drugs slowly parenterally (e.g. vancomycin).
- feed patients parenterally.

## Equipment

- *IV cannulae* (have at least two available): Most IV cannulae consist of an outer, non-irritant plastic cannula with a central needle. These must be of a gauge appropriate to deliver the fluid at the required rate. In gen-eral, use the largest possible cannula, to ensure an adequate flow (see next section). Blood transfusion necessitates gauge 18 or wider.
- Sterile swabs, antiseptic solution, tourniquet.
- Syringes, needles and local anaesthetic solution.
- Adhesive tape (cut into at least four strips of good length), bandages or netting and a splint.
- Syringe and specimen tubes for blood sampling.
- Syringe with 2–5 mL normal saline flush.

## Sites (Fig. 10.2, p. 523)

A large diameter straight arm vein away from a joint is best used, and in the non-dominant arm.

*Forearm veins* are usually very suitable for cannulation. The cephalic vein at the level of the radial styloid process (prominent when the forearm is pronated and the hand pulled into the ulnar deviation) is best, as splints are not usually necessary and the patient can move the arm freely.

*Antecubital fossa* veins are the easiest sites for insertion of cannulae, but a splint is required, for elbow flexibility, and mobility of the arm is reduced.

*Veins of the dorsum of the hand* are useful, as mobility of the limb is retained, but these veins are not easy to access as they are small and venepuncture is also painful there. It is best to avoid this site if drugs, or irritant solutions such as dextrose, or large volumes are to be given.

⚠ Avoid veins of the lower limb, as there is a risk of thrombophlebitis and of deep vein thrombosis. Only use these in cardiac arrest.

## Asepsis

Introduction of micro-organisms may result in suppurative thrombophle-bitis, or septicaemia, with serious consequences. Therefore, always:
- wash hands and nails thoroughly;
- wear gloves;
- use strict asepsis.

## Technique

⚠ If a 'renal' patient is involved, ask the Renal Unit to carry out the procedure, as the veins and especially any arteriovenous fistulae, are very precious.

- *Cleanse* the skin with an isopropyl alcohol swab.
- *Give local anaesthetic* (0.2–0.5 mL of 1% lidocaine without adrenaline) intradermally over the cannulation site, if the patient is nervous or the cannula large (gauge 18 or over).
- *Place the tourniquet* and identify a good vein that you can palpate.
- *Insert the needle* obliquely through the skin and enter the vein; blood will be seen tracking up the cannula. Without inserting the needle further, push the plastic outer cannula gently into the vein, remove the needle and take a blood sample (keep in mind that blood may haemolyse if the cannula is too small) for storage of serum in case blood transfusion becomes needed.
- *Place the cap seal* at the back of the cannula. While the open end of the cannula is unsealed, keep the arm slightly raised and place gentle pressure over the vein to prevent blood spillage (there is no valve at this opening).
- *Flush* cannula with 2–5 mL sterile normal (isotonic) saline (through the second opening of the cannula, which has a one-way valve allowing administration of drugs, even while a drip is running). If the cannula has been inserted correctly and the tourniquet removed, the flow should be unobstructed. If resistance is felt and injecting fluid causes pain and creates a lump under the skin, then the cannula is not in the vein (it is 'tissued'). Slight withdrawal and re-advancement may be successful but, in most cases, you will need to remove the cannula, put pressure on the injection site to avoid/reduce haematoma, and try again at a different site. If this fails again, be kind to the patient and seriously consider asking a colleague for help.
- *Tape the cannula* in place and give the required drugs or fix the giving set for IV fluids to be started (see Fig. 10.3, p.523).
- If the cannula has been placed in the antecubital fossa, a splint is required to keep the elbow extended, as otherwise the cannula may kink or pierce the vein.

# Setting up an IV infusion

## Equipment

Intravenous giving sets ('drip' sets) are available as disposable units of two types:

- *Type 1*—for blood and blood products, has two chambers, the lower containing a plastic ball valve. Blood can therefore be hand-pumped, from the lower chamber into the patient.
- *Type 2*—for non-sanguinous solutions, has a single chamber only.

You will need a bag of sterile normal saline and an IV giving set, ready filled, with air locks removed. Find out how the system works before inserting the cannula.

Even though the 'drip' might be required for giving other fluids, always start with isotonic saline, as any accidents in setting up the 'drip' will then be less harmful to the patient and will not result in the wastage or spillage of other fluids.

▶The use of two- or three-way taps, or of burette type infusion apparatus, is particularly susceptible to infection.

## Procedure (Fig. 10.3)

*Checking the infusion fluids:* Inspect clear fluids for haziness or turbidity in a good light against a dark background, while the container is inverted and gently shaken. A slight swirl of contaminating material may be seen at this time, but should be undetectable once the container has been shaken. If the fluid is not crystal clear or free from particles, it should not be used as it could be infected. The supernatant plasma of blood bottles should show no haemolysis of fibrin web. The clear fluids include water used to reconstitute dried plasma as well as solutions of dextrose, sodium chloride, etc. When satisfied with the fluid, change the saline drip.

*Changing equipment and cannulae:* Change equipment connected to an IV cannula every 48 h. When giving a slow infusion over a prolonged period, use a small needle and change every 48 h to a new site. Change dressings as often as necessary to keep site dry.

*Injections into giving sets* should be reduced to a minimum. Check first that what you are about to inject is compatible with the solution in the infusion set. Before injecting into the tubing, clean the injection site with chlorhexidine in 70% spirit and allow to dry.

*Rapid infusion* of IV fluids may be required to maintain life. The first essential then is that a large cannula is inserted into a large vein (doubling the size of the cannula will increase the flow rate 16 times; increasing the head pressure to four times the normal will only double the flow rate). Blood or fluid may be given rapidly either by squeezing or pumping the lower chamber of a blood transfusion giving set, or by using a pressure bag around the IV fluid. If large amounts of stored blood are to be given rapidly, the temperature of the blood should be raised by first circulating the blood through a blood warmer.

⚠ Beware of causing air emboli when squeezing in fluids rapidly. This especially applies towards the end of each infused unit and with changing of IV fluid bags.

*Monitoring:* Check urea and electrolytes daily.

Cephalic vein
Basilic vein
Left hand
Radial border
Ulnar border
Right arm

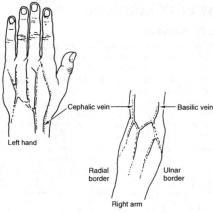

**Fig 10.2** Hand and arm veins

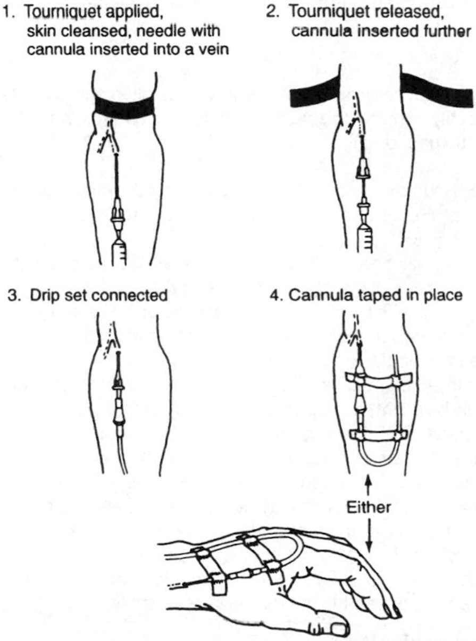

1. Tourniquet applied, skin cleansed, needle with cannula inserted into a vein
2. Tourniquet released, cannula inserted further
3. Drip set connected
4. Cannula taped in place
Either

**Fig 10.3** Setting up an intravenous infusion

# Complications of IV infusions

## Difficulty setting up IV infusions

*Obese patients:* As with venepuncture, you need patience, palpation and correct pressure. Very often the site of a previous successful venepuncture gives a clue. The patient may know from previous experience!

*Hypotensive patients:* The sphygmomanometer is most useful as a tourniquet. Inflate to diastolic pressure (some non-invasive BP [NIBP] machines have a venostasis option). Allow adequate time for the veins to fill and use good lighting. Palpate the veins prior to cannulation.

*The patient with 'no veins':* Although unlikely to occur, you may feel that this is the case with some patients. The patient may know from previous experience, and those with problems arising because of vein loss from IV drug abuse may offer to help themselves! When a suitable vein cannot be found:

- Go systematically through the sites of venepuncture both looking and feeling. Use a sphygmomanometer.
- Imersion of the hand (the patients!) in warm water (40°C) may reveal veins for a short period.
- Ask a colleague to help.
- In an emergency, an ordinary 20 gauge needle may be inserted into a small vein and enough fluid pumped through this to maintain life, or ask for help to do a cut-down on other sites, such as saphenous, jugular or subclavian veins.

## 'Drip' failure

If you see that the drip is not working but the arm is swollen and tender, the cannula has probably pierced the vein and fluid infused into the subcutaneous tissues (a 'tissued' drip).

- Remove the drip.
- If the arm is inflamed, send the cannula tip for bacteriological examination.
- If IV fluids are still required, put another up in another site.
- If the drip has not 'tissued':
  - Check that the drip has been fully opened and that there is nothing constricting the arm (e.g. sphygmomanometer cuff).
  - Inspect the site. If it is inflamed, is the vein tender, or is thrombophlebitis present? In either case, take the drip down immediately. Again, send the cannula tip for culture.
  - If the site is not inflamed, it is likely that the vein has clotted or is in spasm. If the clot is recent, it may be dislodged by gentle pressure from a syringe containing either sterile saline or citrate solution. Use even and firm pressure and a small quantity of fluid (<10 mL), because of the danger of embolism. The use of low dose heparin (50 units of Hepsal or 200 units of Hep Flush) injected every 6 h will reduce drip failure without producing identifiable anticoagulation, but should be avoided if there is a bleeding tendency.
  - If the drip is just going slowly, flush out the cannula with citrate solution or raise the bottle of IV fluid as high as possible.

## Superficial thrombophlebitis

- Mostly caused by chemical irritation.

- Presents with local pain, swelling and erythema.
- Remove the cannula and apply warm (50°C) saline packs to the area.

## Fever

⚠ Septicaemia uncommonly can develop in patients receiving IV therapy but the consequences may be serious or even fatal.

Micro-organisms may be introduced in several ways:
- Contamination before use (rare).
- Contamination during the setting up, or course of the infusion.
- Infected material introduced into the drip. Some Gram-negative bacilli grow rapidly in solutions at room temperature. Some solutions are particularly liable to grow micro-organisms—the anaesthetic, propofol is a good example. Do not use multidose containers more than once if for IV use.
- Infection may occur where the cannula enters the skin, especially if this area remains moist or if the cannula is not inserted aseptically.
- The cannula may cause venous thrombosis, which may become infected and be a source of septic emboli.

When a patient receiving IV fluids develops a pyrexia for no apparent reason, the IV apparatus should be considered a possible source of infection. Then:
- Take a bacteriological swab from the injection site.
- Send to the microbiology laboratory in a polythene bag, the infusion bottle, drip set and cannula, plus any recently used containers of IV fluids or drugs, which have been injected.
- Take a blood culture.
- If the patient is seriously ill, or if it is suspected that the fluid in the container may be contaminated, inform a consultant microbiologist urgently.

## Embolization of catheter material

Take great care not to divide the cannula and cause an embolus.

## Circulatory overload

Fluids infused too rapidly or in large quantities, particularly to elderly patients or those with cardiac failure, may cause circulatory overload. This may precipitate congestive cardiac failure with pulmonary oedema (persistent cough; frothy, sometimes pink blood-stained sputum; dyspnoea), visibly distended neck veins, and crepitations on chest auscultation.

*Avoid fluid overload by:*
- infusing slowly;
- using CVP line in ill patients;
- using packed red cells rather then whole blood;
- giving a diuretic (e.g. 20–40 mg furosemide).

*Manage any fluid overload by:*
- stopping the infusion;
- giving a diuretic such as furosemide 20–40 mg IV;
- giving subcutaneous morphine 15 mg;
- administering oxygen;
- nursing in the sitting position.

# Blood transfusion

## Caution

Blood transfusion must not be undertaken lightly. Many patients have concerns about the possibility of transmission of blood borne agents, not unreasonably as there is a history of transmission of hepatitis viruses, HIV and prions; and some (e.g. Jehovah's witnesses) have religious objections.

▶Wherever possible, the patient's own blood should be used (autologous transfusion).

## Indications for transfusion

Loss of <10% of blood volume may well be compensated naturally, and no transfusion required. However, if losses >20%, or if the haemoglobin level falls <7 g/dL, blood transfusion is usually required.

Failure to transfuse may lead to:
• persistent hypotension;
• hypovolaemic shock;
• acute renal failure.

Dental patients who could need a blood transfusion include those who:
• have suffered severe trauma;
• undergo major surgery, particularly around the carotid;
• undergo surgery to vascular disorder (e.g. large haemangioma);
• have bleeding tendencies;
• are severely anaemic preoperatively.

▶Packed red blood cells are preferred for non-acute transfusions, as they reduce the possibility of fluid overload.

## Grouping and cross-matching

Where possible, blood should be obtained from the patient several weeks before surgery for later autologous transfusion, or grouped and cross-matched before major surgery as required. Otherwise, full blood grouping and cross-matching, are essential. This can take up to 3 h but, in an emergency, rapid cross-matching can be done in 20–40 min. This may be less reliable.

### Taking the blood sample

The chief danger in blood transfusion is the administration of the wrong blood. This should be minimized by ensuring that (see also Chapter 3):
• blood specimens for grouping and matching are taken from the correct patient and fully labelled with the patient's first and second names and hospital number;
• blood to be transfused is carefully double checked for the patient's name and number;
• the request form for blood transfusion and the details on the blood specimen bottle are completed by the person taking the sample;
• details should never be copied from the request form on to the sample bottle label (when collecting specimens from several patients, it is easy to make a mistake, particularly if there are two patients of the same name, but with slightly different details).

**Administering blood or blood products** (Table 10.19, page 526)

- Blood will usually be supplied as packed cells (plasma, platelets and white blood cells removed).
- One unit (250–300 mL) of blood will approximately raise the Hb by 1g/dL.
- Make a final check of identity by the patient's wrist bracelet. It is occasionally necessary to remove a patient's identity bracelet, for example, in the operating theatre to gain access to the veins in the wrist. This is a potentially dangerous situation, as the patient is unconscious and separated from his/her case notes. It is therefore important that, in such circumstances, the identification label should be removed from the old bracelet, put in a new one, and attached to the patient as soon as possible.
- A second person should check the blood with the patient's identity.
- As a general rule, routine transfusions should be given during the daytime as they can be more readily constantly observed.
- A small cannula, preferably a plastic type, is less traumatic than the needle and should be used, particularly for prolonged transfusions.
- Avoid flexures; try to preserve veins and avoid 'cutting down'.
- Care of veins, particularly in repeated or prolonged transfusion, is of paramount importance, particularly in renal patients.
- Monitor urine output and blood urea (and fibrin degradation products if using stored blood).
- 10 mL of 10% calcium gluconate IV may be necessary to correct for the chelating action of the citrate anticoagulant, but it may cause cardiac irregularities and therefore should be given slowly with EGC monitoring. Calcium gluconate should not be used where <3 L of blood have been given.
- Never add any drug to blood intended for transfusion. If a drug is to be administered at the same time as blood, give the drug through a Y-tube inserted into the transfusion apparatus.
- Dextrose solutions are irritant; do not give these through the same giving set as blood, or sludging or thrombophlebitis can occur.
- Incompatibility reactions may be masked by GA; therefore, always monitor the patient's temperature.
- In rapid transfusion of packed cells remember to include normal saline or colloid solution in the regimen (1L of normal saline or 500 mL of colloid solution to 2 units of packed cells).
- Monitor Hb, Plt, clotting screen, acid–base status, $K^+$ and $Ca^{2+}$.

**Table 10.19** Blood and blood products[a]

| Source | Product | Used in | Comments |
|---|---|---|---|
| Whole blood | Autologous blood | Elective surgery | Avoids cross-infection and transfusion reactions |
| | Whole blood | Acute blood loss of more than 1 L | With massive transfusions there might be citrate-induced bleeding tendency or citrate intoxication. Stored blood may cause hyper-kalaemia and has relatively few platelets. Whole blood may cause circulatory overload. |
| Red blood cells | Packed red cells | All non-acute transfusions | Less likely than whole blood to cause circulatory overload. More economic since plasma is saved for other uses. |
| | Washed red blood cells | Patients who have had repeated hypersensitivity reactions to blood or components | |
| | Leukoreduced red blood cells | Patients who have experienced two or more non-haemolytic febrile transfusion reactions | |
| | Paediatric/ divided RBC Units | Infants who require small amounts of red cells | |
| Platelets | Platelet concentrates | Bleeding tendency caused by thrombo-cytopenia or platelet dysfunction (including leukaemia) | Limited shelf life (3–5 days depending on storage conditions). Do not administer without consulting haematologists. |
| Leucocytes | Granulocytes (neutrophils) | Patients with severe neutropenia (<200/µL) and a documented life-threatening bacterial or fungal infection | |

**Table 10.19** Contd.

| Source | Product | Used in | Comments |
|---|---|---|---|
| Plasma | Human plasma protein fraction | Severe burns | Unsuitable for use in bleeding tendency. |
| | Fresh frozen plasma (FFP) | Patients with multiple coagulation defects (e.g. liver disease) | Contains all clotting factors. |
| | Cryoprecipitate (CRYO) | Hypofibrino-genaemia | Contains factor VIII and von Willebrand factor and fibrinogen with some factor XIII and fibronectin. Less effective than factor VIII in haemophilia A. |
| | | Haemophilia | |
| Factor concentrates | Factor VIII | Haemophilia A and von Willebrands disease | |
| | Factor IX | Haemophilia B | |
| | Antithrombin III | Patients with symptomatic, congenital antithrombin III deficiency | |
| CMV Negative, Irradiated, and Leukoreduced Preparations | CMV negative blood and components | Immuno-compromised patients | |
| | Irradiated blood and components | Bone marrow transplant | Irradiation destroys the ability of transfused lymphocytes to respond to host foreign antigens thereby preventing graft versus host disease. |
| | Leukoreduced blood and components | To restrict leucocyte sensitization | |
| | | | Used mainly in aplastic anaemia, thalassaemia, or where there are antibodies from pregnancies or earlier transfusions. |

[a] Blood products are preferred to whole blood since they are less likely to transmit diseases such as hepatitis B; hepatitis C; HIV, prions; better patient management is achieved by giving only the desired and/or essential component; they have a greater shelf life; and they can often be infused regardless of blood group.

# Complications of transfusion

## Minor transfusion reactions

*Presentation*

Pyrexia ± urticaria.

*Management*

- Slow the rate of transfusion.
- Administer an antihistamine, e.g. chlorphenamine 10 mg IM.
- If no improvement within 30 min, stop the transfusion.
- Keep the blood and kit for testing.

## Severe incompatibility reactions

*Presentation*

Pyrexia, rigors, backache, vomiting, collapse, oliguria and haemoglobinuria, facial flushing, angioedema, hypotension and bronchospasm.

*Management*

- Stop the transfusion.
- Summons a physician for advice.
- Check the details of the patient with the labels on the blood pack.
- Take blood samples from the patient, from a vein away from the infusion site (preferably another limb), for:
  - Grouping, crossmatching, and assay for incomplete antibodies;
  - Hb estimation.
- Keep the blood and kit for testing. Send the remaining donor blood and any remains of previously transfused blood to the laboratory for:
  - re-crossmatching;
  - Gram-stain;
  - culture.
- There is no specific treatment, but the patient's BP must be maintained by the use of vasopressor agents, IV hydrocortisone and a suitable volume expander, until more blood can be cross-matched.
- Check urine output, specific gravity (SG) and haemoglobin. Low output or persistent SG <1.01 indicates renal damage; consult a physician as a matter of urgency.

## Delayed incompatibility reactions

Should jaundice appear on 1st–3rd day following transfusion, associated with an unexpected fall in the patient's haemoglobin level, inform the laboratory and supply clotted blood samples for detection of antibodies.

## Bacterial contamination of blood

- Some bacteria, e.g. *Eschericha coli*, can survive at refrigerator temperature (4°C). They multiply at higher temperatures and therefore, never leave blood out of the refrigerator for more than 30 min before use.
- Never give blood if the supernatant plasma is red rather than yellowish, as this implies haemolysis, possibly from infection.
- Never transfuse from a damaged blood pack.

- Accidental transfusion of infected blood is extremely dangerous and causes bacteraemia or septicaemia, with pyrexia, vomiting, diarrhoea hypotension and sometimes haemorrhages.

For measures to avoid the risk of infection from IV infusions, see pages 522 and 524.

### Circulatory overload (see earlier in this chapter)

The danger of this can be reduced by:
- transfusing slowly;
- transfusing packed red cells rather than whole blood;
- giving a diuretic, e.g. furosemide 20–40 mg.

### Citrate toxicity

Massive transfusions, particularly to patients with liver disease, may cause citrate toxicity, manifesting with tremors and ECG changes.
*Avoid by* giving a slow injection IV of 10 mL 10% calcium gluconate with every second bottle of blood, in long continuous transfusions—and monitor the ECG.

### Potassium toxicity

Stored blood tends to haemolyse, releasing potassium. Therefore, a massive transfusion of stored blood may produce hyperkalaemia and can affect cardiac function, even producing cardiac arrest. Hyperkalaemia may be combated by administering non-potassium sparing diuretics (eg. Furosemide), ± bicarbonate and reducing $K^+$ intake.

### Bleeding tendency

*Massive transfusions*

Stored blood also has low levels of platelets and coagulation factors. Therefore, massive transfusions of stored blood (15 units plus) need the addition of platelet concentrates (6 units) and fresh frozen plasma (4 units) to restore haemostatic activity. Send blood for clotting screen and ask haematologist to advise.

*Incompatible blood*

When incompatible blood is given during operation, there may be unexplained hypotension or sudden diffuse and spontaneous bleeding. In this event, 500 mL fresh frozen plasma may be of value in replacing missing coagulation factors.

### Late complications

See Chapter 4 on HIV and viral forms of hepatitis transmitted by blood transfusion.

# Discharge of hospital patients

## Routine discharge

- The patient, partner and relatives should be forewarned as accurately as possible of the date and time of intended discharge.
- Inform the Admissions Officer and, if transport is needed, also the Ambulance Officer, well in advance of the planned discharge (1–2 days at least, where possible). The Ward Sister may agree to do this for you.
- On, or before, the day of discharge, write a discharge letter and give to the patient for delivery to their GP, briefing the GP on the patient's condition and treatment, including the following information:
  - Date of admission.
  - Diagnosis on admission.
  - Operation carried out (and date).
  - Subsequent progress.
  - Date of discharge.
  - Condition on discharge/medications.
  - Follow up treatment required (e.g. suture removal).
  - Any special points of note (e.g. complications).
  - Date of follow up appointment at out-patients.
- Arrange for community care, where necessary, with the district nurse.
- Arrange an out-patient follow-up appointment.
- Arrange for the patient to take or collect from the GDP or GP any necessary long-term medication.
- Give a sick-note if required.
- Tell the patient what they should expect; for example, how long is any pain or swelling likely to persist and what should be done if there are complications or uncertainty.
- Discharge patients only with the express consent of the specialist responsible.

## Convalescence

Recommendation for convalescence is the responsibility of the consultant in charge of the patient and should be made as early as possible. Referrals are usually made in consultation between the Ward Sister and the Convalescence Secretary or Medical Social Worker.

The medical information given to the Convalescence Home Secretary must be up-to-date with details of all treatment, and must include particulars of any co-existing disease. All drugs needed must be listed and sent with the patient to the Convalescent Home.

## Irregular discharge

- Although it is no part of a dental surgeon's duty to detain patients who are mentally well, against their will, any patient who wishes to take his/her own discharge against medical advice should have the consequences politely explained to them, in the presence of a witness such as the Ward Sister, and this recorded in the case notes.

- Try to contact your immediate senior to see if he can be more persuasive. If you are really concerned because, for example, the patient is postoperative and not in a fit state to discharge themselves, speak immediately to the responsible specialist.
- If the patient still insists on leaving, ask them to sign a statement accepting responsibility for their own discharge, in the presence of a witness. Record the event in the case notes.
- If he/she takes his/her own discharge but refuses to sign such a declaimer, again record the events in the case record, and also ask the witness to sign the case notes, stating that the patient is 'leaving against medical advice'.

### Deaths in hospital

- Inform your consultant immediately.
- All deceased patients must be seen as soon as possible, by a medically qualified individual, in order that the death may be certified.
- The GP should be notified by a medically qualified person at the same time as the death certificate is completed.

USEFUL WEBSITES
www.nhsla.com
(http://www.cdc.gov/handhygiene/).
http://www.emedicine.com/med/PERIOPERATIVE_CARE.htm

# Oral and maxillofacial trauma surgery

# General considerations

Maxillofacial trauma includes injuries to any of the bony or fleshy structures of the face.

The main causes include:
- interpersonal violence associated with the consumption of alcohol (the major cause);
- road traffic accidents (RTAs);
- participation in sports, fights, and other violent acts.

Those most at risk include anyone who drives a vehicle or rides in one, those who do dangerous work or engage in aggressive types of behaviour, those who drink excessive amounts of alcohol, and sportspeople.

Maxillofacial trauma can be prevented by avoiding risk activities and using safety equipment such as:
- Vehicle seatbelts;
- Car air bags;
- Child safety seats;
- Helmets for riding motorcycles or bicycles, skateboarding, ski-ing, snowboarding, car-racing and other sports;
- Safety glasses;
- Mouthguards, masks, and goggles.

## Management of the traumatized patient

The definitive management of maxillofacial fractures, despite the frighteningly severe initial disfigurement, actually comes low on the list of priorities.
- Keeping the patient alive is the main priority.
- Immediate life-threatening problems are mainly:
  - airways embarrassment;
  - blood loss;
  - rising intracranial pressure (because of intracranial bleeding).
- Cervical spine damage may be present; take care not to extend the neck as this may cause paraplegia or death.

Patients with maxillofacial trauma can be divided into those with:
- Fractures of the middle or upper third facial skeleton, commonly because of severe trauma (particularly RTAs or assaults), who are more likely therefore to have their life threatened because of associated:
  - airways obstruction;
  - head injury;
  - serious trauma to other parts, particularly chest injuries, ruptured viscera, eye injuries, fractured cervical or lumbar spine, and fractured long bones with serious internal bleeding.
- Fractures of the mandible, commonly from a simple blow to the jaw, who can be managed by open reduction and internal fixation (ORIF) and who less commonly have associated serious injuries to other parts.

Remember:
- **P:** Posture
- **A:** Airways
- **T:** Tongue traction

- **T**: Tubes/tracheotomy
- **E:** Examination
- **R**: Reassurance of patient
- **N**: Notification of specialists, e.g. neurosurgeons

Record immediately, and every 15 min:
- Conscious state (see Glasgow Coma Scale [GCS], page 558)
- BP (falling may mean haemorrhage or shock; rising may mean intracranial bleeding)
- Pulse rate
- Respiration
- Temperature

▶Remember to keep clear and accurate records, including of timing of events and procedures: medico-legal proceedings are increasingly common.

# Indications for hospital admission

Patients with maxillofacial injuries should be admitted to hospital if there is:
- a danger to the airways (e.g. laryngeal trauma, etc.);
- a child with head injuries;
- any neurological damage
  - any loss or depression of consciousness;
  - post-traumatic amnesia greater than 15 min;
  - local neurological symptoms or signs;
- fractures in the head and neck
  - skull or neck fracture;
  - middle third facial fracture;
  - mandibular fracture (unless undisplaced and treatable conservatively);
  - zygomatic fracture with, or where there is danger of, ocular damage;
- serious internal injury or bleeding;
- a patient living alone, without a responsible companion, or of ↓ responsibility;
- any other indication (see page 478).

▶If patients are not admitted to hospital, they and their partner/relatives must be warned the patient must return immediately to hospital if there is any feature suggesting a neurological complication such as:
- conscious level deteriorating;
- restlessness increasing;
- headache—severe or increasing;
- neck stiffness;
- fits;
- vomiting;
- dizziness;
- ocular symptoms.

# Treatment priorities

Surgical problems following severe injury should be addressed in the following order (NAOM):

- **N**eurosurgical intervention for intracranial bleeding; an urgent neurological opinion is needed if there are any of the following:
  - conscious level deteriorating (deteriorating Glasgow Coma Scale [GCS]);
  - restlessness increasing;
  - headache;
  - neck stiffness;
  - fits or focal signs;
  - vomiting;
  - dilatation of pupils;
  - bradycardia;
  - rising BP.
- **A**bdominal surgery to establish haemostasis, etc.
- **O**rthopaedic surgery.
- **M**axillofacial surgery:
  - soft tissue; repair of wounds and lacerations;
  - fracture; temporary fixation if needed;
  - fractures; definitive care.

# Early management

All traumatized patients should be assessed along the lines of the Advanced Trauma Life Support scheme (ATLS), which is:

*Primary survey*
- **A**: Airways
- **B**: Breathing
- **C**: Circulation, and control of haemorrhage
- **D**: Disability and neurological assessment, including pupils
- **E** : Exposure

The primary survey should be repeated at regular intervals.

*Secondary survey*
A full head to toe examination to identify any other serious or life-threatening problems such as:
- **A**bdominal injuries
- **B**urns
- **C**ranium, CNS injuries, CSF leaks, chest and cervical spine injury
- **D**entoalveolar injuries
- **E**ye and ear injuries
- **F**acial lacerations fractures and foreign bodies
- **G**unshot wounds.

Special attention should be paid to:
- History of events
- Drugs (including alcohol)
- Infection control
- Environmental control (protect the patient from further damage and from hypothermia)

All the above will be discussed in more detail in the following sections.

## History
- The history may be directly relevant in revealing the cause of the maxillofacial injury (e.g. epilepsy).
- In children, remember the possibility of child abuse (non-accidental injury; see page 588).
- Drugs (e.g. anticoagulants) may influence patient management.
- Many patients involved in RTAs and personal violence have been drinking alcohol (a blood alcohol level may be needed) or taking other recreational drugs (check and keep serum sample).
- Unconsciousness after a head injury is usually, but not always, caused by traumatic brain damage—but consider other causes such as diabetics who may lapse into coma if not given their medication or food.

▶It is essential that every patient involved in an assault or accident be examined carefully clinically and radiologically and precise records kept in case notes. Photograph the wounds; they may be of forensic value in subsequent litigation.

# Airways

▶The most important consideration in any maxillofacial fracture is airway preservation—cerebral hypoxia can kill a patient within ~3 min.

## Mechanisms of airways obstruction

The airways can readily obstruct, from a blood clot, a foreign body within (e.g. denture) or, rarely, by displacement of a fractured maxilla down and backwards towards the pharynx. Even with mandibular fractures alone, fragmentation of the anterior part (to which the genial muscles are attached) can allow the tongue to fall back and occlude the airways.

## Management to prevent airways obstruction

▶A crucial part of the initial airways establishment involves securing the cervical spine with a hard cervical collar, until radiology has excluded cervical spine damage.

- Removable obstructions must be cleared immediately.
- Suck the mouth and pharynx clear.
- Simple manoeuvres such as jaw thrusts and chin lifts may help establish an airway.
- Backward displacement of the maxilla (rare) should be reduced by hooking the fingers round the posterior border of the palate and pulling the maxilla forward, steadying the head with the other hand.
- An oropharyngeal airway placed over the tongue will prevent it falling backwards and occluding the air passages. A nasopharyngeal tube is useful if the lumen can be kept patent.
- Frequent suction of the mouth and pharynx may be necessary to keep the airways clear of blood, vomit or secretions.

### Patient position

In the patient without respiratory problems (whether conscious or un-conscious), the simplest way to maintain a clear airway is by correct positioning, prone or semi-prone, with the foot of the bed elevated. In this position the tongue falls forward and any saliva, blood or gastric content will dribble out rather than be aspirated into the trachea. Patients with maxillofacial injuries must therefore, be placed and trans-ported in the tonsillectomy (head down) position (Fig. 11.1) to allow fluids to drain out of the mouth.

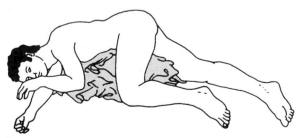

**Fig. 11.1** The tonsillar or head injury position

*Stridor*

Stridor is the inspiratory sound produced by turbulent flow of air through a narrowed segment of the respiratory tract, and may be due to:
- spasm or paralysis of the vocal cords;
- a foreign body or plug of mucus in the larynx;
- laryngeal oedema (may result from trauma, but this can take up to 12–24 h to develop).

In any patient with stridor, laryngoscopy must be carried out as an emergency procedure.

*Laryngoscopy*
- Stand behind the supine patient.
- Spray the fauces and pharynx with 4% lidocaine.
- Insert the laryngoscope.
- Check the vocal cords and their movements.

# Endotracheal intubation

In patients with acute respiratory obstruction, or in whom cardiac arrest has occurred, endotracheal intubation is one of the most important and life-saving measures.

## Equipment
- Macintosh laryngoscope.
- Magill forceps.
- Endotracheal tubes (orotracheal and nasotracheal). For females, a number 7–9 tube is usually adequate; for males, size 8–11 are suitable, depending on the build of the patient. Synthetic plastic tubes are better for long-term use.

## Procedure
- If the patient is unconscious, it is rarely necessary to use muscle relaxants before intubation.
- If the patient is conscious, expert care is required from a clinician experienced in intubation. An IV GA with a muscle relaxant such as 50 mg suxamethonium to relax the vocal cords will need to be administered. Consideration of the possibility of a full stomach must be made. Intubation in this situation is a potentially hazardous procedure and the clinician should ensure that they are able to ventilate the patient by mask before proceeding, and be capable of securing an airway surgically if it is not possible to pass the endotracheal tube. Ventilation thereafter must be assisted. The houseman/intern therefore must never attempt to carry out this procedure on his/her own.
- Stand behind the supine patient.
- Remove any dentures.
- Insert the laryngoscope and push the tongue to the left (Fig. 11.2). Aspirate the mouth and pharynx. Orotracheal intubation is the usual method for emergencies. Nasotracheal intubation is usually used when the patient is to be intubated to allow oral procedures.
- Hold the endotracheal tube ready lubricated (with lidocaine gel) in the right hand and with the left hand pull the laryngoscope upwards to expose the epiglottis and vocal cords (see Fig. 11.2). As the cords come into view, slip the tube into the trachea using Magill forceps.
- Inflate the cuff and connect the tube to an inflation bag. If the tube is properly inserted, the chest should move uniformly with manual ventilation and both lung fields should be auscultated with a stethoscope. The cuff ensures that the trachea is air-tight and prevents aspiration of gastric contents, blood or saliva.

An endotracheal tube should not be left in position for more than about 48 h. With the newer PVC tubes, this period may be extended slightly, but tracheostomy must be considered if intubation is required for more than 7 days.

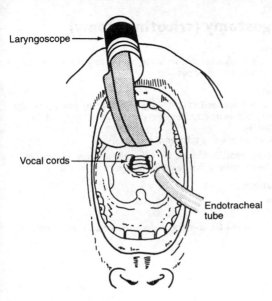

**Fig. 11.2** Endotracheal intubation

# Laryngostomy (cricothyrotomy)

### Indications

Acute laryngeal obstruction or acute respiratory failure when an endotracheal tube cannot be passed.

### Technique

- Thrust a wide bore needle (12–14-gauge), or cricothyrotome, through the cricothyroid membrane, between the thyroid cartilage and the cricoid cartilage.
- Connect this needle to a cylinder of oxygen.

This *temporary* procedure must be followed, as soon as possible, by formal tracheostomy and closure of the laryngostomy wound.

### Complications

- Laryngitis
- Laryngeal stenosis

However, if used as a life-saving procedure, these risks are justifiable.

# Tracheostomy: procedure

### Indications (Fig. 11.3)

Tracheostomy (tracheotomy) is reserved for patients in whom intubation is expected to be needed for more than 7 days. It should be done as an elective procedure, in the operating theatre or intensive care unit, under a GA and with an endotracheal tube in position before starting. It should not be done as an emergency procedure because:

- it is not easy or quick to perform;
- division of the thyroid isthmus during the procedure may lead to dangerous bleeding;
- if improperly sited, it may require revision.

### Tracheostomy tubes

Modern tracheostomy tubes are sterile packed single use polyvinyl chloride or silicone with a double lumen changeable inner tube to facilitate cleaning. These tubes have low pressure cuffs to minimize tracheal trauma.

For the average male, French gauge sizes 36–39 should be suitable, and for females, sizes 33–36. To aid selection, the surgeon should consult the anaesthetist as to the size of the endotracheal tube used during the GA.

### Procedure

- Warn the patient, partner and relatives that the patient will be able to speak after the tracheostomy only once a speaking tube is inserted.
- Use sterile technique in theatre.
- Make a transverse 4–5 cm incision in the neck skin, midway between the cricoid cartilage and the suprasternal notch. Divide the tissues down to the deep fascia. Divide the strap muscles vertically in the midline, retract them to expose the trachea. All bleeding must be stopped before making further incisions.
- It is imperative that the first tracheal cartilage is not incised, or tracheal stenosis will occur. It may not be possible to see tracheal rings 2–3 because of overlying thyroid tissue. If this is the case, retract or divide the thyroid isthmus. Clamp either side of the thyroid gland and divide it to expose the trachea.
- At this point it is worthwhile comparing the size of the trachea with the proposed tracheostomy tube.
- Withdraw the endotracheal tube a little before opening the trachea, usually between the second and third rings so that if difficulties arise, the tube may be replaced rapidly.
- Select the appropriate tracheostomy tube and check the connections to the anaesthetic equipment, as well as patency of the cuff.
- Cut out a circular hole in the trachea, after placing artery or tissue forceps on the cartilage so that there is no change of the portion removed falling into the trachea, or use an inferiorly based flap (Bjork flap), suturing the tracheal cartilage to the skin.
- Insert the tracheostomy tube as rapidly as possible. If the patient is anaesthetized and paralysed, there will be no oxygen reaching the lungs during this time; intubation must therefore be carried out with speed.

- Inflate the cuff of the tracheostomy tube and loosely suture the ends of the wound. Knot the tapes of the tube securely at the back of the neck.
- The tracheostomy tube itself may then be sutured to the skin.

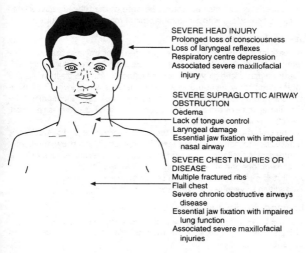

SEVERE HEAD INJURY
Prolonged loss of consciousness
Loss of laryngeal reflexes
Respiratory centre depression
Associated severe maxillofacial injury

SEVERE SUPRAGLOTTIC AIRWAY OBSTRUCTION
Oedema
Lack of tongue control
Laryngeal damage
Essential jaw fixation with impaired nasal airway

SEVERE CHEST INJURIES OR DISEASE
Multiple fractured ribs
Flail chest
Severe chronic obstructive airways disease
Essential jaw fixation with impaired lung function
Associated severe maxillofacial injuries

**Fig. 11.3** Maxillofacial surgical indications for tracheostomy

# Tracheostomy: care

### The conscious patient and the tracheostomy tube

Some conscious patients with a tracheostomy tube or endotracheal tube rapidly adapt to the situation, even if assisted ventilation is being used. Reassurance and explanation may then be all that is required.

Other conscious patients get restless because of the tube, and associated injuries. Sedation (e.g. with a benzodiazepine) may then be required.

### Care of the tracheostomy

- At least initially, the patient will require frequent tracheal toilet to remove retained secretions. This must be a sterile procedure, carried out using masks and gloves. Insert the catheter into the trachea using forceps and apply suction only as the catheter is withdrawn. The catheter is inserted into one main bronchus, then the other. Depending on the clinical state of the patient, suction is repeated as often as required (which may initially be every 15–30 min).
- As the cuff of the tracheostomy tube causes pressure on the trachea, it is necessary to deflate it for at least 5 min every 2 h to prevent ulceration/necrosis. Deflation often induces coughing; therefore, suck out the trachea before and after deflation, and after re-inflation.
- Aspirate hourly—and every 48 h send aspirate for culture.
- Humidified oxygen will prevent secretions hardening.

### Changing the tracheostomy tube

- Cut the tapes securing the tube and remove the dressings.
- Using sterile technique, suck out the tracheostomy, deflate the cuff and use suction again.
- Gently remove the tube and insert a new one of similar size. A smaller tube must always be available in case the tube cannot readily be inserted.
- Repeat the suction.
- If the tracheostomy is likely to be required for more than 2–3 days, ensure that a double lumen tube is used, as the inner sleeve can easily be changed to keep the lumen patent. In prolonged tracheostomies, an inner speaking tube can be used.

### Finally removing the tracheostomy tube

- Remove the tube at the earliest possible moment compatible with the clinical state of the patient, to minimize the complications associated with long-term tracheostomy (see below).
- Before removing the tube, a fenestrated tube should be exchanged, and over the following 2–3 days the external stoma should be capped for increasing periods of time, to encourage speech and breathing through the upper airways.
- The tube should be removed first thing in the morning, for staffing reasons.
- If the trachea and upper air passages are patent, the patient should then be able to speak and breathe normally.

- As with the changing of the tracheostomy tube, always have a second, smaller tube available in case there is laryngeal obstruction, or obstruction at the stoma.
- The patient must be closely observed over the first few hours after tube removal, for any increasing respiratory difficulty or stridor. If these occur, immediately re-intubate. A lateral soft tissue radiograph of the neck may be needed, to exclude obstruction higher up in the trachea, for instance an area of granulation tissue above the tube, which, on tube removal, may block the tracheal lumen.
- After successful removal of the tube, it is usually unnecessary to suture the wound; just place a simple dressing.

## Complications of tracheostomy

- Obstruction of tube: deflate cuff and replace tube.
- Tube displacement: re-locate.
- Bleeding from tracheal ulceration: remove the source of pressure.
- Infection: avoid by using an aseptic technique; treat with antimicrobials.
- Tracheal stenosis.
- Tracheo-oesophageal fistula due to ulceration/erosion.

## Other factors affecting breathing

Airways patency does not guarantee adequate ventilation; good gas exchange is required. Each component of ventilation (lungs, chest wall, diaphragm) should be examined, if problems with the tracheostomy cannot explain a compromised gas exchange.

The following injuries will impair ventilation and must be identified and treated:

- tension pneumothorax;
- flail chest with pulmonary contusions;
- open pneumothorax;
- haemothorax or chylothorax;
- fractured ribs with pulmonary contusion.

# Bleeding

## Sources of serious bleeding

Serious internal bleeding may be concealed, for example into the abdomen from a ruptured viscus (particularly the spleen) or into the thigh from a fractured femur.

Nose bleeds that do not cease spontaneously after pressure or after packing with 0.5 inch ribbon gauze, may be controlled with a postnasal gauze pack or by using a Foley balloon catheter passed through the nose into the nasopharynx, softly inflated and then pulled gently against the posterior nasal choanae.

Maxillofacial injuries alone, unless associated with a split palate or gunshot wounds rarely cause severe haemorrhage. A ruptured inferior alveolar artery usually stops bleeding spontaneously, but bleeding may recur if, for example, there is traction on the mandible. Severe maxillofacial bleeding may be tamponaded with craniofacial fixation. If bleeding recurs, the damaged vessel must be ligated, at open operation if necessary.

## Possible serious consequences

- Severe haemorrhage (especially abdominally) can lead to shock and:
  - cardiac failure;
  - renal failure;
  - cerebral hypoxia (fatal).
- Haemorrhage into the pleural cavity from fractured ribs can embarrass respiration.
- Haemorrhage into the cranial cavity can be life-threatening by pressure on higher centres.

## Assessment

Rapidly assess the haemodynamic status by:
- pulse;
- BP;
- conscious level;
- skin colour.

Latent haemorrhage can be recognized by:
- skin colour;
- increasing pulse rate;
- falling BP;
- increasing pallor;
- air hunger;
- restlessness;
- decreasing consciousness;
- abdominal rigidity and increasing girth (if there is intra-abdominal bleeding).

▶A rising BP and slow pulse, by contrast, may indicate rising intracranial pressure produced by cerebral bleeding or oedema.

## Management

If severe haemorrhage occurs, or is suspected:
- Establish an IV line (see page 520).
- Take blood for grouping and cross-matching.
- Seek a surgical opinion and begin a thorough secondary survey.
- Organize quarter-, or half-hourly, observations of:
  - pulse rate,
  - BP,
  - respiratory rate,
  - conscious level.
- Organize daily observations of:
  - urine output,
  - fluid balance.
- Blood transfusion is not needed to replace losses of less than 1000 mL in an adult, unless there was pre-existing anaemia, deterioration of the general condition, or ongoing significant blood loss. (see Chapter 10.)

# Head injuries

- Head injuries are usually associated with some degree of brain damage.
- The brain is invariably damaged to some degree when consciousness has been lost, even briefly, and sometimes when it has not.
- Head injuries with severe primary brain injury can cause death before the patient reaches hospital, or within the first few days.
- Head injuries are also the main cause of permanent disability in patients with maxillofacial injuries.
- Prolonged or increasing loss of consciousness is indicative of serious brain damage (or of other disease interfering with brain function).
- Many patients, even if not comatose, are confused after the injury. Witnesses are needed to give an account of events. Relatives or friends may be able to fill in the patient's medical background.
- Skull fractures and even mild head injuries can cause extra- or subdural haematomas (see page 234), causing increased intracranial pressure, secondary brain damage and possible death.
- Several other factors can contribute to secondary brain damage:
  - airways obstruction;
  - hypotension;
  - meningitis;
  - concomitant causes of coma.
- It is crucial to establish a baseline level of neurological function and monitor progress with regard to 'neurological observations' using a chart such as in Fig. 11.4.
- For analgesia avoid opiates, as they mask clinical signs and cause respiratory depression, but rather give codeine phosphate 10–20 mg IM.

## Examination of the head

Examination of the head is extremely important and may reveal:
- fractures,
- scalp wounds (particularly in the occipital region),
- leakage of cerebrospinal fluid (nose, ears or throat).

## Important investigations

- Radiographs (see Chapter 3).
- CT scan.
- Blood analyses (particularly glucose).
- Urinalysis.

Skull radiography may particularly be indicated in:
- loss of consciousness;
- amnesia;
- CSF leaks (see page 560);
- suspected or known penetrating wounds;
- scalp bruising or swelling;
- fits.

## Neurological observations

See next section.

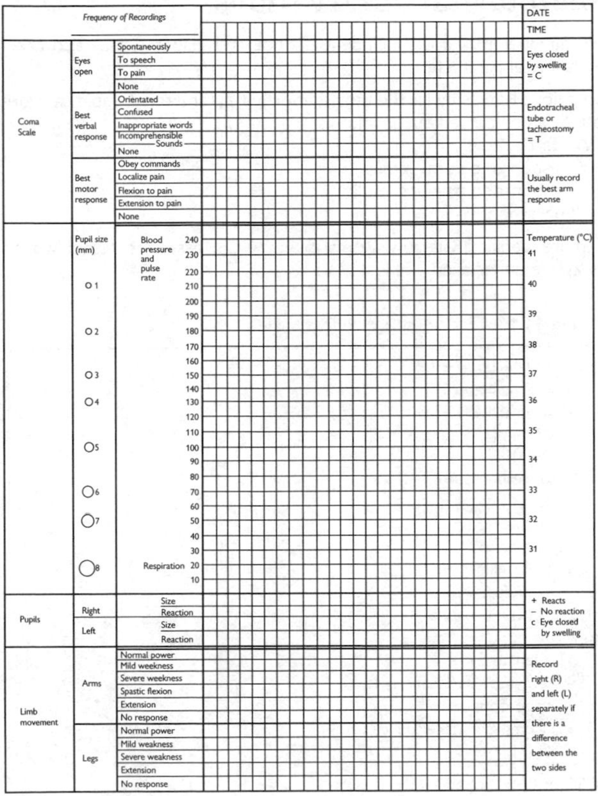

| | | | Frequency of Recordings | DATE |
| | | | | TIME |

| Coma Scale | Eyes open | Spontaneously | | Eyes closed by swelling = C |
| | | To speech | | |
| | | To pain | | |
| | | None | | |
| | Best verbal response | Orientated | | Endotracheal tube or tacheostomy = T |
| | | Confused | | |
| | | Inappropriate words | | |
| | | Incomprehensible Sounds | | |
| | | None | | |
| | Best motor response | Obey commands | | Usually record the best arm response |
| | | Localize pain | | |
| | | Flexion to pain | | |
| | | Extension to pain | | |
| | | None | | |

Pupil size (mm)
O 1
O 2
O 3
O 4
O 5
O 6
O 7
O 8

Blood pressure and pulse rate
240 230 220 210 200 190 180 170 160 150 140 130 120 110 100 90 80 70 60 50 40 30
Respiration 20 10

Temperature (°C)
41 40 39 38 37 36 35 34 33 32 31

| Pupils | Right | Size | | + Reacts |
| | | Reaction | | – No reaction |
| | Left | Size | | c Eye closed by swelling |
| | | Reaction | | |

| Limb movement | Arms | Normal power | | Record right (R) and left (L) separately if there is a difference between the two sides |
| | | Mild weekness | | |
| | | Severe weekness | | |
| | | Spastic flexion | | |
| | | Extension | | |
| | | No response | | |
| | Legs | Normal power | | |
| | | Mild weakness | | |
| | | Severe weakness | | |
| | | Extension | | |
| | | No response | | |

**Fig. 11.4** Neurological observation chart

# Neurological observations

▶Remember that drugs including alcohol, and diabetes, may also affect neurological parameters.

Conscious level is by far the most important parameter. A rapid categorisation can be carried out as follows:
- **A**: alert
- **V**: response to vocal stimuli
- **P**: response to painful stimuli
- **U**: unresponsive

A more detailed Glasgow Coma Scale (GCS) assessment should then always be undertaken (Table 11.1).

**Table 11.1** GCS or Responsiveness Scale

- Eye opening *(E: 1–4)*
  - spontaneous (4)
  - to speech (3)
  - to pain (2)
  - nil (1)
- Motor response *(M: 1–6)*
  - obeys (6)
  - localizes (5)
  - withdraws (4)
  - abnormal flexion (3)
  - extends (2)
  - nil (1)
- Verbal response *(V: 1–5)*
  - orientated (5)
  - confused conversation (4)
  - inappropriate words (3)
  - incomprehensible sounds (2)
  - nil (1)

*GCS (or EMV) score: 3–15*

15: normal, 13–14: minor head injury, 9–12: moderate head injury, <8: coma

More detailed examination is warranted when the history or the GCS are suggestive of head injury (Fig. 11.4, see p.557).
- Pupil reaction, pupil size and cranial nerve function
- Pulse
- BP
- Respiratory rate and pattern

Signs and symptoms that suggest development of neurological complications and indicate the urgent need for a neurosurgical opinion include:
- conscious level deteriorating;
- coma continuing after resuscitation;
- increasing restlessness and behavioural changes;

- depressed fracture of skull vault;
- penetrating injury to brain;
- fracture of the skull base (CSF leak, haematoma over mastoid [Battle's sign]);
- headache;
- vomiting;
- focal signs (e.g. hemiparesis, dysphasia, focal epilepsy);
- dilatation of pupil(s);
- bradycardia;
- rising BP.

# Cerebrospinal fluid leaks

CSF leaks occur in up to 25% of patients with middle third fractures involving the naso-ethmoidal complex because of dural tears. CSF leak should be assumed in all high-level facial fractures.

▶ CSF leaks predispose to meningitis, with serious consequences.

### Diagnosis of CSF leaks

CSF leaks may occur either from the nose or into the nasopharynx (CSF rhinorrhoea) or from the ear (CSF otorrhoea). If a CSF leak is not visible, but the patient complains of an intermittent salty taste, place him/her prone, tipped with the face downwards, to provoke an obvious flow of CSF from the nose. CSF is a watery, clear fluid, often disguised in the early stages by bleeding. CSF can be differentiated by its high sugar (use Clinistix) and low protein content (electrophoresis) from serous nasal discharge or lacrimal fluid (which both have a high protein content). The gold standard for laboratory diagnosis of CSF fistulae is beta-2-transferrin. Radionuclide cisternography using technetium 99-labelled albumin (half-life 6 h) and indium 111-labelled DTPA (half-life 2.8 days) may be useful when a CSF leak is in question.

### Management if CSF leak present or suspected

- Medical management consists of elevation of the head of bed and avoidance of coughing, sneezing, blowing the nose or straining at stool.
- Reduction of the fracture is the most effective method of treating the CSF leak. Indeed, a CSF leak in a patient who has facial fractures may spontaneously close when the fractures are reduced.
- The use of prophylactic antibiotics is controversial, with no evidence of efficacy, and the possibility of inducing resistant pathogens. Rifampicin (600 mg 12-hourly for 2 days) is used by some, as it reaches the CSF in adequate concentrations and is effective against most of the bacterial causes of post-traumatic meningitis. Metronidazole is used by some. Penicillin is inadequate as prophylaxis against meningitis. The traditional use of sulphadiazine is no longer indicated, because of the many resistant bacteria, particularly *Neisseria meningitidis*.
- If persisting for more than 10 days, CSF leaks demand a neurosurgical opinion, as dural repair may be necessary.

# Other important injuries

### Cervical spine injuries

- Cervical spine injuries are not infrequent in RTAs and some contact sports (especially rugby).
- Never extend the neck of a traumatized patient until it has been established that the cervical spine is indeed intact, otherwise you may cause spinal cord damage → paralysis or death.

### Chest injuries

If there has been trauma to the chest, careful examination and radiographs are required to exclude:

- cardiac or great vessel damage;
- fractured ribs;
- pneumothorax;
- haemothorax;
- lung collapse;
- mediastinal shift;
- air under the diaphragm (suggests rupture of an abdominal viscus)

If the airways are unobstructed, difficulty in breathing associated with paradoxical movements of the chest and cyanosis may indicate a flail chest. Obtain a medical/surgical opinion, as intermittent positive pressure artificial respiration via an endotracheal tube is then needed.

### Abdominal injuries

Traumatic injuries, particularly from RTAs or personal violence may well be associated with serious abdominal or other injuries, which can be life-threatening.

Gathering of evidence for abdominal injury may involve the following:

- Elicit the history to discover evidence of a blow, stab or gunshot to the abdomen, loins or lower back.
- Examine carefully the abdomen, loins and lower back.
- Measure the girth.
- Radiography, ultrasound or peritoneal lavage may help confirm the diagnosis.

Rupture of an abdominal viscus may cause:

- pain,
- abdominal bruising,
- tenderness and guarding,
- increasing girth,
- falling BP,
- rising pulse,
- respiratory embarrassment.

Urinary retention may cause pain or, in the semi-conscious patient, restlessness. However, do not catheterize a patient who is passing only blood per urethram as he/she may have a ruptured urethra. Instead, consult the urologist.

## Eye injuries

- Ophthalmological help should be obtained:
  - Immediately—if there are lacerations of cornea or sclera, ocular concussion, orbital blow-out, or any injury involving internal bleeding or external vitreous leakage.
  - Early—if deep lacerations of the eyelids involving the conjunctiva or extending to the palpebral fissures need to be sutured, if there is any suggestion of loss of visual acuity or of diplopia pre- or postoperatively, or if ocular lesions are suspected from the history or examination. Better safe than sorry!
- Obtain radiographs if there is any possibility of a foreign body having entered the orbit or eye.
- Corneal damage or swollen contused eyes should be treated in the interim with chloramphenicol 1% ointment. An ophthalmologist should be asked to see the patient. Do not apply an eye pad to the traumatized eye as the pad may mask other injuries, or aggravate an existing injury due to pressure

### Diplopia

Diplopia following maxillofacial trauma may be caused by:

- Ocular or orbital oedema;
- Ocular or orbital haemorrhage;
- Ocular or orbital displacement (e.g. blow-out fractures);
- Damage to or entrapment of extra-ocular muscles;
- Damage to cranial nerves III, IV or VI.

Determine whether diplopia is mon- or bin-ocular, as monocular diplopia is most often caused by ocular damage (e.g. lens dislocation).

►Obtain an ophthalmological surgeon's opinion if there is any suggestion of loss of visual acuity or of diplopia pre or postoperatively.

## Ear injuries

- Blood in the external auditory meatus may signify a basal skull fracture, or, more likely, a condylar fracture.
- CSF otorrhoea indicates a basal skull fracture, as may bruising behind the ear (Battle's sign).

# Facial lacerations

## Immediate care

- Facial lacerations can cause profuse haemorrhage, but often appear worse to the patient, partner, relatives and operator than they are.
- Ask relatives and partners, who may be more distressed and upset than the patient, to wait elsewhere.
- Always ask about the accident and any known foreign bodies in the tissues.
- Control bleeding with pressure, diathermy or ties.
- Check for damage to important structures such as the:
  - eyes and eyelids
  - nasolacrimal ducts
  - facial nerve
  - parotid gland or ducts.
- Examine, probe and consider imaging lacerations carefully for foreign bodies such as road dirt, plastic, glass and metal.
- Consider whether you are the best person to repair the wound. The ophthalmologist may be the best person to repair ocular or eyelid wounds. Lips and vermilion borders should be repaired by a specialist.
- In some cases, especially when there is tissue loss, primary closure may not be possible. Consult your senior if in doubt.
- Facial lacerations can, if necessary, because of other more serious injuries, be left for up to 24 h for closure, as long as they are cleaned and dressed with saline packs after haemostasis has been achieved.
- Antimicrobials (e.g. flucloxacillin 250 mg 6-hourly for 5 days) may be needed, particularly if lacerations are old, dirty, or through-and-through.
- Tetanus prophylaxis may be needed (see page 573).
- Photograph the wounds; they may be of forensic value in subsequent litigation.

## Cleaning, debridement and closure of wounds

### Abrasions

- Simple, relatively uncontaminated superficial abrasions should be cleaned with Savlon and sterile saline, and dressed with water-rinsable petrolatum gauze and then dry sterile dressings.
- Abraded skin contaminated with dirt may heal leaving a tattoo, unless thoroughly cleaned. Such lesions should be scrubbed clean under anaesthesia, using a soft brush, irrigating with 10% hydrogen peroxide.

### Lacerations

- Areas suspected of being non-viable by virtue of a bluish colour and diminished capillary return on pressure should be excised until bleeding occurs, along with damaged muscle. Nevertheless, in the face, the good blood supply and significant consequences from losing skin, dictate that as much skin as possible is retained, especially if clean.
- All foreign bodies and dirt should be carefully and thoroughly removed (by scrubbing if necessary). Tattoos and other long-term complications are often caused by failure to remove debris.

- Clean wounds by washing with a mild antiseptic solution such as aqueous chlorhexidine (Savlon; an aqueous solution containing 0.3 g chlorhexidine gluconate and 3 g cetrimide as active ingredients per 100 mL and 2.84% m/v n-propyl alcohol and 0.056% m/v benzyl benzoate as preservatives) and irrigating copiously with sterile normal saline. Do not use hydrogen peroxide; surgical emphysema could result.
- Wounds, except those from high velocity missiles, should then be immediately closed as detailed below.
- Only close lacerations over fractures after first ensuring that they will not be required as access for exploration.

# Suturing of facial lacerations

## Procedure

- LA is often sufficient for suturing, but consider GA if the wounds may:
  - be difficult to anaesthetize with LA,
  - take more than 30 min to repair,
  - involve tissue loss,
  - be large (especially in children or females),
  - involve arterial haemorrhage,
  - involve foreign bodies.
- Facial suturing may be facilitated by the use of operating loupes.
- For most wounds, the placement of deep subcutaneous sutures (3/0 or 4/0 undyed Vicryl [polyglactic acid] on a cutting needle) to approximate severed layers correctly is the most important part of the procedure. The closure of the skin or mucosal layers is then considerably aided, with better function and aesthetics. This is especially important in areas such as the lips and vermilion borders.
- For skin wounds, tissue adhesives and skin tapes (Steri-strip) may be valuable in certain cases (especially in children) where the wound edges are not under great tension.
- For skin suturing, a monofilament non-resorbable material such as 5/0 or 6/0 nylon on a fine cutting needle is associated with less skin scarring and a lower rate of wound infection compared with multifilament sutures.
- Take mucosa bites of ~3 mm from the wound edge and space sutures by ~5 mm so that the edges lie correctly together, and aim for slight eversion of the edges.
- Corners need a special closure technique to avoid ischaemia (ask an experienced colleague to demonstrate).
- The lip vermilion border and eyebrows need very careful alignment.
- For most oral wounds, insert sutures of 3/0 vicryl ~5–10 mm apart.

### Care of sutures

- Clean wounds twice daily (except the first 2 days, when the wound should be left undisturbed) with Savlon.
- Apply Polyfax ointment (polymyxin B sulphate, bacitracin, zinc) or chloramphenicol 1% ointment, twice daily to prevent scab formation and wound infection, facilitate suture removal and reduce scarring.

### Suture removal

- Facial skin sutures should be removed within 4–6 days, to minimize scarring.
- Mucosal sutures can be removed at 1 week.
- Many patients are apprehensive and need reassurance about removal.
- Clean the wound and surrounding mucosa or skin with an antiseptic solution such as Savlon.
- Lift the suture with sterile forceps and cut the stitch on one side, as close to the skin or mucosa as possible (this avoids pulling contaminated suture material through the wound).

- Pull the suture out using traction on the long end, across the wound so as to avoid pulling apart the edges.
- Remove alternate sutures first to see if wound has healed adequately. If not, remove the remaining sutures 2–3 days later. If skin wounds still tend to gape a little, use tapes (not in the mouth).
- Clean the area again with an antiseptic solution such as Savlon.

# Challenging wounds

## Gunshot wounds (Table 11.2)

Facial gunshot wounds typically also involve facial bone damage and tissue loss in the majority and, in about one-quarter, also involve intracranial wounds and/or injury to major blood vessels.

- Low velocity handgun bullets damage only the tissue they touch and thus inflict wounds that can be managed by conventional surgical methods.
- High velocity rifle bullets or explosive blast fragments produce small entrance wounds hiding extremely severe wounds with extensive necrotic tissue contaminated with clostridial spores (danger of gas gangrene), other bacteria, clothing and debris. They have a mortality 4–5 times higher than low velocity injuries and require special attention.

### Management

- Secure the airways,
- Control haemorrhage,
- Identify other injuries,
- All patients should be radiographed to locate the missiles. CT is often helpful to maintain a proper three-dimensional relationship
- Definitively repair the facial deformities
- To avoid gas gangrene, high velocity wounds must be treated by:
  - excision of damaged tissue;
  - delayed primary closure (4–5 days later) and, if necessary, skin grafts;
  - antibiotics.

**Table 11.2** Gunshot wounds

| Type of gun | Comment |
| --- | --- |
| Airgun | Missile can be left *in situ* if deep and not in orbit, or causing damage |
| 0.22 rifle | Missile can be left *in situ* if deep and not in orbit, or causing damage |
| 0.410 shotgun | May cause considerable damage at close range |
| Twelve-bore shotgun | Dangerous even from a distance; widespread damage |
| High velocity bullets | Cause damage more extensive than initially evident |
| Explosive bullets | Cause damage more extensive than initially evident |

## Stab wounds

- Stab wounds should always be treated with suspicion as there may be extensive damage beneath an apparently trivial wound.
- The wound may need to be explored, especially if in the chest, neck, back, or abdomen.
- Radiographs are indicated.

- Consider tetanus prophylaxis.
- Photograph the wounds; they may be of forensic value in subsequent litigation.

## Foreign bodies

Common foreign bodies include:
- glass from windscreen lacerations or assaults;
- plastic from car components;
- metal projectile fragments;
- gravel, dirt, wood and other materials.

### Management

- If there is any suggestion of ocular involvement, immediately ask an ophthalmologist to see the patient.
- Explore all wounds with a sterile probe and take relevant soft tissue radiographs—some glass is radio-opaque.
- Photograph the wounds; they may be of forensic value in subsequent litigation.
- Retain all foreign bodies; they may be of forensic value in subsequent litigation.

▶Be very meticulous with your exploration and cleaning of such wounds. Your best chance of clearing all F.B.s is at initial presentation; so obtain adequate analgesia (or GA) and carefully explore all wounds (including trivial scrapes) to their full depth.

# Burns

Burns can be serious injuries. Children with burns affecting more than 10% of the body surface area, and adults with over 15% burns (Fig. 11.5), are at special risk because of fluid loss and should be treated in Burns Units.

*Management*

First aid treatment of burns includes the following:

- Ensure adequate airways.
- Give oxygen if there are respiratory burns or smoke has been inhaled.
- Cool the area to reduce tissue damage and pain.
- Treat superficial (no blisters) or partial thickness (blisters) burns by:
  - On the face, leaving exposed.
  - On the extremities, dressing with silver sulfadiazine cream and enclosing in plastic bag.
- Treat full thickness burns or those over 15% by:
  - Calling the Burns specialist.
  - Taking blood for grouping and cross-matching.
  - Putting up an IV line.
  - Giving plasma substitutes (e.g. gelatin [Gelofusine or Haemaccel]) or plasma or blood, or 5% dextrose initially.
  - Giving analgesia IV (morphine 5–15 mg for adults).

Photograph the burns; they may be of forensic value in subsequent litigation.

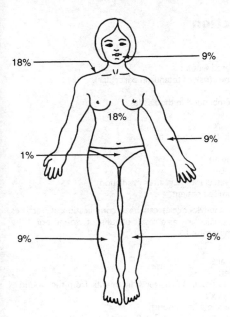

**Fig. 11.5** Calculations of the area involved in burns by Wallace 'rule of nines'

# Wound infection

*Risk factors*
- Complex trauma
  - Open contaminated wound.
  - Penetrating injuries (risk of tetanus in particular).
  - Gunshot wounds.
  - Foreign bodies embedded in the tissues.
  - Major trauma.
  - Compound fractures.
  - Teeth involved in the fracture line.
  - CSF leakage.
- Bites (human or animal).
- Impaired host defences
  - Impaired tissue vascularity (e.g. after irradiation).
  - Immunocompromised patient.

Osteomyelitis (often staphylococcal) can be a complication, if fractures are open to the skin, particularly as a result of gunshot wounds, or if the patient is immunocompromised.

*Prevention*
The main precautions are:
- prompt wound toilet;
- removal of foreign bodies, including teeth fragments, from the wound;
- antimicrobial prophylaxis
  - benzylpenicillin 600 mg IM, 6-hourly
  - co-amoxiclav 1.2 g IV or 625 mg PO, 8-hourly
  - flucloxacillin 250 mg IV or PO, 6-hourly
- good nutrition.

## Meningitis

- Bacterial meningitis may arise if there are:
  - dural tears (as indicated by CSF leaks);
  - skull fractures compound to the exterior or into paranasal sinuses;
  - scalp wounds.
- Meningitis may occur early or late (even years after the injury) if dural tears remain unrepaired (consult a neurosurgeon).
- Prophylactic rifampicin is indicated if there is risk of meningitis (see page 560).

## Tetanus

Management depends on the patient's immunity to tetanus, and the nature and amount of contamination of the wound (Table 11.3).

**Table 11.3** Prophylaxis against tetanus in the wounded patient

| Clean superficial wound or abrasion | | Tetanus-prone wounds (deep wound; puncture wound; bite; burns; wound contaminated with soil or manure; delayed [>6 h] surgical toilet) | |
|---|---|---|---|
| Immune patient* | Immune status uncertain | Immune patient* | Immune status uncertain |
| Wound toilet | Wound toilet; tetanus booster or vaccine[a] + complete course (if non-immunized) | Wound toilet; anti-tetanus immunoglobulin[b]; antibacterial prophylaxis (benzylpenicillin, co-amoxiclav or metronidazole) | Wound toilet; tetanus booster or vaccine[a]; anti-tetanus immunoglobulin[b]; combination antibacterial prophylaxis |

* Patient who has in the past 5 years been vaccinated (completed course) or had a booster (following a completed initial course).
[a] Tetanus toxoid 0.5 mL IM or deep SC.
[b] Anti-tetanus globulin 250 units IM if seen before 24 h have elapsed; otherwise give 500 units IM.

# Maxillofacial fractures

## Diagnosis

Facial fractures are diagnosed primarily from the history and clinical examination, supplemented where required by radiographic examination. Photograph the patient; they may be of forensic value in subsequent litigation.

*Radiographs* for maxillofacial and head injuries may include:
- occipitomental views (10° and 30°);
- lateral skull view;
- postero-anterior view of skull;
- postero-anterior view of mandible;
- panoramic view or lateral obliques of mandible;
- reverse Townes view;
- submentovertex view;
- CT scans.

See Chapter 3 and Table 11.4 for more details on investigations for maxillofacial fractures.

## Classification of fractures

- *Closed (simple):* no skin or mucosal penetration.
- *Open (compound):* skin or mucosal penetration (or compound into the periodontium or paranasal sinus).
- *Comminuted:* bone fragmented (can also be simple or compound).
- *Greenstick:* occur in children.
- *Displaced or undisplaced,* depending on the:
  - severity of the fracture,
  - angulation of fracture,
  - effect of muscle action,
  - presence of erupted teeth,
  - intactness of the periosteum.

## Communication with colleagues

Information to give a specialist or his/her deputy regarding a patient with maxillofacial injuries should include:
- patient's name, age, occupation and social circumstances;
- patient's gender;
- type of accident or assault;
- involvement of alcohol or other drugs;
- the current state of the airways;
- the present Glasgow Coma Scale, whether it is changing, and whether the patient is, or has been, unconscious at any point;
- other features suggestive of neurological damage;
- relevant medical history;
- any other injuries—particularly those which are serious;
- facial fractures—description;
- facial injuries involving the eyes, eyelids, nasolacrimal duct, parotid duct or facial nerve;
- any other facial injuries;

- state of dentition—general care and injuries;
- anything which may necessitate urgent operation.

*Other information to record*
- Photographs for medicolegal purposes.
- Results of investigations.
- Treatment.

**Table 11.4** Radiographs for maxillofacial fractures

| Fracture site | Radiographs recommended initially |
|---|---|
| Mandibular | Panoramic or Bilateral oblique laterals<br>Postero-anterior view of mandible (or reverse Townes)<br>Occlusal (for anterior mandible) |
| TMJ and condyle | Conventional and high OPT plus<br>Reverse Townes, and consider CT scan |
| Zygomatic arch | Submentovertex (exposed for zygomatic arches, not<br>base of skull) |
| Middle third | Occipitomental 30°<br>Occipitomental 10°<br>Lateral face |
| Skull | Postero-anterior view of skull<br>Lateral skull (brow up)<br>Submentovertex (exposed for base of skull)<br>CT scan |
| Nasal | Soft tissues lateral view for nasal bones<br>Occipitomental 30° |

# Malar (zygomatic) fractures

## Diagnosis

- History of trauma to the cheek.
- Depression of the cheek (may be masked by oedema).
- Haematoma and lateral subconjunctival haemorrhage with no posterior limit.
- Step deformities on the orbital rim.
- Pain on palpation.
- Tenderness and haematoma in the buccal sulcus.
- Restricted eye movements.
- Diplopia.
- Enophthalmos or exophthalmos.
- Change in visual acuity, variation in pupil size and reactivity.
- Infra-orbital nerve anaesthesia, hypoaesthesia or paraesthesia.
- Restriction of mandibular movements, especially lateral excursions (zygoma interfering with movement of coronoid).

## Radiological features (see also Chapter 3)

- Fracture lines.
- Step deformities of orbital rim.
- Distracted zygomatico-frontal (Z-F), zygomatico-maxillary (Z-M), or zygomatico-temporal (Z-T) sutures.
- Fluid in antrum.
- Hanging drop sign in the roof of the antrum.

## Management

- All patients with an injured malar process, even if evidence of fracture cannot be found, must be advised to avoid blowing their nose for 1–2 weeks (to avoid surgical emphysema). Some patients with undiagnosed malar fractures (following an indolent injury) present for the first time with sudden swelling usually of the lower eyelid, following nose blowing. Such emphysema resolves slowly and needs antibacterial prophylaxis (e.g. Co-amoxiclav).
- Undisplaced fractures with no ocular or aesthetic complications may need no treatment.
- For others, reduction ± retention (fixation) are indicated.

*Reduction* is by:
- elevating it from the temporal region (Gillies approach);
- using a hook applied from the face;
- an intra-oral approach;
- exposing the fracture and reducing it directly (usually by a Z-F and infra-orbital approach).

*Fixation* (if needed) is by:
- plating (most commonly);
- direct wiring;
- pin fixation;
- Kirschner wire.

## Complications

### *Ocular complications*

- Optic nerve damage.
  - *A potential cause of blindness.*
  - May be caused by direct trauma if there is fracture of the optic foramen.
  - Examine the consensual reflex.
- Retrobulbar haemorrhage.
  - *A potential cause of blindness.*
  - Presents with pain, proptosis and paralysis of eye movements.
  - Always check visual acuity. Also check as soon as the patient has regained consciousness after operation for reduction, then half-hourly for 6 h and hourly for 12 h.
- Periorbital oedema.
  - Do not allow this to prevent careful examination of the eye.
- Periorbital surgical emphysema.
  - Occurs when patient blows nose in fractures involving antral or nasal walls (see above).
  - May occasionally occur following operation (surgical emphysema).
- Enophthalmos.
  - May indicate orbital blow-out.
- Diplopia.
  - Often caused by oedema and haemorrhage, when it settles within about 10 days (but see above: Retrobulbar haemorrhage).
  - If not, this may be caused by muscle entrapment, nerve damage, or eye or orbit displacement.

*Malunion* may leave a cheek depressed or jaw movements restricted.

*Sensory changes* may persist over the ipsilateral cheek (infraorbital nerve distribution).

*Compensation neurosis* may affect anyone sustaining injury, especially from interpersonal violence.

# Mandibular fractures

## Diagnosis

- History of trauma to mandible.
- Pain.
- Swelling.
- Haematoma (particularly sublingually).
- Bleeding (usually intra-orally from, or through, gingival lacerations).
- Step deformity of lower dentition.
- Mobility of fragments (and possible crepitus).
- Deranged occlusion.
- Paraesthesia/anaesthesia/hypoaesthesia of nerves involved in the site (usually ipsilateral lower lip and chin anaesthesia).

## Radiological features (see also Chapter 3)

- Fracture lines.
- Step deformities.
- Widening of periodontal space (if teeth are involved).

## Management

- Simple undisplaced fractures may occasionally be treated conservatively with a soft diet, especially if they do not involve the teeth.
- Condylar fractures, even if displaced, are often treated conservatively, unless there is significant malocclusion with worsening symptoms. This is because open reduction may be associated with ↑ complications, particularly with high condylar neck fractures, while prolonged intermaxillary fixation may be associated with long-term stiffness of the TMJ.
- Definitive treatment of displaced fractures involves:
  - prevention of infection;
  - reduction and fixation.

### Fixation

- Direct fixation:
  - Open reduction and internal fixation (ORIF) is now used, with bone mini-plates fixed with screws. These are usually made of titanium and do not need removal unless infected or fractured. Absorbable plates and screws are also available for use.
  - Lag screws.
  - Direct (transosseous or interdental) wire, on the upper or lower borders of the mandible (or mid-alveolar).
- Indirect fixation (stabilizing mandible against maxilla—intermaxillary fixation [IMF]):
  - Eyelet and tie wires (where there is a substantial dentition).
  - Arch bars and tie wires (where several teeth are missing or there are bilateral fractures).
  - Splints (cap splints on teeth, or Gunning's splint if edentulous).
  - IMF screws and tie wires.

## Complications

### Body fractures

- Deformity.
- Limitation of movement.
- Malocclusion and inadequate mastication.
- Inferior alveolar nerve hypoaesthesia, anaesthesia, paraesthesia, or dysaesthesia.
- Infection (early infection of fracture or delayed infection of plates).
- Dental complications.

### Condylar fractures

- Impaired growth (children).
- Chronic traumatic arthrosis.
- Ankylosis.
- Limitation and abnormality of movement.
- Dislocation.
- Malocclusion.
- Asymmetry of chin.
- Mandibular division of trigeminal nerve hypoaesthesia, anaesthesia, paraesthesia, or dysaesthesia.

### General

- Malunion—anatomically incorrect healing, delayed union, or non-union due to a variety of local or systematic problems.
- Compensation neurosis.

# Mid-facial fractures

## Classification

Despite its inadequacies the Le Fort classification of facial fractures has persisted (Fig. 11.6):

- Le Fort III: high level;
- Le Fort II: pyramidal;
- Le Fort I: low level or Guérin's fracture.

The variations are many in different patients and on opposite sides of the mouth. They are often closed fractures.

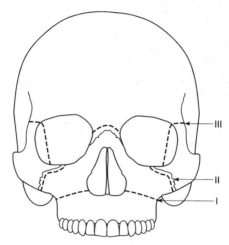

**Fig. 11.6** Le Fort lines of middle third facial fractures

## Diagnosis

- History of severe trauma to the face, usually in a backward and downward direction (often an RTA).
- Swelling of the upper lip in Le Fort I, and massive swelling of face (ballooning or Panda facies) in severe Le Fort II and III fractures.
- Haematoma—bilateral black eyes common; buccal sulcus also affected. Subconjunctival ecchymoses. Bruising in the palate over the greater palatine foraminae.
- Bleeding (usually from the nose).
- Pain.
- Mobility, sometimes gross (floating face). Grasp the upper jaw and elicit movement, while observing and feeling along the Le Fort lines.
- Posterior gagging of occlusion and lengthening of the face (anterior open bite).

- Percussing teeth may elicit a 'cracked-pot' sound in dento-alveolar as well as in any of the Le Fort types of fracture.
- Anaesthesia/hypoaesthesia/paraesthesia of the infra-orbital nerves.
- Double vision/restricted eye movements.
- CSF rhinorrhoea (leakage of CSF through the nose or into nasopharynx) in high level fractures.

## Radiographic features (see also Chapter 3)

- These fractures are mainly diagnosed clinically.
- Fractures around the orbital apex or medial wall may be undetectable on radiography.
- Damage to the orbital walls, floor or roof, and displacement or entrapment of orbital soft tissues is often identifiable only on CT scans.

## Management

- Nearly all middle-third facial fractures are now treated by open reduction and internal fixation (ORIF), with bone plates (mini, low-profile, and micro), in order to accurately reduce and fix all fragments. In the minimally mobile fractured maxilla, internal fixation with titanium mini-plates across the functional buttresses of the mid-face is usually used.
- There is occasionally a place for simple IMF. External fixation is maintained for 3 weeks, when union is tested.
- Alternative methods of fixation and immobilisation, now rarely used, include:
  - craniomandibular fixation (e.g. by means of a box- or halo frame);
  - craniomaxillary fixation (e.g. by means of supra-orbital pins and a Levant frame or a halo frame);
  - intermaxillary fixation using arch-bars with internal suspension from frontozygomatic wires or circumzygomatic wires to lower arch-bar.

## Complications

*Nose:* Deformity; deviation; obstruction; anosmia.

*Orbit:* Diplopia (muscle or fibrous entrapment/nerve injury); lacrimal duct damage (fractures of medial orbital wall may damage duct and produce swelling, pain and oedema, sometimes with epiphora—may not be clinically obvious until 10 days after trauma); enophthalmos; optic nerve injury; ruptured globe; retinal damage.

*Maxilla and zygomatic bones:* Delayed union (occasionally encountered, with the maxilla retaining a degree of mobility [springiness], which is not in itself clinically significant—non-union is virtually never seen); deformity; malocclusion; zygomatic interference with mouth opening.

*Maxillary division of trigeminal nerve:* Hypoaesthesia, anaesthesia, paraesthesia, or dysaesthesia.

*Cerebral:* CSF leak (± meningitis); headaches; aerocoele; pneumocephalus; cavernous sinus thrombosis; epilepsy; compensation neurosis.

# Postoperative care of facial fractures

### General observations

- Airways
- Respiration
- Conscious level and neurological observations
- BP
- Pulse
- Temperature
- Fluid balance

*Obtain a neurological/neurosurgical opinion* if:

- consciousness deteriorating;
- behavioural changes;
- headache;
- neck stiffness;
- ophthalmic or neurological signs, (?aerocele ?intracranial haemorrhage);
- CSF leak still present 7–10 days after fixation of fracture.

*Obtain an ophthalmological surgical opinion* if there is:
any risk of retrobulbar haemorrhage. During or after elevation of a fractured zygoma or surgery around the orbit, there is a small risk. Retrobulbar haemorrhage is an emergency. It presents with pain, proptosis, poor vision and loss of pupil reflexes. Always do half-hourly observations for 6 h then hourly for the next 12 h. In a few cases, high dose corticosteroids may obviate the need for surgical intervention.

### Care of airways

ORIF has the main advantage that IMF is not required. However, if IMF has been used, in case there is sudden and unexpected respiratory obstruction by vomiting, bleeding or oedema:

- show the nurses how to remove IMF;
- have adequate suction always at the bedside;
- have available, in order to undo fixation,
  - wire cutters,
  - wire holding forceps,
  - box spanner.

### Antimicrobials

- Give penicillin for 5 days after fracture fixation, and rifampicin for 7 days, or until 2 days after a CSF leak stops.
- Chloramphenicol eye drops 0.5% (or ointment 1%) may be used if there is conjunctival damage. Chloramphenicol ointment is also useful in lubricating incision wounds (bd application).

### Oral hygiene

- Blood clots and dried blood should be cleaned away with a bicarbonate mouthwash.
- 0.2% aqueous chlorhexidine mouthwashes at least twice daily are valuable.
- The mouth and any intra-oral fixation should be cleaned gently with a soft toothbrush.

## Feeding

- Food should be liquidized, but a dietician should be consulted to avoid a monotonous diet.
- The patient with IMF can feed with a straw, plastic suction tubes, etc.
- Clean the mouth after meals.

## Sutures, intraoral fixation, splints, pins and screws

- Do not permit crusts to remain on these.
- Clean twice daily with chlorhexidine and then apply Polyfax (not intraorally).
- Cover wire ends with soft wax.

## Splint or wire/bar removal

- When union is assured, remove splints and wires
- Cast splints if used are removed with splint removal forceps or old extraction forceps. Remove as much cement as possible, and then clean the teeth with an ultrasonic scaler, or ask a hygienist to help.
- Eyelet wires and arch bars can be simply removed under local anaesthesia.

## The wider care of trauma patients

Trauma, particularly from assaults, may produce social and psychological effects, which may necessitate social or psychiatric care or help from victims support schemes, especially for advice about compensation, alcohol and drug dependence, and compensation neuroses.

# Jaw dislocation

Dislocation of the mandible is usually anterior and caused by trauma, sometimes by extreme opening (yawning), or predisposed by a disorder such as Ehlers–Danlos syndrome. Some people (especially women) have a tendency for repeated jaw dislocations and are often said to have a subluxated joint. The cause is often unidentifiable, but it usually occurs following a yawn in the late evening or early morning hours. Dislocation may be classified as acute, chronic, or recurrent.

## Management

### Acute dislocation

- Give sedation (e.g. midazolam IV), if unsuccessful in reducing the mandible following the first attempt.
- Stand facing patient and grip molars and lower mandibular border, with thumbs over teeth or external oblique ridge, and the rest of the fingers beneath mandible extra-orally.
- Press down with thumbs and rotate fingers upwards and forwards to push the condyle under the anterior articular eminence of the glenoid fossa and relocate the mandible.
- Immediately move behind the patient and hold the mouth closed instructing them not to try speaking, as the mandible has a tendency to re-dislocate (explain in advance). Put an elastic bandage around the head and chin and retain for 1–2 days to keep the mouth from opening excessively and prevent recurrence. Alternatively, splint or use elastic IMF (if reduction done under GA).

### Chronic dislocation

Is usually diagnosed in elderly or demented patients in nursing homes. The dislocation is often not manually reducible and open operation is then required.

### Recurrent dislocation

This is recurrence of acute dislocation in susceptible patients. Prolonged inter-maxillary fixation is usually not effective or a reasonable treatment. Surgical treatment includes either increasing or reducing the articular eminence or the use of sclerosing solutions.

# Traumatized teeth

Following oral and maxillofacial injuries, establish the whereabouts of dentures, lost teeth or fragments thereof, as they may have been lost into the tissues, swallowed or, far more seriously, inhaled (see page 278). Radiography may be indicated.

The immediate management of traumatized teeth is shown in Table 11.5. Avulsed permanent teeth should be handled by the crown, washed or stored in saline or milk, and replanted with splinting, as soon as possible.

**Table 11.5** Management of traumatized incisors

| Trauma | Management |
|---|---|
| *Deciduous teeth* | |
| Coronal fracture | If pulp exposed: pulp treat or extract<br>If pulp not exposed: acid etch composite or leave |
| Root fracture | If slightly mobile leave alone<br>If coronal fragment very loose: remove and leave apical fragment |
| Loosened tooth | Usually leave alone |
| Displaced tooth | If tooth interferes with occlusion or germ of underlying permanent tooth, or is loose: extract<br>Otherwise, leave |
| Intruded tooth | Remove if pressing on germ of underlying permanent tooth. Wait and see |
| Avulsed tooth | Check tooth not in chest; do not replant |
| *Permanent teeth* | |
| Fractured enamel only | Leave alone |
| Fractured enamel and dentine but no pulpal exposure | Restore crown (acid-etch composite, veneer or crown) |
| Fractured enamel and dentine with pulpal exposure but pulp vital | Partial pulpotomy |
| Fractured enamel and dentine with pulpal exposure but pulp non-vital | Root canal treatment |
| Root fractures | If fracture not involving gingiva: splint[a] rigidly for 4 weeks<br>If fracture communicating with mouth: remove coronal part<br>If fracture longitudinal: remove tooth |
| Slightly mobile (subluxated) teeth | Soft diet |
| Mobile teeth | Splint[a] semi-rigidly for 1 week |
| Intruded tooth | Leave alone |
| Extruded tooth | Seat tooth back and splint[a] semi-rigidly for 1 week |
| Avulsed teeth | Clean tooth; replant and splint[a] semi-rigidly for 1 week; follow-up in case endodontics needed |
| | Dirty tooth: wash in saline, replant and splint[a]; check tetanus immunity; give antibiotics. |

[a] Splint with a polythene occlusal splint or metal foil or epimine resin (Scutan) or acrylic resin (e.g. Trim). Alternatively, acid-etch and splint with composite resin wire strengthener; however, this is difficult to remove. Resin placed between the teeth makes immobilization rigid.

# Non-accidental injury (NAI)

NAI (or child abuse) refers to a condition in young children, usually under the age of 3 years, who present with injuries received as a result of non-accidental violence, inflicted (usually) by a parent or guardian.

## Recognition

- Inexplicable delay between injury and medical attention.
- Obvious discrepancy between the nature of the injuries and the explanation offered by the parent.
- The child is often the only one in the family to receive repeated assaults (frequently the youngest, and often unwanted or rejected).
- The child may often have been seen elsewhere or previously, for other injuries.
- The child appears quiet or frightened when parent in question is present.
- Predominantly a lower social class, Anglo-American-Nordic phenomenon.
- Sixty per cent recurrence—10% eventual fatal injury.

### Lesions

- Bruising, especially around the arms (child has been gripped and shaken), on the scalp, face, around the mouth, around the joints of the upper limbs, back of thighs (almost impossible to explain by a fall or 'bumping into' furniture), neck, chest, and abdomen.
- Lacerations of upper labial mucosa, often with torn fraenum.
- Bite marks are common, on the face and upper limbs.
- Fracture of ribs, long bones (commonly at epiphyses) and skull.
- Other lesions include cigarette burns, ruptured viscera (lacerated liver, torn bowel), eye injuries, periostitis over facial bones or limbs.

## Action in suspected battering

- Record the history, and clinical and radiographic findings (complete skeletal survey needed). Photographs can be useful.
- Admit the child with severe injuries suspected to have been non-accidental, under a specialist appropriate to its injuries, or under a paediatrician, for standard medical and surgical care.
- The child should not be discharged from hospital until appropriate enquiries have been made.
- If the injuries do not warrant admission and the parent is not prepared to allow the child to be admitted, it is essential that the social services be contacted by the medical social worker in the hospital.
- Teamwork is essential; general practitioners, health visitors, child care services, paediatricians and other medical specialists must work together.

⚠ *It is not enough merely to treat the acute injuries and then return the child to a dangerous domestic situation.*

USEFUL WEBSITES
http://pubs.ama-assn.org/cgi/collection/oral_maxillofacial_trauma
http://www.baoms.org.uk/ce/ce_trauma.html

# Oral and maxillofacial non-trauma surgery

# Extraction of teeth in children

Dental extractions can have a profound effect upon the developing dentition, so an orthodontic opinion should be sought for non-urgent cases.

## Extraction of deciduous teeth

There is seldom a case for the removal of only one deciduous tooth, unless it is close to being shed naturally, or has been retained so long that it impedes the eruption of its successor, or is submerging.

Enforced extractions of deciduous canines or molars should usually be balanced by extraction of a contralateral tooth in the same arch, to prevent a centre line shift. The balancing extraction need not be exactly the same tooth contralaterally; a first deciduous molar extraction for example, can be balanced by removal of the contralateral C, D, or E.

Radiographs should be taken to ensure that there are no other problems (e.g. a mid-line supernumerary tooth), which may also require attention.

## Extraction of permanent teeth

Although many orthodontic treatments include the extraction of premolars, there may be indications for the removal of a different tooth. Particularly check the following.

*At assessment:*
- all successional teeth are present;
- teeth (e.g. first molars) other than those scheduled for removal are of good prognosis.

*Before extraction:*
- the correct tooth to be removed is written down clearly in the notes;
- both patient and parent understand that a permanent tooth is being removed—and the reason;
- informed consent has been obtained;
- any orthodontic appliance is being worn satisfactorily before any orthodontic extractions are performed.

# Tooth impactions

These are:
- usually due to soft tissue, bone, or adjacent teeth;
- most commonly involve third molars, followed by canines, second premolars and mandibular second molars;
- often ectopic and can cause considerable difficulties for the patient, including;
  - infection (pericoronitis) when they are exposed into the oral cavity,
  - caries of, or displacement of, adjacent teeth,
  - dentigerous cysts, rarely;
- in general should be managed either by allowing teeth to functionally erupt, leaving them alone (observing them), exposing them to allow eruption, or removing them.

There is no evidence to support the routine removal of asymptomatic unerupted third molars (see NICE guidelines, page 638), as many remain asymptomatic for years, or forever.

## Assessment of impactions is by:
- thorough clinical examination;
- palpation of the region of the impacted tooth;
- assessment of the axial inclination of adjacent teeth (for instance, with an impacted maxillary canine tooth, if the crown of the adjacent lateral incisor is displaced labially then its root will be displaced palatally, indicating that the impacted canine tooth is labially positioned);
- radiography—including an OPTG, periapical, occlusal, cephalometric radiography and, in selected cases, CT scans, demonstrating the root pattern and relationship to structures such as the inferior alveolar nerve or antrum.

## Exposure of impacted teeth

Exposure is commonly used for canines and second premolars whose eruption is impeded. Maxillary canines are commonly impacted either labially or palatally, second premolars in a palatal or lingual position.

Exposure is normally undertaken in combination with orthodontic management, ensuring that there is adequate space for eruption of the impacted tooth. Orthodontic traction is often required.

### Techniques

*Palatally impacted teeth*
- After appropriate anaesthesia, raise a palatal flap preserving the gingival tissues around erupted teeth and, using a sharp 3 mm chisel and mallet or burr, expose the greater circumference of the tooth along with the incisal tip.
- Excise the mucosa overlying the tooth, taking care to control bleeding from the greater palatine artery, often using diathermy.
- Pack the mucosal defect with Coepak or ribbon gauze soaked in Whitehead's varnish.
- Remove the pack approximately 10 days later.

- If the tooth is not impacted against the adjacent teeth it can be allowed to erupt passively prior to orthodontic repositioning.
- If the tooth is impacted against adjacent teeth then orthodontic traction should be applied at an early stage to disimpact it.

*Labially impacted teeth*
Expose either:
- with an apically repositioned flap, bringing gingival tissue around the cervical margin of the impacted tooth, or
- by placing an orthodontic bracket and chain at the time of surgery to allow traction to be applied, so that the tooth erupts through the keratinized gingival tissues.

## Removal of impacted teeth

### Hazards
Removal of impacted teeth may cause significant morbidity, particularly:
- temporary
  - pain and swelling
  - haemorrhage or bruising
  - trismus
  - infection
- longer-lasting
  - damage to nerves (usually the inferior alveolar and lingual);
  - damage to the crown or roots of adjacent teeth;
  - damage to the periodontium of adjacent teeth;
  - displacement of roots, or sometimes the tooth, into adjacent soft tissue spaces, i.e. the floor of mouth, infratemporal fossa, or antrum;
  - communication with the maxillary antrum (oro-antral fistula).

### Technique
- Adequate anaesthesia and exposure are essential.
- A gingivo-buccal (sometimes gingivo-palatal or gingivo-lingual) incision is made over the tooth.
- Adequate bone should be removed to visualize the tooth.
- Depending on the nature of impaction, the tooth may then be delivered, or surgically divided to relieve the impaction and then delivered.
- After debridement, the flap is sutured back.

### Complications and their prevention
- Pain is almost inevitable; analgesia is indicated.
- Postoperative swelling is common; usually caused by oedema, sometimes by haematoma, or rarely by infection (there is no evidence to support the routine use of perioperative antibiotics). Nevertheless, antimicrobials and/or corticosteroids are often used to reduce complications.
- With mandibular third molar impactions, care must be taken to avoid injuring the lingual nerves, by avoiding disto-lingual bone removal, or if disto-lingual bone removal is essential, taking care not to damage the soft tissues. Placing a lingual retractor such as a Howarth's periosteal elevator between the bone and periosteum should prevent permanent severe injury to the lingual nerve, although it may in fact cause some traction injury to the nerve, resulting in paraesthesia, which is usually temporary.

# Odontogenic infections

Odontogenic infections may arise from non-vital teeth, pericoronitis, or as post-surgical infections, and are:

- commonly polymicrobial (caused by a mixture of oral bacteria including both anaerobes and aerobes);
- usually minor, and localized to the alveolus or sulcus, resolving promptly with appropriate management;
- sometimes severe and life-threatening, particularly if they are necrotizing or spread. Fascial space infections endanger the airways and may spread to the mediastinum. Infections may spread into blood vessels.

### Spread of infections

Infections may spread:

- from mandibular teeth into the
  - floor of mouth,
  - submandibular space,
  - submental space,
  - lateral pharyngeal spaces,
- from maxillary infections into the
  - infra-orbital region,
  - cavernous sinus,
  - maxillary sinus,
  - infra-temporal space
  - lateral pharyngeal space.

## Management

*The principles* of management of odontogenic infections are:

- establish and maintain drainage;
- remove cause;
- give supportive therapy, including antibiotics, hydration and nutrition.

*Patients with severe infections* who have trismus and a fever in excess of 39°C may present significant airways problems and may require:

- advanced intubation techniques such as fibreoptic intubation or occasionally tracheostomy;
- exploration of the involved fascial spaces and placement of drains;
- high doses of penicillin or cephalosporins, plus metronidazole;
- microbiological analysis—mandatory, although most patients will recover before the results are known.

# Periapical pathology

Periapical pathology usually results from pulpal necrosis typically due to dental caries or trauma. A periapical granuloma will often form initially, but may progress onto a periapical (radicular) cyst and can eventually achieve significant size. Either of these lesions commonly become infected and give rise to periapical abscesses.

## Management

- The non-vital tooth should be endontically managed or removed. There is increasingly a case for removal and implant replacement.
- Small periapical granulomas or cysts (<10 mm diameter) will often resolve following endodontic treatment.
- Larger periapical granulomas or cysts (>10 mm diameter) should be removed, either in association with removal of the tooth or following conventional endodontic treatment.
- Apicectomy is sometimes needed to treat periapical pathology although, if the endodontic treatment is satisfactorily completed, there are limited indications.
- Retrograde root fillings are indicated when the root canal has been inadequately obturated.
- Historically, amalgam has been used for an apical seal, although this has been largely superceded by composite materials.

## Odontogenic cysts

- Most common are periapical (radicular) cysts.
- Incomplete removal of periapical cysts may leave a residual cyst.
- Dentigerous cysts are the next most common.
- Keratocysts are less common but liable to recur.
- Other odontogenic cysts are rare.

### Assessment

Includes:
- clinical examination;
- radiographs;
- CT scans for larger lesions or those involving the maxillary sinus;
- if there are still doubts about the diagnosis, an aspiration biopsy or incisional biopsy should be considered:
  - aspiration of a keratocyst will usually show the presence of keratin and a total protein level <4 g/dL;
  - the problem with incisional biopsy is that, unless definitive surgery follows soon after, there is a moderate risk of cyst infection.

### Management

- Enucleate—most periapical, residual and dentigerous cysts.
- Keratocysts—require more thorough removal as they tend to recur and, if they are large and perforating bone, or multiply recurrent, they should be resected with a margin of normal bone. Cryosurgery may be used. Patients should be followed-up long-term.

# Pre-prosthetic surgery

Pre-prosthetic surgical procedures include:

### Soft tissue procedures
- fraenectomy;
- tuberosity reduction;
- vestibuloplasty
  - submucosal or
  - supraperiosteal with a mucosal or skin graft.

### Hard tissue procedures
- alveoloplasty;
- mylohyoid ridge reduction;
- removal of bony prominences;
- tuberoplasty;
- ridge augmentation (Table 12.1);
- osseointegrated and other dental implants (see next).

**Table 12.1** Materials for repair of bone defects and for ridge augmentation

| | | |
|---|---|---|
| Autogenous bone | Intra-oral origin<br>Extra-oral origin | Limited availability of material<br>Two operations required |
| Allograft bone | Donor<br>  Cadaver<br>  Freeze-dried | Possibility of infection or rejection |
| Xenograft bone | Porcine usually | Limited success |
| Ceramics | Hydroxyapatite<br>Tri-calcium phosphate | Biocompatible but resorbed rapidly unless sintered |
| Guided tissue regeneration membranes | | Useful for augmentation of implant sites |
| Expanded polytetrafluoroethylene (PTFE) | | Must be removed later |
| Resorbable collagen membranes | | As PTFE but can be left |

# Dental implants: general principles

Various endosseous implants are available, but osseointegrated implants have virtually replaced every other type, because of their considerable success: up to 95% of mandibular and 85% of maxillary implants should be functional at 5 years, and still 90% and 80% by 10 years. Most are titanium implants, which appear to be extremely biocompatible. They are inserted as a one- or two-stage procedure (Table 12.2).

**Table 12.2** Main implants in current use

| Type | Comments |
|---|---|
| Endosseous | Embedded in maxillary or mandibular bone and projects through ridge mucosa, usually a two-stage procedure. |
| | Cylindrical threaded endosteal osseo-integrated titanium implant is the version of most proven success (Branemark: Nobelbiocare). Many variations in design, including non-threaded press fit types are available. |

## Principles

- Materials used must be:
  - biocompatible;
  - of adequate strength.
- Bone must be of adequate:
  - quantity;
  - quality.
- Surgery should be:
  - atraumatic;
  - aseptic.
- Implant should:
  - be biomechanically of sound design;
  - be stable;
  - usually not be loaded for at least 3–6 months;
  - have adequate gingival tissue;
  - have adequate oral hygiene.

## Criteria for success of implants

(Adapted from Bolender C. L., *J Dent Educ*, 1988; 757–759)
- Bone loss:
  - no greater than one-third of the vertical height of the implant;
  - less than 0.2 mm annually after 1st year;
  - no evidence of peri-implant radiolucency.
- Implant:
  - good occlusal balance and vertical dimension;
  - mobility <1 mm in any direction.
- Any gingival inflammation (peri-implantitis) should be amenable to treatment.

- Absence of symptoms of infection.
- Absence of damage to adjacent teeth.
- Absence of paraesthesia, anaesthesia or violation of inferior dental canal, antrum or nasal passage.

## Advantages of implants
- Independent of, and no need to damage, adjacent teeth
- Prosthesis is retentive
- Improved masticatory function
- Low morbidity
- Aesthetic
- Immune to caries.

## Disadvantages of implants
- Invasive: surgery is required
- Costly
- Time-consuming
- An adequate amount of bone is required
- Must be precisely positioned.

# Dental implants: clinical procedures

## Patient selection

Patient selection is crucial to success and includes:
- Ability to co-operate with the procedure
- Ability to maintain good oral hygiene
- Absence of any smoking
- Absence of any contraindications (see below)
- Adequate bone quantity
- Adequate bone quality

## Contraindications

### Absolute
- Lack of adequate training or skills of operator
- Poor co-operation between implant placer and prosthetist
- Poor patient co-operation
- Poor patient motivation
- Poor patient oral hygiene
- Inadequate minimum requirements for quantity or quality of bone
- Hypersensitivity to any components of implants

### Relative
- Cigarette smoking
- Alcoholism
- Bleeding tendency
- Bone disease in the jaws
- Diabetes mellitus
- Drug abuse
- Immunocompromised patient
- Pregnancy
- Psychiatric disorders
- Radiotherapy involving the implant site
- Susceptibility to infective endocarditis

## Assessment

Co-operative planning between implant placer and restorative dentist is required for optimal results and includes:
- clinical examination;
- study models;
- radiography
  - intraoral
  - OPTG
  - tomography
  - possibly sinus, paranasal and zygomatic views;
- CT or denta-scan.

## Procedure

- After the provision of adequate anaesthesia; local, local with sedation or general.

- Raise a mucoperiosteal flap.
- Prepare receiving channel using a spiral drill at low speed with cooling.
- Countersink the hole.
- Screw fixture in receiving channel.
- Place cover screws.
- Replace and suture flap.
- After 4–6 months, excise overlying mucosa to expose fixtures.
- Remove cover screws.
- Insert abutment.
- With single stage procedures, the abutment is placed instead of a cover screw, and the gingival tissues sewn around the abutment.

## Adjunctive procedures (mostly to improve quantity of bone at site)

- Bone grafting
- Sinus lift procedures
- Nasal floor augmentation
- Inferior alveolar nerve lateralization
- Guided tissue regeneration
- Alveolar ridge augmentation.

## Follow-up

Check implants at least yearly to ensure:

- individual implant is immobile;
- no radiological evidence of peri-implant resorption;
- <0.2 mm annual vertical bone loss, after 1 year of initial functional load;
- no prolonged symptoms in connection with implant;
- peri-implant soft tissues free from inflammation on at least 85% of checks.

# Orthognathic surgery

**The aim** of orthognathic surgery is to provide an ideal occlusion within a pleasing facial form, maximizing both aesthetics and masticatory function.

## Assessment
- Includes both orthodontic and surgical planning
- Principally clinical
- Cephalometry (see Appendix 3) and jaw radiographs
- Study models
- Sometimes computer modelling

Face, jaws and dentition must be assessed in three dimensions, balancing the skeletal and dental relationships with the orofacial soft tissues.

## Management
### Presurgical orthodontics
Aims within 12–18 months to:
- decompensate tooth angulation;
- align and level the dental arches;
- create root divergence adjacent to surgical sites for segmental osteotomies.

### Surgery
A wide range of procedures is available (Figs. 12.1–12.5).
- Le Fort I osteotomies are commonly carried out in the maxilla (Fig. 12.1).
- Bilateral sagittal split osteotomy is the commonest procedure used in the mandible (Fig. 12.2). Vertical sub-sigmoid osteotomy (Fig 12.3) and sometimes body osteotomy (Fig 12.4) are also used, but usually only for posterior movement.
- A sliding genioplasty may be added to correct chin deformity (Fig. 12.5).
- Fixation is with mini-plates and screws or bicortical screws.

### Post-surgical orthodontics
May take 6–12 months to finalize occlusal adjustments.

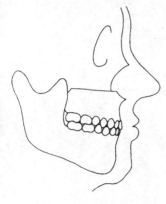

**Fig. 12.1** Le Fort I maxillary osteotomy (reproduced by kind permission of Professor G. R. Seward)

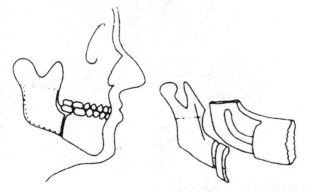

**Fig. 12.2** Sagittal split osteotomy (Obwegeser-Dal Pont)

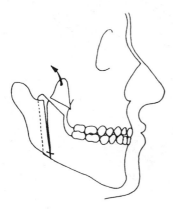

**Fig. 12.3** Vertical sub-sigmoid osteotomy (Caldwell and Letterman)

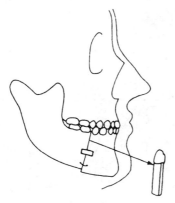

**Fig. 12.4** Body ostectomy (Dingman)

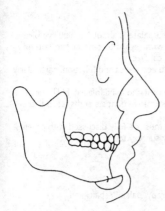

**Fig. 12.5** Sliding genioplasty

# Cleft lip or palate

- The worldwide incidence of cleft lip/palate is about 1 in 800 live births.
- The neonate should be examined with regard to orofacial and other possible associated anomalies, e.g. cardiac.
- The aim of treatment is to improve aesthetics and function, particularly speech.
- Interdisciplinary management with oral and maxillofacial, ENT and plastic surgeons, orthodontists, restorative dentists and speech therapists is indicated (Table 12.3).
- The treatment plan and prognosis must be fully discussed with parents.
- Aesthetic defects are corrected by surgery to:
  - lip,
  - palate,
  - alveolus,
  - nose.
- Speech is improved by speech therapy, palatal repair, and pharyngoplasty.

**Table 12.3** Schedule for management of patients with cleft lip and palate

| Approximate age | Schedule[a] |
|---|---|
| Birth | Assess with photographs, impressions and radiographs. Discuss with team and parents. Feeding advice. Possible presurgical orthodontics. |
| 3 months | Repair cleft lip. Possibly myringotomy and tubes. |
| 9–18 months | Repair cleft palate. Oral hygiene instruction to parents. |
| 30 months | Assess speech. |
| 4 years + | Consider surgical revision of lip and/or plate. |
| 5 years + | Consider surgery for correction of speech defects. Speech therapy. Preventive dentistry. |
| 8 years + | Simple orthodontics. |
| 10 years + | Alveolar bone graft. |
| 12 years + | Definitive orthodontics. |
| 16 years + | Maxillofacial surgery may be needed for correction of maxillary hypoplasia or nasal deformity. Restorative dentistry. |

[a] Preventive dental care required throughout.

# Soft tissue surgery

A range of instruments is available to facilitate soft tissue surgery.

## Scalpel

Use the following disposable surgical scalpel blades, number:
- 11—for incising abscesses;
- 15—for intraoral and small skin inclsions, incising mucoperiosteum, and excision of soft tissue lesions;
- 10—for larger skin incisions.

## Cutting diathermy and electrosurgery

These may be used for extensive oral incisions, or removal of soft tissue as they reduce haemorrhage from wound edges.
Avoid in people with cardiac pacemakers.

## Cryosurgery

### Advantages
- Can sometimes be used without analgesia.
- No haemorrhage.
- Little postoperative infection.

### Disadvantages
- No biopsy specimen.
- Depth and extent of tissue damage difficult to predict.
- Substantial postoperative oedema.

### Indications; useful in:
- Control of intractable facial pain (cryoanalgesia to peripheral nerve).
- Removal of
  - leucoplakias (keratoses). The diagnosis should be established by histology prior to cryosurgery, lest there be malignancy.
  - warts, papillomas and condylomas.
  - mucus extravasation cysts.
  - haemangiomas.
  - premalignant skin lesions (e.g. actinic keratosis).
  - keloid scars.
- Palliation of
  - Severe erosive lesions.
  - Malignant neoplasia.

### Procedure
The probes are either liquid nitrogen ($N_2$) or nitrous oxide ($N_2O$). The low temperatures achieved using liquid $N_2$ make this particularly useful in the management of recalcitrant lesions and it is perhaps better than $N_2O$, but large volumes are required, and liquid $N_2$ probes and sprays are quite capable of full thickness skin necrosis, and therefore, when the cosmetic result is an important consideration, dosage is limited to 15- or 30-s applications. The $N_2O$ apparatus is prone to breakdown, and cylinders and scavenging are needed.

- Give local analgesia if required.
- Ensure good contact of the cryoprobe with the lesion by coating it with a jelly such as KY jelly.
- Select a cryoprobe tip of adequate size to cover the lesion.
- Freeze the lesion. Dosage in cryosurgery is largely empirical, but $N_2O$ cryoprobes are usually applied for at least two periods of 30 s.
- Turn the freezing off. Leave the cryoprobe on the lesion until it thaws and defrosts.
- Multiple freezes, with thawing between each freeze to maximize the tissue damage produced by ice recrystallization and hypertonicity.

## Laser surgery

The hard laser, especially the carbon dioxide laser, is the most useful.

*Advantages*; Laser surgery usually:
- causes little bleeding. Haemostasis occurs during vaporization, 2° to coagulation of small vessels in the wound bed.
- is followed by less pain and swelling than that which follows surgical excision or cryotherapy.
- leaves little postoperative scarring.
- is particularly helpful for surgery close to important anatomical structures, e.g. lesions affecting the floor of the mouth.

*Disadvantages*
- Treatment is usually best under GA.
- Histopathological diagnosis should be obtained preoperatively.
- Laser equipment is expensive.
- Laser can damage eyes and teeth.
- Laser travels in straight lines, making access to some lesions difficult.

*Potential hazards*
- Damage to the eyes and other tissues from reflection of the laser beam from retractors, mouth props, or anaesthetic tube couplings.
- Vaporization of anaesthetic tubes, leading to ignition of inflammable anaesthetic agents.

*Indications*
- Leucoplakias.
- Early neoplasms.
- Haemangiomas.

*Procedure*
The carbon dioxide laser is a cutting laser and can be used to excise, much as does a scalpel, or to fulgurate the lesion.
- Follow laser safety recommendations.
- Use non-inflammable general anaesthetic agents.
- Avoid reflections from instruments or other metal objects. (e.g. by covering them with gauze).

# TMJ surgery

TMJ surgery is not generally indicated for temporomandibular pain/dysfunction syndrome. However, surgery can produce relief in some patients suffering intractable internal derangement or where there is organic disease affecting the joint.

## Surgical techniques

*Arthrocentesis*—two wide-bore needles are passed into the TMJ (usually under GA) to allow irrigation of the joint with normal saline and occasionally a sterioid injection (see Chapter 8). The jaw can be manipulated at the same time. Arthrocentesis is a relatively conservative procedure that may be indicated in patients with moderate to severe symptomatology from the TMJ and a limited mouth opening, where disc pathology cannot clearly ne demonstrated (e.g. on MRI).

*Arthroscopic surgery*—performed through a small stab incision to permit an arthroscope access, to loosen adhesions in the joint or in some cases reposition a displaced disc with the assistance of a laser and operative or surgical arthroscopic techniques. Arthroscopy has recently fallen out of favour in many centres in the UK, as outcomes have generally been less than satisfactory.

*Open arthroplasty*—performed through an incision in a skin crease in front of the ear and aimed at repairing or repositioning a displaced disc (meniscus) but sometimes can result in disc removal (meniscectomy).

*Total joint replacement* (for severe and chronic conditions failing to respond to other treatments)—performed through two incisions, one in front of the ear and the other under the angle of the mandible.

## Complications

Surgery of the TMJ is almost always performed as a day case procedure and most patients suffer only moderate discomfort and trismus in the immediate post-operative period. A soft diet and exercises are needed for six to eight weeks.

# Parotid surgery

### Indications

The common indications for parotidectomy include:
- a tumour,
- chronic infection, or
- chronic salivary obstruction.

#### Surgical techniques

Parotidectomy is usually performed under GA, the amount of gland to be removed often being determined at the time of surgery, dependent on the location, size and nature of the lesion.

Benign superfical lesions are treated with excision of the superficial lobe of the gland (superficial parotidectomy) or conservative lumpectomy.

For malignant neoplasms, surgical excision is also the preferred treatment, with superficial or total parotidectomy depending on the state and histology of the tumour. Small low-grade neoplasms are treated with a superficial parotidectomy when possible. Deep tumours may require a total parotidectomy or excision of the portion of the tumour that is deep to the facial nerve. Every effort is made not to damage the facial nerve. Postoperative radiation therapy is often used when surgical margins are positive, neoplasms are high grade or larger than 4 cm, or local extension is noted.

Neck dissection should be considered when evaluating node positive disease. A locally invasive neoplasm may require resection of the facial nerve, skull base, or mandible. Chemotherapy has not proved effective.

#### Complications

- For 2–3 days after the surgery, it is common to have some pain or difficulty on swallowing.
- Bleeding.
- Infection.
- Numbness of the earlobe and outer edge of the ear in many, which may resolve over time.
- A thick scar or keloid in some.
- A depression or a 'dent' at the site in some.
- A salivary fistula, rarely, or a sialocele (fluctuant lump caused by accumulated saliva produced by residual gland tissue, which has had its drainage disrupted—usually resolves with time).
- Frey's syndrome (gustatory sweating)—in a few patients the face on the side of the parotidectomy sweats while eating (produced when during the healing phase, disrupted secretomotor parasympathetic fibers form anastomoses with vasoactive sympathetic fibres innervating the skin over the parotid gland). This usually goes essentially unnoticed but, if bothersome, medication, botulinum injections and sometimes surgery are available.
- Facial palsy—the most disabling complication and the patients should always be warned about this before surgery. Even if the nerve is not permanently injured, there may be decreased motion of the facial muscles as the nerve recovers from the surgical procedure. If facial movement does not fully return, nerve anastomosis may be indicated.

# Oral cancer: diagnosis and staging

- Tumours of the mouth and jaws may be benign or malignant, primary or metastatic, or according to their cell type of origin, i.e. epithelial, salivary gland, odontogenic, or bone lesions.
- Cancer is the term applied mainly to the most common malignant tumour of epithelium—squamous cell carcinoma (SCC).
- Cancer may supervene in potentially malignant lesions (see page 626).
- Carcinoma has the greatest incidence among the over-50s, especially males.
- Smoking, alcohol use and betel chewing are the main lifestyle habits that predispose to cancer.
- Patients with oral cancer are at risk from second *primary* tumours in the mouth or upper aerodigestive tract.
- The incidence of oral carcinoma in many societies is currently rising.
- Early diagnosis carries the best prognosis but patients continue to present late, mainly because they ignore symptoms.
- Reconstruction has improved significantly over the past 25 years but mortality has not.

## Diagnosis

Diagnosis requires the recognition of pathology from the history and examination. SCC on the lip and anterior tongue is easy to detect but in the posterior tongue needs very careful examination. Every attempt should be made to ensure a diagnosis as early in the course of the disease as possible. The diagnosis may not always be simple. Early tumours may be symptomless. Suspicion should be greatest in the patients most at risk, namely

- Over 50s
- Males
- Smokers or tobacco users
- Alcohol drinkers
- Betel users.

*The clinical presentation* may include:

- A sore on the lip or in the mouth that does not heal
- A lump on the lip or in the mouth or throat
- A white or red patch on the gums, tongue, or lining of the mouth
- Unusual bleeding, pain, or numbness in the mouth
- A sore throat that does not go away, or a feeling that something is caught in the throat
- Difficulty or pain with chewing or swallowing
- Swelling of the jaw that causes dentures to fit poorly or become uncomfortable
- Pain in the ear
- Enlargement of a neck lymph gland
- Loosening of the teeth
- Paraesthesia or hypoaesthesia involving a trigeminal nerve branch.

⚠ Any persistent ulcer must be suspected as being a cancer until proved otherwise. The patient should be referred to a specialist, with an indication of the possible diagnosis, without delay. A false alarm is better than a false diagnosis. Unfortunately, about 50% of patients present for treatment with late stage tumours.

*A definitive diagnosis* is made with a biopsy, which should include some of the affected tissue, along with some normal tissue, particularly for mucosal carcinomas, so that the origin of the lesion can be identified. Biopsy is usually incisional except for very small lesions, which may have an excisional biopsy (see Chapter 3).

*TNM staging* (Tables 12.4, 12.5, and 12.6) is essential to treatment planning.

*Assessment* is discussed on page 626.

## Prognosis

Prognosis depends on several factors including:
- Neoplasm
  - clinical staging (especially presence of metastases),
  - histopathological grading,
  - site.
- Patient
  - age,
  - general health status.

**Table 12.4** TNM classification of malignant neoplasms[a]

| Primary tumour (T) | |
|---|---|
| T0 | No evidence of primary tumour |
| Tis | Carcinoma *in situ* |
| T1, T2, T3, T4 | Increasing size of tumour[b] |
| Regional lymph nodes (N) | |
| N0 | Regional lymph node not clinically demonstrable |
| N1 | Unilateral movable |
| N2[c] | Large, multiple or contralateral |
| N3 | Massive (>6 cm) or fixed nodes |
| Nx | Regional nodes cannot be assessed clinically |
| Distant metastases (M) | |
| M0 | No evidence of distant metastases |
| M1 | Evidence of metastatic involvement, including distant nodes |

[a] Several other classifications are available, e.g. STNM (S = site).
[b] T1 maximum diameter 2 cm; T2 maximum diameter of 4 cm; T3 maximum diameter over 4 cm; T4 massive or invading adjacent structures (e.g. muscle, bone).
[c] N2a >3 cm but <6 cm; N2b multiple ipsilateral <6 cm; N2c contralateral <6 cm.

**Table 12.5** TNM staging system

| Tumour (T) | Nodes (N) | Metastases at a distance (M) |
|---|---|---|
| 0 — | No cervical nodes enlarged | No detectable metastases |
| 1 <2 cm diameter | Single node <3 cm diameter | Metastases present |
| 2 2–4 cm diameter | Single node 3–6 cm diameter, or multiple ipsilateral nodes or contralateral | — |
| 3 >4 cm diameter | Single ipsilateral node >6 cm diameter or fixed | — |
| 4 Massive or invading adjacent structures | — | — |

**Table 12.6** Staging of lip and oral cancer

*TNM definition*

Primary tumour (T)

TX:   Primary tumour cannot be assessed

T0:   No evidence of primary tumour

Tis:   Carcinoma *in situ*

T1:   Tumour 2 cm or less in greatest dimension

T2:   Tumour more than 2 cm but not more than 4 cm in greatest dimension

T3:   Tumour more than 4 cm in greatest dimension

T4:   (lip) Tumour invades through cortical bone, inferior alveolar nerve, floor of mouth, or skin of face, i.e. chin or nose

  T4a:   (oral cavity) Tumour invades adjacent structures (e.g. through cortical bone, into deep [extrinsic] muscle of tongue [genioglossus, hyoglossus, palatoglossus, and styloglossus], maxillary sinus, skin of face)

  T4b:   Tumour invades masticator space, pterygoid plates, or skull base and/or encases internal carotid artery

Regional lymph nodes (N)

NX:   Regional lymph nodes cannot be assessed

N0:   No regional lymph node metastasis

N1:   Metastasis in a single ipsilateral lymph node, 3 cm or less in greatest dimension

N2:   Metastasis in a single ipsilateral lymph node, more than 3 cm but not more than 6 cm in greatest dimension; or in multiple ipsilateral lymph nodes, none more than 6 cm in greatest dimension; or in bilateral or contralateral lymph nodes, none more than 6 cm in greatest dimension

**Table 12.6** Contd.

| | |
|---|---|
| N2a: | Metastasis in a single ipsilateral lymph node more than 3 cm but not more than 6 cm in dimension |
| N2b: | Metastasis in multiple ipsilateral lymph nodes, none more than 6 cm in greatest dimension |
| N2c: | Metastasis in bilateral or contralateral lymph nodes, none more than 6 cm in greatest dimension |

N3:   Metastasis in a lymph node more than 6 cm in greatest dimension or fixed

Distant metastasis (M)

MX:   Distant metastasis cannot be assessed

M0:   No distant metastasis

M1:   Distant metastasis

*Stage grouping*

Stage 0

Tis, N0, M0

Stage I

T1, N0, M0

Stage II

T2, N0, M0

Stage III

T3, N0, M0

T1, N1, M0

T2, N1, M0

T3, N1, M0

Stage IVA

T4a, N0, M0

T4a, N1, M0

T1, N2, M0

T2, N2, M0

T3, N2, M0

T4a, N2, M0

Stage IVB

Any T, N3, M0

T4b, any N, M0

Stage IVC

Any T, any N, M1

Lip and oral cavity. In: American Joint Committee on Cancer: AJCC Cancer Staging Manual, 6th edn. New York, NY: Springer, 2002, pp. 23–32.

# Oral cancer: management principles

### Discussing the disease

It is always a problem to know how much to tell a patient who has cancer. If a patient asks a direct question, using the word cancer or a more technical synonym, one must presume that they have considered the implications and expect a truthful answer. Few patients do actually ask the direct question, and it is usually wrong to volunteer too much pathological information; however, do ask them whether there is anything that they would like to ask.

It is usually wise to explain that there are many kinds of tumour, some of which can be completely eradicated and others quite effectively treated. It is best to refer such questions to senior colleagues.

In many instances, investigations are carried out on patients to exclude the presence of a cancer, and if cancer is excluded from the differential diagnosis, it is part of good management to tell patients and their relatives that they need no longer worry about cancer. At least the partner or one of the responsible relatives should always be told the complete truth.

### Choice of treatment

Patients with oral cancer are best managed in specialized centres with access to all modern surgical, radiotherapy, dental and rehabilitative facilities, with high volumes of patient throughput, and where the best results can be reliably achieved.

Treatment, depending on the stage and other factors, may be directed towards:
• a cure,
• local disease control, or
• palliation only.

Treatment of choice may be:
• surgery (the treatment most commonly used);
• radiotherapy (as effective as surgery in small localized lesions);
• chemotherapy (not very effective against oral cancer in isolation, but often used in combination with radiotherapy).

Combinations of the above methods are used, e.g. post-surgical radiotherapy or chemo-radiation are often used if surgical clearance is doubtful, or patients have presented with advanced disease, and deeply invasive tumours.

Choice of treatment depends upon:
• option that gives best chance of a cure;
• adverse effects of treatment (see below);
• patient choice.

*Palliative therapy* may include various combinations of radiotherapy, chemotherapy, and occasionally debulking surgery.

*Effects of treatment on the oral tissues* (Table 12.7)
- Surgical treatment of malignant neoplasms in the head and neck is inevitably disfiguring to some degree, but cosmetic results are continually being improved and much can be offered.
- Rapidly proliferating epithelium such as the oral mucosa is highly susceptible to the cytotoxic action of radiation or chemotherapeutic drugs → mucositis (epithelial thinning, erythema, sloughing and a susceptibility to ulceration and infection). Mucositis is usually painful but self-limiting, healing in 2–3 weeks without scarring. Salivary and other tissues may also be damaged.
- Chemotherapeutic agents and their effects on the oral mucosa are discussed in Chapter 4.

**Table 12.7** Oral complications of cancer therapy

|  | Acute | Chronic |
| --- | --- | --- |
| Surgery | Pain<br>Disfigurement | Pain<br>Neuropathy<br>Disfigurement<br>Eating and speech difficulties |
| Radiotherapy | Pain<br>Mucositis<br>Xerostomia<br>Infection; candidosis;<br>herpes viruses | Pain<br>Osteoradionecrosis<br>Xerostomia; caries;<br>candidosis; sialadenitis<br>Fibrosis |
| Chemotherapy | Pain<br>Mucositis<br>Xerostomia<br>Infection<br>Nausea/vomiting | Pain<br>Neuropathy<br>Xerostomia<br>Infection |

# Oral cancer: preoperative management

**Preoperative assessment** (see also Chapters 1, 2, 3 and 10)

- A full history, physical examination, and examination of the head, neck, mouth and perioral tissues, including bimanual palpation of the lesion, and staging.
- Lesional biopsy.
- Assess tumour invasion, especially bone and nodes.
  - Examination of the neck for the presence of any enlarged lymph nodes or masses (are they fixed or mobile?).
  - Fine needle biopsy of equivocal neck lymph nodes with ultrasound control, or sentinel node biopsy (biopsy of the main draining lymph node).
  - Radiographic investigations—may include an OPTG and bitewings or oblique lateral mandibles for lesions involving or close to the jaw bones, and CT or MRI scanning of the head and neck. CXR; important as a pre-anaesthetic check especially in patients with known pulmonary or airways disease and to demonstrate metastasis to lungs or hilar lymph nodes, ribs or vertebrae.
  - MRI or CT—of suspected sites of distant metastases, and MRI scans of the neck to delineate the extent of cervical node metastases. MRI scanning particularly for lesions involving the sinuses.
  - Endoscopy to detect second primary tumours in the upper aerodigestive tract.
  - Radionucleotide bone scans where bone involvement is suspected.
  - PET (positron emission tomography) scans, which have a specificity for malignant tumours.
- Blood tests
  - full blood examination
  - grouping and cross-matching
  - clotting assays
  - urea and electrolytes
  - liver function tests
  - blood gases (if indicated)
- ECG is usually indicated as well as the above investigations.

**Preoperative management** (see also Chapter 10)

- Take blood for group and cross-match . There is seldom time in cancer treatment for autologous donation.
- Book intensive care unit bed.
- Check that informed consent has been given—extends to warning the patient that he/she will have procedures such as tracheotomy and will awaken in ITU with swelling and deformity.
- Plan care of dentition (see below).

### Management of the dentition

The newly diagnosed patient who has just been told that he/she has cancer will be in a state of mental turmoil, may not be able to assimilate much of what is said, and may fail to appreciate the importance of the oral examination.

It is not right to be judgemental of the patient who has poor oral hygiene, but it is absolutely essential that he/she understands the risks and discomfort that may ensue unless meticulous oral hygiene is maintained.

Quality of life is important. Elimination of pain and infection, and even provision of dentures, can make a great difference to the patient's psychological state. Discuss the prognosis with the responsible specialist. Heroic removal of teeth and bridge-planning may be inappropriate for a patient who has a poor life expectancy.

### Oral hygiene

Gentle, constant reiteration or oral hygiene with instruction and supervision by a dental hygienist, and scaling and polishing, will be not only valuable but will be appreciated as part of the general care. The patient should be provided with 0.2% aqueous chlorhexidine mouthrinses.

### Pain

Potential sources of pain, e.g. carious teeth, should be treated or extracted, as appropriate. Pain from mucositis and ulceration can be relieved by warm bicarbonate or saline mouthwashes, lidocaine 2% or benzydamine 0.15% mouthrinses 1-hourly, reducing to 2–3-hourly as the pain abates.

Deep pain needs systemic analgesia; do not hesitate to prescribe to patients with terminal malignancy, narcotics such as morphine sulphate.

Refer patients to a pain relief clinic or hospice as required.

# Oral cancer: surgery

Surgery is the mainstay of treatment for most oral carcinomas, unless small and in soft tissues only. Surgical treatment includes excision of the tumour (resection) and reconstruction to restore function and aesthetics.

**Principles in excision (resection)** include:
- Excision of the neoplasm with a margin of clinically normal tissue. A 2 cm three-dimensional margin is ideal for carcinoma. Intra-bony lesions may require a greater anatomical margin due to the tendency of neoplasms to spread along cancellous spaces.
- A marginal resection preserving the lower border of the mandible, or the superior part of the maxilla may be appropriate for small lesions.
- Larger lesions require a partial mandibulectomy, or maxillectomy, along with the soft tissues and lymphatics where tumour has spread.

The benefits of complete and radical excision, which may effect a cure must always be balanced against the inevitable mutilation of surgery.

**Reconstruction of defects** may involve:
*Bone grafts*—which provide structural replacement, and may later permit osseointegrated implants to be used, to replace teeth.
- For the mandible,
  - for small defects <5 cm, bone grafts can be harvested from rib, iliac crest, or calvarium. Bone grafts are seldom used for cancer reconstruction as the soft tissue bed may be compromised, and the grafts do not easily tolerate postoperative radiotherapy
  - for larger defects, free vascularized bone flaps including soft tissue can be used.
- For the maxilla,
  - an obturator can be utilized to close the oroantral communication;
  - the defect may be able to be closed surgically.

*Soft tissues* are reconstructed with a flap:
- In small defects, using local tissues, such as tongue, buccal fat pad, or mucosal flaps, or skin grafts (split thickness).
- In larger defects, using either
  - regional flaps such as nasolabial, or neck skin flaps, which require division later, or temporalis muscle flaps; or
  - distant myocutaneous flaps, which may be pedicled, i.e. pectoralis major, and latissimus dorsi muscle flaps. These require division later and are fairly bulky but useful.

*Free tissue transfer flaps* established with microvascular anastomosis are commonly used for oral reconstruction. They include:
- radial forearm flaps based on the radial vessels (fasciocutaneous or composite radial flaps with bone);
- composite fibula free flaps based on the peroneal vessels;
- composite deep circumflex iliac flaps based on this artery;
- rectus abdominis flaps based on the inferior epigastric vessels.

**Postoperative management** (see also Chapter 10)

Postoperatively, careful attention must be given to management of:

- the airways, often with a tracheostomy;
- pain;
- fluid and blood replacement;
- nutrition, often with nasogastric (NG) or percutaneous endoscopic gastrostomy (PEG) feeding;
- mental health state (delirium is not uncommon postoperatively; symptoms and signs of alcohol withdrawal should be expected in those that misuse alcohol; symptoms of depression are common, especially following prolonged hospitalization).

# Oral cancer: radiotherapy

### Uses of radiotherapy

- Radiotherapy alone may be used for small cancers involving the soft tissues only.
- Adjuvant radiotherapy is indicated for:
  - large cancers;
  - cancers with poor prognostic factors, i.e. perineural spread, lymphatic infiltration, close or positive surgical margins (i.e. where there may have been incomplete tumour excision);
  - the management of lymph nodes enlarged because of metastasis, particularly those with evidence of extra-capsular spread.

### Oral effects of radiotherapy (see also Chapter 4)

Radiotherapy can affect the mucosae, salivary glands, bone and muscles, and developing tissues. Recent advances in radiation therapy technology (see below) and the use of amifostine, have allowed a reduction in the occurrence and/or intensity of these complications.

- Mucositis is a troublesome adverse effect if radiotherapy includes the oral mucosa. Painful red and then erosive oral lesions appear early and may cause severe discomfort as well as difficulty in eating.
- The salivary glands, if in the field of radiation, are directly affected, resulting in saliva of:
  - ↓ volume;
  - ↓ pH;
  - ↑ viscosity;
  - altered composition.
- Salivary gland injury is slow in onset, but correspondingly much longer in recovery, with the possibility of permanent damage. Many patients then adopt a soft carbohydrate diet, which leads to a greatly increased caries rate. Cervical margin and cuspal caries are common.
- Endarteritis obliterans in the bone (especially the mandible) → risk of osteoradionecrosis—a serious late problem affecting the irradiated bone, and necessitating careful planning of any dentoalveolar surgery that may be needed.
- Endarteritis obliterans in muscles may cause trismus.

*Management* of the oral complications of radiotherapy is outlined in Table 12.8.

### Dentoalveolar surgery in those receiving radiotherapy

Teeth in the radiation field should be assessed for periodontal and dental disease. Teeth that should be removed include those:

- with furcation involvement;
- with periodontal pockets >4 mm;
- which are impacted;
- of doubtful prognosis.

Tooth extraction, or other surgical procedures should ideally be done well before radiotherapy is started, preferably at the time of cancer resection, because of the risk of osteoradionecrosis if surgery is carried out later. It is better to complete surgery at least 1 week before starting radiotherapy or shortly after completion of the course. It is unwise to delay surgery for longer than 3 months after radiotherapy, as endarteritis obliterans will have reached a peak effect by 6 months, which is non-reversible (although treatment with hyperbaric oxygen may help)—osteoradionecrosis is then a risk.

## Quality of life

Quality of life is crucial after cancer treatment; some 30% of patients suffer from depression. Counselling and medical care may be indicated. Smoking and other risk habits should be abandoned as the patient is at risk from second primary tumours.

**Table 12.8** Management of oral complications of radiotherapy

| Complication | Management |
|---|---|
| Mucositis | Prophylaxis: mucosal protection with blocks and amifostine |
| | Warm normal saline or benzydamine or aqueous chlorhexidine mouth baths |
| Ulcers | Aqueous chlorhexidine or benzydamine mouth baths four times daily |
| Candidosis | Nystatin suspension 100 000 u/mL as mouth wash four times daily, or fluconazole if immunocompromised |
| Xerostomia | Saliva substitute (see Chapter 8) |
| | Frequent ice cubes, popsicles or sips of water |
| Caries | Topical fluoride applications (see Chapter 7) |
| | Avoid sugary diet |
| Dental hypersensitivity | Fluoride applications |
| Periodontal disease | Oral hygiene |
| | Aqueous chlorhexidine mouth baths |
| Loss of taste | Consider zinc sulphate |
| Trismus | Jaw-opening exercises three times daily |
| Osteoradionecrosis/ irradiation-induced osteomyelitis | Avoid by planned pre-radiotherapy extractions or extractions within 3 months of radiotherapy |
| | When needed, use hyperbaric $O_2$ treatment and atraumatic extractions under antibiotic cover, with primary wound closure |

# Advances in radiation therapy

### Intensity-modulated radiation therapy (IMRT)

- IMRT (also known as conformal radiation) is one of the most advanced treatment methods available in external beam radiation therapy.
- IMRT uses computer-controlled X-ray accelerators to deliver precise radiation doses to a cancer. The radiation dose is designed to conform to the 3D shape of the tumour by modulating or controlling the intensity of the radiation beam to focus a higher radiation dose to the tumour while minimizing radiation exposure of surrounding normal tissues.
- The dose of radiation to the tumour is thus increased, while more adjoining normal tissue is spared.
- Rather than using a single large radiation beam as in conventional radiotherapy, with IMRT the radiation is broken up into thousands of tiny pencil-thin radiation beams which, with millimetre accuracy, enter the body from many angles and intersect on the cancer.
- IMRT can allow treatment of tumours to a higher dose, retreat cancers, which have previously been irradiated, and safely treat tumours that are located close to delicate organs such as the eye.
- Adverse effects from IMRT are the same as with conventional radiation therapy, but are less frequent and less intense.

# Potentially malignant lesions and conditions

These are listed in Table 12.9.

**Table 12.9** Oral lesions and conditions with the potential of malignant transformation

| Approximate malignant potential | Lesions/conditions | Known aetiological factors | Main clinical features |
|---|---|---|---|
| Very high (85%+) | Erythroplasia | Tobacco; alcohol | Red plaque |
| High in some instances (30%+) | Actinic cheilitis | Sunlight | White plaque/erosions |
| | Chronic hypertrophic candidosis (candidal leucoplakia) | *Candida albicans* | White or speckled white and red plaque |
| | Dyskeratosis congenita | Genetic | White plaques |
| | Leucoplakia (non-homogeneous) | Tobacco; alcohol | Speckled white and red plaque or nodular plaque |
| | Proliferative verrucous leucoplakia | Tobacco; alcohol; human papilloma-virus (HPV) | White or speckled white and red or nodular plaque |
| | Sublingual keratosis | Tobacco; alcohol | White plaque |
| | Submucous fibrosis | Areca nut | Immobile pale mucosa |
| | Syphilitic leucoplakia | Syphilis | White plaque |
| Low (<5%) | Atypia in immunocompromised patients | ? HPV | White or speckled white and red plaque |
| | Leucoplakia (homogeneous) | Friction; tobacco; alcohol | White plaque |
| | Discoid lupus erythematosus | Autoimmune | White plaque/erosions |
| | Lichen planus | Idiopathic | White plaque/erosions |
| | Paterson–Kelly–Brown syndrome (sideropenic dysphagia; Plummer–Vinson syndrome) | Iron deficiency | Post-cricoid web |

# Benign tumours

- The most common benign tumours affecting the mouth and jaws are epithelial lesions such as papillomas, fibroepithelial polyps, salivary gland tumours such as pleomorphic adenomas, and odontogenic tumours such as ameloblastomas and myxomas.
- The principle of management is that the lesion should be completely excised with a margin of normal tissue.
- Intra-bony tumours, such as ameloblastoma and myxoma present more significant problems with regard to achieving this, due to the tendency for the lesions to spread along the cancellous spaces in the mandible and spread into the soft tissues from the maxilla.
- Patients with odontogenic tumours are usually in a younger age group from those with oral squamous cell carcinoma and, as such, have different requirements for reconstruction and rehabilitation.

USEFUL WEBSITES
http://www.baoms.org.uk

# Being a professional

# Evidence-based dentistry

*Definition of evidence-based healthcare*
The use of the best evidence to make a decision regarding healthcare.

*Why is it important?*
There is a large amount of evidence available, but much is scattered and sometimes of questionable quality. Therefore, practice has traditionally had to be based on 'authority'. An evidence-based approach optimizes the effective use of available data, allows clinicians to keep up-to-date with rapid changes, raises patient and professional expectations, and more effectively regulates competing pressures on resources.

*What does it involve?*
Evidence-based healthcare can work on different levels—whether it is individual clinicians undertaking their own reviews of specific clinical decisions, departments reviewing the literature to produce protocols or health services producing national clinical guidelines.
The steps to establishing an 'evidence-base' remain the same whatever the scale of the review; the systematic location, appraisal and implementation of evidence into clinical practice.

## Levels of evidence

When deciding whether to implement evidence from a study, it is important to look at the type of study design employed, which determines the 'strength' of evidence on which to base the clinical decision.

### The 5 levels of evidence

**1a.** Systematic review of multiple randomized controlled trials (RCTs)
**1b.** Individual well-designed RCT
**2a.** Systematic review of cohort studies
**2b.** Individual cohort study, or low quality RCT
**3a.** Systematic review of case–control studies
**3b.** Individual case–control study
**4.** Non-analytical studies (case series)
**5.** Opinions of expert committees or respected authorities

These levels can be seen to represent a 'hierarchy', with more weight given to evidence from RCTs compared with expert opinion.

### Evidence-based dentistry resources

The Cochrane Collaboration conduct systematic reviews of evidence from RCTs and have a specific oral health group that have conducted reviews in many aspects of dentistry:

USEFUL WEBSITES
http://www.cochrane.org
http://www.cochrane-oral.man.ac.uk
http://www.ihs.ox.ac.uk/cebd/
http://www.cebm.net/levels_of_evidence.asp#levels

# Clinical governance

### Definition
Actions and systems put in place to monitor and enhance the quality of clinical services.

### Background
Quality of healthcare in some areas of the NHS came under the political spotlight in the 1990s after public confidence was undermined by some serious clinical 'scandals'. Clinical governance was introduced to make lines of accountability more explicit and organize quality improvement activities in a coordinated way.

Every NHS organization, whether a hospital, Primary Care Trust (PCT) or a general dental practice, has the responsibility for ensuring that clinical governance is in place. The Healthcare Commission (organization also known as CHAI—Commission for Healthcare, Audit and Inspection) is responsible for monitoring clinical governance arrangements and collecting information to enable performance rating of NHS organizations.

## The '7 pillars' of clinical governance
Clinical governance is an umbrella term for everything that helps maintain and improve standards of patient care. It has been described as having '7 pillars':

*1. Patient and public involvement* This can be demonstrated by the use of patient satisfaction surveys and Patient Advice and Liason Services (PALS)—which exist in every NHS trust (see http://www.dh.gov.uk).

*2. Risk management*—a four-stage process:
• Identify risks, using screening, checklists, etc.
• Assess frequency and severity of risks.
• Eliminate risks where possible.
• If risk elimination is impossible, reduce the risk, and plan for damage limitation.

*3. Clinical audit* See page 642.

*4. Staffing and management* Having a quality improvement approach to human resource management including staff appraisals, and mechanisms to deal with poor performance (such as 'whistle-blowing') rather than ignoring such practices.

*5. Clinical effectiveness* Concerned with how to implement and apply effective clinical practice (see evidence-based dentistry and clinical guidelines).

*6. Continuous Professional Development (CPD)*
• Each registered dentist has to declare their CPD activities to the General Dental Council. A random sample of dentists is monitored. Failure to comply may result in removal from the Dentists Register (see: http://www.gdc-uk.org/lifelong/LifelongNew/).
• Dentists should undertake 250 h of CPD every 5 years, of which 75 must be 'verifiable'.

- To count as verifiable CPD, an activity must have educational aims and objectives, clear anticipated outcomes and an evaluation procedure. Examples include courses organized by Postgraduate Dental Deans, the British Dental Association (BDA) and other specialist and professional bodies, participation in regional clinical audit meetings, etc. Documentary proof of attendance must be obtained from the organizer, and retained.
- General (non-verifiable) CPD activities are those that contribute to professional development as a dentist, but do not fulfill all criteria for verifiable CPD (e.g. journal reading, staff training and private study).
- Personal development plans are recommended, to identify training needs and plan attendance at courses etc accordingly.

**7. Information** Use information to support clinical governance. Provide information on the patient experience.

# Clinical audit

### Definition of clinical audit

The comparison of current practice against previously agreed standards and criteria.

*Examples* of clinical audit include reviewing the quality of operations, radiographs or cross-infection control protocols.

## The steps are

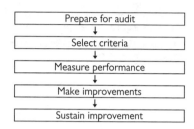

### Prepare for audit

- Choose a topic—start with a topic of concern to staff.
- Set aside time to conduct the audit.
- Ensure the support of colleagues.

### Select criteria

Explicit criteria such as guidelines or reviews of evidence are best (see Clinical Guidelines, page 644).

### Measure performance

- Collect data on current practice. Depending on the topic, this may be from clinical records and/or department/hospital databases. Using several data sources helps overcome problems of incomplete records.
- Performance is reviewed against the criteria.

### Make improvements

- In the light of findings, devise a plan for implementing improvements.
- Discuss improvements with colleagues and take account of potential barriers to change.

### Sustain improvements

Monitor and reinforce the improvements, and keep up-to-date.

# Clinical guidelines

### Definition of clinical guidelines

Systematically developed statements, which assist in decision-making about appropriate healthcare for specific clinical conditions.

### Why set clinical guidelines?

Clinical guidelines are developed using an evidence-based approach to encourage best practice and limit unsatisfactory treatment variations. Some clinicians feel guidelines are an infringement on professional judgement and autonomy but, with risk management strategies in place, there is already an inevitable move towards a reduction in clinical freedom.

## Who develops clinical guidelines?

*The National Institute for Clinical Excellence (NICE)* is one of the main organizations that develop healthcare guidelines for the NHS in England and Wales (http://www.nice.org.uk/). For example,

- in 2000 NICE produced guidance on the removal of impacted third molars (see box below), and
- guidelines on the recall interval between routine dental examinations, and improving outcomes in head and neck cancer appeared in 2004.

*The Scottish Intercollegiate Guidelines Network (SIGN)* develops guidelines for Scotland.

*The Royal College of Surgeons of England (RCSEng)* has produced the 'Faculty of Dental Surgery National Clinical Guidelines 1997', a document that contains clinical guidelines for five of the dental specialties (http://www.rcseng.ac.uk/dental/fds/clinical_guidelines/).

- *Oral and maxillofacial surgery:* e.g. 'Management of pericoronitis', 'Management and prevention of dry socket', 'Management of unilateral fractures of the condyle'.
- *Orthodontics:* e.g. 'Management of the palatally ectopic maxillary canine', 'Management of unerupted maxillary incisors'.
- *Paediatric dentistry:* e.g.'Prevention of dental caries in children', 'Continuing oral care—review and recall'.
- *Restorative dentistry:* e.g. 'Screening of patients to detect periodontal diseases', 'Guidelines for selecting appropriate patients to receive treatment with dental implants; priorities for the NHS', 'Restorative indications for porcelain veneer restorations'.
- *Dental public health:* e.g. 'Turning clinical guidelines into effective commissioning'.

*Specialist societies* may publish their own guidelines, e.g.:
'Paediatric Dentistry Clinical Guidelines' have already been published and include 'Treatment of avulsed permanent teeth in children', 'Treatment of traumatically intruded permanent incisor teeth in children', etc.

## Implementation of clinical guidelines

Guidelines are not mandatory and implementation is the concern of the individual clinician, if self-employed, or the employing NHS organization (e.g. hospital or Community Dental Service) as part of their clinical governance plan.

## NICE guidance on the removal of third molars (wisdom teeth)

- The routine practice of prophylatic removal of pathology-free impacted third molars should be discontinued in the NHS.
- The standard routine programme of dental care by dental practitioners and/or paraprofessional staff, need be no different, in general, for pathology-free impacted third molars (those requiring no additional investigations or procedures).
- Surgical removal of impacted third molars should be limited to patients with evidence of pathology. Such pathology includes unrestorable caries, nontreatable pupal and/or periapial pathology, cellulitis, abcess and osteomyelitis, internal/external resorption of the tooth or adjacent teeth, fracture of tooth, disease of follicle including cyst/tumour, tooth/teeth impeding surgery or reconstructive jaw surgery, and when a tooth is involved in or within the field or tumour resection.
- Specific attention is drawn to plaque formation and pericoronitis. Plaque formation is a risk factor but is not in itself an indication for surgery. The degree to which the severity or recurrence rate of pericoronitis should influence the decision for surgical removal of a third molar remains unclear. The evidence suggests that a first episode of pericoronitis, unless particularly severe, should not be considered an indication for surgery. Second or subsequent episodes should be considered the appropriate indication for surgery.

# Critical appraisal of literature

A key part of reviewing evidence is sifting through the often huge quantities of published literature to identify what should inform practice and what is unreliable. This is where appraisal of the quality of a paper is important. The appraisal should consider research design and conduct.

Critical appraisal can be done informally by asking yourself a few simple questions as you read the paper:

- *What clinical question were the authors addressing?* Look for a brief review of the published literature leading on to realistic aims and set of objectives.
- *What type of study was done?* Does the paper describe research first hand ('primary research') or review existing studies ('secondary research')?
- *Was this design appropriate to the research?* Different research questions are best answered by different types of study. For example, if the study was to test the efficacy of a surgical procedure or drug regime, the preferred study design is an RCT.

Alternatively, critical appraisal can be carried out by the use of an 'off-the-shelf' *structured checklist*. The Critical Appraisal Skills Programme (CASP) has a useful website (http://www.phru.nhs.uk/~casp/appraisa.htm). These checklists include 10 questions that systematically guide the reader through the issues pertinent to the study design in question.

*Further reading* on critical appraisal:
'How to read a paper' (http://bmj.bmjjournals.com/collections/read.shtml).

# Dental specialty training

### General professional training (GPT)

Anyone wishing to train as a specialist in UK must first complete at least 2 years of GPT in approved posts, covering at least two disciplines. At least 1 year in total must be spent in hospital or community practice, and each post must be occupied for a minimum of 3 months. During this period, the trainee is graded as a senior house officer (SHO), clinical assistant, or house officer (if they occupy a post at a dental teaching hospital).

#### Member of the Faculty of Dental Surgery (MFDS) exam

During or after GPT, trainees are also required to complete all parts of the MFDS Examination of one of the Royal Colleges.

- Part A may be taken after 12 months of training. The exam is composed of written examination papers.
- Parts B may be taken after 20 months of training and is another written exam.
- Part C may also be taken after 20 months of training (if successful in part B) and consists of clinical and oral examinations.

### Specialist training (Higher professional training; HPT)

After completing the MFDS exam and 24 months of GPT, the next step is to gain an appointment as a Specialist Registrar (SpR). These posts are for a defined period of training → Certificate in Completion of Specialist Training (CCST). All SpRs are registered with the appropriate Specialist Advisory Committee (SAC) of the Royal College of Surgeons, which is responsible for monitoring the trainee's progress and the quality of training received. Progress is monitored by appraisal from a trainer, with an annual assessment (Record of In-Training Assessment [RITA]).

### Dental specialties

The recognized dental specialties in the UK and training periods are summarized in Table 13.1. There is growing political pressure for ↓ training times and ↑ number of 'Specialists'; therefore, the training length in certain specialties (especially Oral & Maxillofacial Surgery) is likely to change.

**Table 13.1** Dental specialties in the UK

| Specialty | Length of training |
| --- | --- |
| Oral and maxillofacial surgery | 5 years (after medical school and 2 foundation years) |
| Oral surgery (academic) | 5 years |
| Surgical dentistry | 3 years |
| Endodontics | 3 years |
| Periodontics | 3 years |
| Prosthodontics | 3 years |
| Restorative dentistry | 5 years |
| Dental Public Health | 5 years |
| Orthodontics<br>—specialist<br>—consultant | <br>3 years<br>5 years |
| Paediatric dentistry<br>—specialist<br>—consultant | <br>3 years<br>5 years |
| Oral medicine | 3 years (after medical school) |
| Oral microbiology | 5 years |
| Dental and maxillofacial radiology | 4 years |
| Oral pathology | 5 years |

# Working as a dentist in the UK

To work as a dentist in the UK requires registration with the General Dental Council (GDC). The GDC website has full details on how to register (http://www.gdc-uk.org).

- For graduates from the UK, Switzerland and the European Economic Area (EEA), registration with the GDC involves completing an application form, providing proof of qualification recognized by the relevant member state, and sending a fee.
- In addition, the dental qualifications awarded by certain countries outside the EEA, e.g. Hong Kong, Australia and Singapore, are also recognized by the GDC for the purposes of registration in the UK.
- For non-UK, non-EEA nationals or those whose dental degree is not recognised by the GDC, the procedure for registering with the GDC involves either seeking temporary registration (see below) or full registration upon completion of the International Qualifying Exam (IQE).

*Temporary registration*

Temporary registration is not appropriate for work in the general or community dental services, but is appropriate for those involved in:

- postgraduate study in a post approved by one of the Royal Surgical Colleges of the UK;
- specialist training;
- teaching at a dental school or hospital;
- clinical research work in a dental school or hospital.

To be eligible to apply, dentists must have an offer of employment. Those with temporary registration can only practise under the supervsion of a named consultant. Temporary registration is granted for between 3 and 12 months at a time, and for a total of no more than 5 years.

*International Qualifying Exam (IQE)*

Dentists whose primary qualifications are not recognized by the GDC, but who wish to have full registration in the UK are required to complete the IQE. To be eligible to sit the exam, a certificate showing a minimum score of 7.0 in each section of the academic International English Language Testing System (IELTS) should be attained.

The IQE consists of three parts (A, B and C) and involves written exams, oral exams, tests in an operative techniques laboratory and practical clinical exams. An information pack about the IQE is available from the GDC.

# Dental services

*Aim of dental services:* 'To provide the opportunity for everyone to retain a healthy functional dentition for life by preventing what is preventable and containing the remaining disease by the efficient use and distribution of treatment resources'.

## Levels of health service

In the UK, dental services, like medical services, are provided on primary, secondary and tertiary levels.

### Primary care

Primary health services are the first point of contact for the public and are locally based. Primary care includes General Medical Practitioners (GMPs), General Dental Practitioners (GDPs), Opticians, Pharmacists etc. Primary Care Trusts (PCTs) are responsible for the planning and securing of primary health services and improving the health of the local population. There are ~300 PCTs in England; they are given the funding to plan and commission primary health services for their local communities.

### Secondary care

Access to secondary services is controlled through referral from primary care—primary care practitioners can be thought of as the gate-keepers to secondary and tertiary care. Secondary care involves specialist services, based mainly in hospitals; for example district general hospitals (DGHs).

### Tertiary care

Tertiary care services are based at centres of clinical excellence provided on a regional or national basis, such as teaching hospitals. Examples include Cleft Lip and Palate Services, Cancer Services, etc.

## Structure of dental services

The dental services in the UK include General Dental Services (GDS), Community Dental Services (CDS), Hospital Dental Services (HDS) and Personal Dental Services (PDS). In dentistry, there is more emphasis on primary care than in medicine (Table 13.2).

**Table 13.2** Dental services and % of professionals working in them

| Service | Dental personnel (%) | Medical personnel (%) |
|---|---|---|
| General | 75 | 40 |
| Hospital | 10 | 50 |
| Community | 10 | 10 |
| Others | 5 | 0 |

The differences between these services are levels of care provided, types of patients seen, funding and contractual arrangements with health commissioners, and methods of payment of the personnel (see next).

# Providers of dental services in the UK

*General Dental Services (GDS)* provide primary care through dentists, hygienists and therapists. In the UK, only 50% of the population are registered with a GDP—but about 99% are registered with the General Medical Service. GDPs, unlike GMPs, run small businesses and are responsible for their own premises and staff.

Currently, most of the income of GDPs is generated through a fee-per-item system. There is a small component for continuing care of patients. The Dental Practice Board (DPB) is a statutory body that currently administers the GDS.

*Community Dental Services (CDS)* have the role to:
- Monitor levels of dental disease through school-based screening and epidemiological surveys.
- Provide a full range of treatments to patients who are unable or unwilling to obtain treatment from GDS. This includes patients that have special needs such as dental phobics and adults and children with learning difficulties. The CDS also has a so-called 'safety net' role in treating patients who have difficulty accessing mainstream services.
- Assist in oral health promotion, including involvement in community projects.
- Provide a specialist referral service for the provision of GA and orthodontics for patients referred from GDPs.

Thus the CDS provides both primary and secondary services and has a contract with the PCT that is monitored by Consultants in Dental Public Health. The CDS dentists are salaried and have a career structure with Community Dental Officers, Senior Dental Officers and Directors of Clinical Dental services.

*Hospital Dental Services (HDS)* provide specialist care, acting as a point of referral for complex cases including oral & maxillofacial surgery, oral medicine, orthodontics and restorative care. The HDS is consultant led and based almost entirely in hospitals. The other aspect is the training of undergraduates and postgraduates. The HDS includes secondary and tertiary care. Dentists working in the HDS are salaried, or honorary and University employees.

*Personal Dental Services (PDS)* pilot schemes were established in 1998 to examine different methods of providing dentistry in order to solve local problems, including provision of GA services and denture services. Dental Access Centres are designed to solve local access problems. Some CDSs have converted to PDS to give them greater flexibility and allow modernization. There are about 600 dentists working in about 100 pilot schemes across the UK. Most PDS dentists are salaried.

*Corporate bodies* are 'companies' that provide dental services. There are 27 corporate bodies in the UK and the 1952 Dentist Act prevented the creation of additional corporates. Examples include 'Oasis', and 'Petrie Tucker and Partners Ltd'.

***Private dentistry*** Current estimates suggest 24% of adult patients receive some or all of their dental treatment privately. Patients can receive both private and NHS treatment from the same dentist in the same course of treatment, although some restrictions exist.

***Other dental services*** include Prison Dental Services and the Armed Forces.

# Future NHS dentistry

*NHS Dentistry: Options for Change* was published in 2002 by the Department of Health (DoH). The key themes were:
- Local commissioning and funding via PCTs
- Different methods of paying general dental practitioners
- Focus on prevention of oral diseases
- More evidence-based dentistry into everyday clinical practice
- Information and Communication Technology
- Dental team approach
- Improving the patient experience

In England, *the Health and Social Care (Community Health and Standards) Act 2003* provided the legislation to make some of the changes suggested in 'Options for Change' legal. Further regulations will follow in 2006. In summary, for primary dental services, PCTs will have responsibility to secure or provide dental services in their area to the extent considered reasonable to do so. In addition:
- All GDPs will have a contract with a PCT
- GDPs will no longer be paid per item of treatment
- The new method of payment will mean a stable monthly income
- The way patients are charged for treatment will change
- The DPB will be abolished

(http://www.bda-dentistry.org.uk)

# Applying for a new appointment

### Finding posts

*Advertisements* for dental posts appear mainly in the professional journals, such as the national dental or medical Journals, and *Lancet* and, in some countries state dental or medical journals. The more junior a post, the more predictable the time of its advertisement. If you are really interested in a specific post, check the journals of the previous year to assess the time it is likely to be advertised.

*Discussions* with colleagues or the Postgraduate Dean may indicate when jobs are likely to appear.

### Deciding to apply

Before applying for a post, *ask the advice of your chief*; do not just announce your firm intent to apply.

It is also good manners to *contact your referees*, preferably by letter, when you have decided to apply, even though many referees will happily give a reference without a prior request. Referees may well be able to advise upon the advantages or otherwise of the advertised position and the appropriateness or otherwise of the application. They may also know of another, more appropriate job. They will need your up-to-date curriculum vitae (CV) (see below).

### Closing dates

There may be only a very brief time between the advertisement and the closing date for applications. If the closing date has passed, no harm is done by telephoning, as they may have had no applicants. Alternatively, your boss may suggest that this is better done by him/her.

### Equal opportunities

Equal opportunity means that in the recruitment, selection, training, appraisal, development and promotion of staff, the only consideration must be that the individual meets, or is likely to meet the requirements of the post. The requirements being met, no employee should be discriminated against on the basis of their sex, sexual orientation, race, colour, ethnic origin, nationality (within current legislation), disability, marital status, caring or parental responsibilities, age, or beliefs on matters such as religion and politics.

### Application procedures

Application procedures are usually given in the advertisement. Apart from the necessary application forms, submit a CV (see next) with a neat and courteous letter of application.

Send your referees a recent CV and photograph; this will help to remind them of you, of all your qualifications, and help to do you justice!

# Curriculum vitae (CV)

The CV is an essential component of most applications. The object is to summarize the qualifications and experience relevant to the post advertised. Brevity, clarity and honesty are required; Keep the CV updated. The following suggestions are adapted from 'Ellis *et al BDJ* 2002 Vol. 192 no. 3', but for some positions, a different format is required.

## Some general rules

- A separate title page bearing your name and qualifications can give a professional first impression.
- A structured lay-out including headings, bullet points and 'line spacing' of text of 1.5 makes a CV easy to read.
- Stick to either chronological or reverse chronological order, when listing qualifications, jobs, publications, etc.
- The CV should be no more that 6 pages long.
- Check spelling and grammar carefully, as mistakes can be taken to indicate a less than thorough attitude.
- Photographs should not be included.

## Contents of the CV

- *Personal details*—full name, date of birth, nationality, address and email address, and telephone numbers.
- *Details of secondary education* are relevant for junior posts. Do mention if you had a position of responsibility such as head boy/girl.
- *University education*—include University attended, qualifications gained, year of qualification and prizes won.
- *Postgraduate education*—include name of qualification, institution and dates.
- *Academic awards and honours.*
- *Membership of societies* including General Dental Council number, whether a member of a medical defence organization as well as membership of national or international dental associations and specialist societies.
- *Publications*—include papers published, papers in press and papers submitted:
  - Original reports
  - Review papers
  - Theses
  - Books
  - Chapters in books
  - Monographs
  - Non-printed materials
- *Presentations*—include title of presentation, date and name of meeting.
- *Research*—include interests and any research grants.
- *Audit*—include audits completed and in progress.
- *Teaching experience.*
- *Committee or administrative experience.*
- *Employment history*—any gaps should be explained.
- *Hobbies and outside interests*—outline briefly.
- A statement of ambitions.
- *Referees*—remember always to politely ask the referee for permission to use them, and (again!) always give the referee a recent CV if you want their help.

## Before the interview

# Before the interview

- 'Forewarned is forearmed'. Find out about the department, staff qualifications and publications (from colleagues, from the website and from
a *Medline* or *Google* search).
- Prepare yourself by making yourself aware of current trends in health
care; governance; etc.
- Check if you can or should visit. Some busy units may receive dozens
of applications and may only appreciate pre-interview visits from
candidates whom they have short-listed. You do not lose anything by
asking; indeed most people will see this as a sign of your interest. A
brief visit will give you a chance to:
  - find out about the clinical and other responsibilities and potential of
    the post,
  - meet potential colleagues and find out about their professional
    interests (try and meet all the persons with whom you hope to
    work),
  - determine conditions of service such as duty rotas, study leave,
    holidays, accommodation (do not leave this until you are inter-
    viewed!).
- Your visit will also give the staff a chance to assess you as a potential
colleague.
- Avoid telling them how suitable you think you are! Do not canvass
(solicit for preferential treatment).
- Try and meet the person you are replacing, as he or she is likely to
have the most useful information about the job.
- Never be dissuaded from applying by rumours about possible better
applicants. Competitors may fail to arrive for interview, may suffer
from a drawback of which you are unaware, may interview badly, or
even withdraw after appointment.
- Many a candidate who was destined (on the grapevine) for assured
success has failed at interview!
- If you are short-listed, you may need to revisit to clear up any points
you are unclear about, but be careful not to appear to canvass.

# At the interview

- Turn up in good time; the interviews may be running early and you will not impress the committee (even if you are on time) if they have to wait for you—catch an earlier train/flight, etc.
- Few applicants enjoy being interviewed (even your apparently relaxed competitors), but a well-prepared applicant invariably finds the ordeal less harrowing and is often more successful.
- If there is a problem in attending interview, make every effort to communicate personally with the principal, head of department and/ or administrator to explain.
- Although there are no regulations concerning dress or personal appearance for an interview, most of the interviewers will be middle-aged or older and are often fairly conservative in their views. Ignore this if you do not care for the job (Fig. 13.1).
- Take along a copy of your CV and a logbook if you have one.
- Think beforehand about obvious questions such as:
  - 'Why do you want this particular job?'
  - 'Where do you see your future career?' or 'Where do you see yourself in 5 years?'
  - 'Why did you take the job at your last hospital or practice?'
  - 'When do you intend to take the .............. examination?'
  - 'How do you see your role in relation to ............ (specific) members of staff?'
  - 'What publications are you preparing?'
  - 'What do you do in your spare time?'
  - 'What would you like to ask the committee?' (be careful!)
  - 'What are your strengths and weaknesses?'
- Less obvious questions may include:
  - 'How would you define clinical audit?'
  - 'What is the definition of clinical governance?'
  - 'What do you understand by evidence-based treatment?'
- The interview is not designed to upset or embarrass the applicant (although it may on occasion do so), but is aimed at finding the most suitable person for the post.
- The main purpose is not simply to gain factual information about the applicant (this is on the application form or CV), but is often the only opportunity to assess the applicant's ideas, personality and ability to relate to colleagues, and to achieve what is required in the post. These are important factors, particularly in a clinical post, and are often far more important than academic factors.
- Act naturally, but be honest and courteous. Discuss points but never argue; you may win the battle, but you will surely lose the war.
- You do not have to agree with everything either, or it may appear as though you have no opinions. Most committees appreciate applicants who know what they want and appear determined (but not arrogant!).
- The interview committee consists of a range of individuals, each with their own personal and professional backgrounds, experiences, interests and prejudices. A hospital or university interview committee usually consists of the head of department, other dental and/or medical

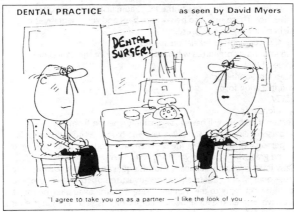

Courtesy of D. Myers and *Dental Practice*.

**Fig. 13.1**

specialists, representatives of the PCT, administration and often university. There may also be lay members and representatives of Higher Training bodies present.

- Equal Opportunities legislation applies.
- The interview committee will have knowledge of the applicant by virtue of the:
  - application letter
  - application form
  - CV
  - references
- Certain members will have additional information from:
  - personal discussions with colleagues who have worked with the applicant
  - personal observation of the applicant at meetings, when visiting, etc.
  - the grapevine (be sure your sins will catch up with you!)
- Many interviews will culminate with the question: 'Have you anything you would wish to ask us about the advertised post?' Think beforehand about a brief reply to this, remembering that, for example, you might not have located the local medical library or Postgraduate Centre on your visit (of course you knew it existed), or discussed the opportunity to attend specific clinics that may help your education.

⚠ Do not, at this time, ask about pay, study leave, time off, or holidays. You should have discussed this before the interview (or save it for later).

- In general, be prepared to accept the post straight away if an offer is made immediately after the interview. For some posts, someone will write subsequently to the candidates to give the result of the appointment procedure. If this mechanism is adopted, it is particularly bad form to decline an offered post at this stage.
- At all times, if applying for more than one post, be frank and have a clear idea of which is your preferred post. Remember the grapevines!

### The attributes of the 'perfect' member of staff

- Appropriate level of clinical knowledge
- Knowledge of evidence-informed practice
- Awareness of own limitations
- Ability to prioritize clinical need
- Ability to organize oneself and own work
- Experience and ability to work in multiprofessional teams
- Communication and language skills (the ability to communicate with clarity and intelligibility in written and spoken English; ability to build rapport, listen, persuade, negotiate)
- Decisiveness/accountability (ability to take responsibility, show leadership, make decisions, exert appropriate authority)
- Interpersonal skills (see patients as people, empathize, work co-operatively with others, open and non-defensive, sense of humour)
- Non-judgemental approach to patients and colleagues regardless of their sexuality, ethnicity, disability, religious beliefs or financial status
- Flexibility (able to change and adapt, respond to rapidly changing circumstances)
- Resilience (able to operate under pressure, cope with setbacks, self-aware)
- Thoroughness (is well prepared, shows self-discipline/commitment, is punctual and meets deadlines)
- Initiative/drive/enthusiasm (self-starter, motivated, shows curiosity, initiative)
- Probity (displays honesty, integrity, aware of ethical dilemmas, respects confidentiality)
- Clear, logical thinking showing an analytical/scientific approach
- Good manual dexterity and hand/eye co-ordination
- Understanding of clinical risk management

# If accepted for a position

- Thank your referees; you will probably need their references again in the future.
- Ensure that your subscriptions to professional bodies and medical insurance are paid.
- Contact the clinic before taking up the post, to determine when they expect you to arrive, where to report to, and whether there are any duties to perform before or shortly after the post is taken up. Ask whether there is a specific booklet about the clinic, department and/or hospital.
- Find out your timetable and any on-call duties. If 'on-call', establish which wards, patients, and other duties are your responsibility.
- Meet the ward sister or senior practice nurse, after asking the best times to visit. This will often greatly enhance cooperation and expedite the carrying out of the duties.
- A member of staff who appears promptly on the first day of a post and is well versed in protocol and responsibilities is obviously better received than one who arrives late and disorientated.
- Always wear a clean clinical coat, and look smart.
- Familiarize yourself with the layout and introduce yourself to those with whom you will be working and those who will need to recognize your signature (e.g. secretaries, technicians) or, in hospital, departments such as radiology, pharmacy and pathology.
- Find out about emergency procedures and where the emergency kits are kept on day 1.
- Check health and safety at work regulations etc.
- You may have to report to the Occupational Health department on the first day (or before you start), regarding your HBV immunization status, etc. It saves time to have any relevant documentation with you. Some hospitals may not allow you to start any clinical work before you get clearance from Occupational health.

# Professional skills

- There is much more to being a successful member of staff than simply knowing all about dentistry, although, clearly, staff should be well-informed.
- Remember you are only one of a team (see page 672); **nobody** is indispensible.
- There is much truth in the saying that the three As are important in making a successful dental surgeon (and note the order!): Availability, Affability and Ability.

## Reliability

There is nothing more irritating than an unreliable member of staff. Reliability includes not only good timekeeping, but also reliability in case note-keeping, carrying out duties, etc.

## Record keeping

It is of paramount importance always to make legible, accurate, dated and signed records in the case notes whenever you check a patient, or when there is an incident involving a patient (e.g. complaint or accident).

Keep a *notebook* with a separate page for each patient, and the details of various procedures.

In addition, ensure that you:

- Enter details of any examination, medication or procedure, patient complaint or discharge.
- File all results of investigations in the correct place.
- Do not lose records, hide records, or take them away from where they should be.

## Referrals

All patients in the hospital service must be in the charge of a consultant, who has personal responsibility for the patient, despite any delegation of duties to other professional staff.

Junior staff must ensure that the consultant knows about patients admitted or seen under him/her and you should not refer patients to another firm unless there is an emergency or you have been instructed to do so by your consultant or his deputy.

## Off-duty rotas

- Proper cover must be arranged for patients, even when the member of staff is out of the clinic and off duty. This is a clear and moral responsibility, if not a legal one.
- When handing over to a colleague, be sure to indicate all patients who may require attention, preferably leaving a written list.

## Hospital annual and study leave

After you have discussed this with your consultant(s), send an Annual/Study Leave form (obtainable from the hospital administrator) to the medical personnel department, as far in advance as possible of the proposed period of leave. Make it clear, in writing, exactly who has agreed to cover your duties when needed.

## Behaviour towards patients

- The psychological welfare of the patient must always be considered, and this is best accomplished by the personal interest and presence of the dentist, largely learnt by example and experience.
- Remember that words and manners may well have great significance to patients. Casual remarks will be analysed and repeated verbatim and phrases may be recalled for a lifetime. The smallest word of encouragement may well lift a patient from despair, or, conversely, lack of compassion may compound their misery.
- Routine is a fertile soil for indifference, but there is nothing routine for patients about their visits to, or time in, a clinic or hospital, and in their view there is no such thing as a 'minor' procedure.
- The reputation of and confidence in the practice, department or hospital, as far as patients are concerned, depend largely upon the attitudes and behaviour of the staff.

## Private patients

- Private patients are usually affable, appreciative and cooperative.
- A minority are difficult, a few highly demanding and unreasonable.
- In any event, make a concerted effort to give the quality of care that you would to any patient and do not be pushed into doing anything against your better judgement.
- Except in general practice, do not mix private treatment with health service care.

# Being part of a team

## Communication

Communication is essential in any teamwork; if it fails, this can lead to endless problems. If in doubt, ask for advice. Unless you have instructions to the contrary, contact the next most senior colleague.

It is a common mistake of junior staff to try too hard to impress their seniors. Nobody expects you to know everything; certainly not when you start a new job. All senior staff are aware of the difficulties that a new member of staff is likely to face, and will be happy to give advice. It is much more preferable to 'embarrass' yourself by asking something 'silly' (they will forget very soon), rather than risking taking up more responsibility than you are expected to (this they will not forget!). As one consultant once put it: 'There is nothing more dangerous than an over-enthusiastic trainee!'

▶If in any doubt, call someone senior.

## Interpersonal relationships

Apart from the obvious need for a good 'bedside manner' with patients, the dental surgeon must behave in a way that is acceptable to other staff and engenders their support. Communication, courtesy and consideration are essential qualities. A sense of humour is also helpful!

## Behaviour towards colleagues and staff

- The new graduate is the most junior member of a team and should be ready to ask questions, but slow to offer opinions or advice.
- It is particularly important to avoid criticism of another practitioner (even if it is competitor).
- If you consider that seniors are in error (and they might be), use the utmost tact when airing this view.
- Do not argue in front of a patient.
- The time to be most cautious is when feeling most confident.
- You are the least experienced member, even if you are brighter than other staff.
- A word of appreciation costs nothing.
- Excessive familiarity with staff is most unwise.
- Never mix business with pleasure!

### Nursing staff

Most disagreements with nurses arise because of different priorities. Almost invariably there will have been an avoidable failure in communication. The following considerations should minimize potential trouble:

- The senior nurse or Sister is responsible for running the clinic, practice or ward (everything from housekeeping and equipment maintenance to administering treatment). This is particularly so in allocating duties to nurses and domestic staff. The junior dentist interferes in these matters at his own peril.
- Avoid telling nurses what do to. Most senior nurses respond to politeness, and are usually willing to impart their considerable knowledge and experience if you ask for advice.

- If you need assistance, politely ask the Sister or senior nurse. The obvious exception is in the case of an emergency.
- Senior nurses often regard their clinics or wards as they would their own house. Visitors, including dental staff, should observe normal social protocol; always ask permission of the nurse in charge if you wish to see a patient, do a ward round, or show a visitor around.

### Telephonists and receptionists
- Good communications are essential in any establishment.
- Answer the 'page' or 'bleep' and telephone calls promptly.
- Receptionists and telephonists talk to everyone and can damage your reputation more quickly than anybody else if they so choose!

### Secretaries and administrative staff
- Secretaries are not impressed by the member of staff who 'knows it all' or criticizes others.
- If they like you, they can be extremely helpful at times when you need a favour, e.g. while working on an audit.
- Secretaries often speak freely with their senior staff, who may value their comments about junior staff, especially at reference time!

### Students
New graduates should recall their immediate past when dealing with students. Despite what staff might like to think, there is only a marginal difference in experience and knowledge. There is no need for arrogance when dealing with students, juniors, or nurses.

### Other ancillary staff
Establish at an early stage the responsibilities of and type of work carried out by ancillary staff such as Professionals Complementary to Dentistry (PCDs). For example:
- Hygienists work only to the prescription of a registered dentist and carry out oral hygiene instruction, scaling and application of fissure sealants.
- Dental therapists can carry out simple fillings and exodontia.
- Both hygienists and therapists are permitted to give local anaesthetic injections by infiltration and, subject to appropriate training, can administer inferior alveolar nerve blocks under the personal supervision of a registered dentist.

## The golden rules are
- Always answer your bleep/page/phone.
- If in doubt, ask.
- Tell the truth.
- Always err on the side of over-communication.
- Inform your colleagues of your whereabouts, holidays, etc.
- Do not upset your colleagues or the telephonist, secretary or nurses.

# Records and confidentiality

## Records

Good clear and accurate records are essential:
- to good practice and patient care
- medicolegally

*Records should be:*
- in ink or type, not pencil;
- legible;
- dated;
- signed clearly (with your name in capitals if the signature is obscure);
- factually accurate (take especial care on tooth notation);
- complete;
- in correct sequence.

*Records should not:*
- be subsequently altered unless the alteration is signed and dated, as in the case of an altered bank cheque;
- contain confusing abbreviations or acronyms;
- contain obscene, sarcastic, politically incorrect or other unprofessional comments.

## Correspondence with other clinicians

Some hospitals have standard proformas for accepting referrals from primary care (Appendix 13), although a self-designed well-written and informative letter is usually just as acceptable. It is useful for the general practitioner to find out the usual arrangements, when starting in a new area, as well as the special interests of the local consultants.

When working in hospitals, clear and reasonably frequent communication with the referring clinician, primary care physician or dentist is essential, not only to ensure care of the patient, but also to maintain and enhance professional relationships. Apart from patient details, this should contain (but see confidentiality, below) the:
- name of the responsible clinician or consultant;
- date the patient was seen;
- relevant history, diagnosis, clinical course, treatment and prognosis;
- information of which the patient should or should not be informed.

## Confidentiality and data protection

It is normal practice to impart medical information to the patient's physician and dentist. It is crucial first to be sure that the patient agrees with this. There is increasing reluctance by some patients to have information divulged, especially when that involves transmissible diseases such as HIV. The Data Protection Act 1984 has now been repealed by the Data Protection Act 1998 c.29, which permits access to all manual health records whenever made, subject to specified exceptions (http://www.hmso.gov.uk/acts/acts1998/19980029.htm).

Information about a patient is sometimes requested by a '*third party*'. Unless you have written permission from the person in question to divulge the information, to do so is an invasion of privacy, is unethical and may be illegal. However, common sense should prevail and clearly the spouse should, for example, normally receive information as to postoperative progress, etc.

▶Such details should never be disclosed to others, such as the press or media.

Messages containing clinical information must not be left on answer-phones or with third parties; simply say 'Please ask X to call Y on ......'

The following are guidelines for dealing with inquiries, but always elicit the policy of your seniors and the institute in which you work.

*Always*

- identify the inquirer;
- check with the patient if information can be imparted and to whom—including whether relatives or partner are to be told, or not;
- give any information to relatives or partner in person and with the patient's express permission, and never over the telephone (you cannot be sure who is calling).

*Never*

- give information to members of the press or media, or the police, without checking with your seniors (indeed, the wise person avoids any voluntary contact with the media!);
- delegate the task of giving information.

### Access to medical reports

Nowadays, patients in many countries have rights of access to their health reports, and are permitted to request the clinician to make altera-tions if they feel the contents are inaccurate.

Likewise, the law often grants patients access to computer-held records.

### Medicolegal reports

Such reports should only be prepared with the express consent of the patient or his/her legal representative. Then give clearly and accurately the:

- patient's full surname and first name, date of birth, address and occupation;
- reason for the report;
- detail of who was the responsible clinician for the clinical care related to the incident involved;
- date, time and place, if the report is from a specific examination of the patient;
- history given by the patient and the history as shown by the clinical records;
- examination findings and results of investigations;
- treatment given;
- clinical course and prognosis;
- possible long-term effects, disabilities and costs.

⚠ Remember that this may involve legal proceedings.

# Logbooks and appraisals

## Logbook

Keeping a logbook enables you to record the experience you have had of various procedures. The logbook can also be used as evidence of this experience when you are applying for jobs or having an appraisal or assessment. Formats for logbooks vary and they can be kept on paper or electronically.

### You need to record:
- Date
- Patient identifier number
- Age of the patient
- Procedure carried out
- Your level of involvement (e.g. P = performed, S = performed under supervision, A = assisted, O = observed)
- Type of anaesthesia (e.g. local anaesthetic = 1, LA/sedation = 2, general anaesthesia = 3)

Summary sheets recording the number of different procedures and the level of involvement are useful.

▶ Gaining signatures from supervisors can strengthen the evidence.

## Appraisals

An appraisal is 'a confidential, educational review process'; it is for your benefit!

The appraisal should review the training and experience you have got so far, give you the opportunity to discuss strengths and weaknesses and plan for the next stage.

Before the appraisal, make sure your logbook is up-to-date and produce a summary sheet of your experience. Review your achievements since the last appraisal, e.g. publications, audits completed, journal clubs, courses attended.

# Administrative points

*Terms and conditions of service*
A copy of the Terms and Conditions of Service of Medical and Dental Staff should be available in the Human Resources Department.

*Contracts of employment*
Employers are usually required to give employees, written information about their main terms of employment.

*Staff health*
Friendly, unofficial arrangements may lead to ethical problems. Treat staff only on a formal basis, and keep proper records.

*Removal expenses for hospital posts*
Details of eligibility and entitlement to assistance with house purchase and removal expenses are available from the Medical Personnel Department.

*Personal property and valuables*
Although health authorities are not responsible for the loss or theft of personal effects, they are often insured against some risks, up to certain limits. Honorary staff not remunerated by the hospital are excluded from these insurance arrangements.

*Reimbursement of telephone rental*
Staff required to participate in formal 'on-call' rotas from home on a regular basis may be eligible to reclaim costs of telephone rental.

*Witnessing of wills*
Members of the administration should normally act as witnesses when a hospital patient wishes to make a will, although members of the dental staff may do so in an emergency.

*Press enquiries*
Routine enquiries about a hospital patient's condition are answered by the Hospital Administrator during office hours and the duty nursing officer out of hours. Do not answer enquiries yourself.

## Leaving a post

- Complete and return outstanding case notes.
- Hand in books and keys.
- Thank your consultant or principal and request him as a future referee.
- Thank colleagues and staff.
- Inviting everyone out or to your house is always a winner.
- Leave a forwarding address.

# Appendices

# Appendix 1   Some commonly used symbols, abbreviations, acronyms and eponyms

| Name | Abbreviation | Multiplier |
|------|--------------|------------|
| atto | a | $10^{-18}$ |
| femto | f | $10^{-15}$ |
| pico | p | $10^{-12}$ |
| nano | n | $10^{-9}$ |
| micro | μ | $10^{-6}$ |
| milli | m | $10^{-3}$ |
| kilo | k | $10^{3}$ |
| mega | M | $10^{6}$ |
| giga | G | $10^{9}$ |
| tera | T | $10^{12}$ |
| peta | P | $10^{15}$ |

| Quantity | Unit | Abbrev | Derivation |
|----------|------|--------|------------|
| Length | Metre | m | |
| Mass | kilogram | kg | |
| Time | seconds | sec, s | |
| Current | Amps, Amperes | A | |
| Temperature | kelvin | K | |
| Luminous intensity | candela | cd | |
| Force | newton | N | kg.m/sec/sec |
| Pressure | pascal | Pa | N/sq m |
| Energy | joule | J | N.m |
| Power | watt | W | J/sec |
| Torque | newton-metre | N.m | N.m |
| Charge | coulomb | C | A.sec |
| Potential | volt | V | J/C |
| Resistance | ohm | R | V/A |
| Capacitance | farad | F | C/V |
| Inductance | henry | H | J/A/A |
| Magnetic flux | Weber | Wb | V.sec |
| Magnetic intensity | tesla | T | Wb/sq m |
| Frequency | hertz | Hz | /sec |
| Disintegration rate | becquerel | Bq | /sec |
| Radiation dose | Gray | Gy | J/kg |

| A&W | Alive and well |
| A&P | Anterior and posterior (repair) |
| A/G | Albumin/globulin ratio |
| aa | Of each |
| abd | Abdomen |
| ABGs | Arterial blood gases |
| ac | Before meals |
| ACC | Ambulatory Care Center |
| ad lib | Freely |
| ADL | Activities of daily living |
| ADME | Absorption, distribution, metabolism & excretion |
| AE | Adverse events |
| AF | Atrial fibrillation |
| AFB | Acid fast bacillus |
| AI | Aortic incompetence or Aortic insufficiency |
| AIDS | Acquired immune deficiency syndrome |
| A-K | Above knee (amputation) |
| alb | Albumin |
| ALK PASE | Alkaline phosphatase |
| ALL | Acute lymphatic leukaemia |
| ALP | Alkaline phosphatase |
| ALS | Advanced Life Suppport |
| ALT | Alanine transaminase |
| am | In the morning |
| AMA | Against medical advice |
| amb | Ambulation |
| AMI | Acute myocardial infarction |
| AML | Acute myeloid leukaemia |
| ANF | Antinuclear factor |
| Angio | Angiology |
| ANK | Appointment not kept |
| AODM | Adult onset diabetes mellitus |
| AP | Apical pulse |
| APTT | Activated partial thromboplastin time |
| ARC | AIDS-related complex |
| ARF | Acute renal failure |
| AROM | Active range of motion |

| AS | Aortic stenosis |
|---|---|
| As Tol | As tolerated |
| ASD | Atrial septal defect |
| ASHD | Arteriosclerotic heart disease |
| ASOT | Antistreptolysin O titre |
| AST | Aspartate transaminase |
| ATC | Around the clock |
| ATS | Antitetanus serum |
| AV | Arteriovenous |
| $B_2m$ | Beta 2 microglobulin |
| BCG | Bacille Calmette Guerin (vaccine against TB) |
| BDA | British Dental Association (also British Diabetic Association) |
| BE | Barium enema |
| Bee | Basal energy expenditure |
| bid or bd | twice a day |
| biw | twice a week |
| B-K | Below knee (amputation) |
| BLS | Basic Life Support |
| bm | Bowel movement |
| BMMP | Benign mucous membrane pemphigoid |
| BNF | *British National Formulary* |
| BP | Blood pressure |
| BPC | British Pharmacopoeia |
| BPH | Benign prostatic hypertrophy |
| BPMF | British Postgraduate Medical Federation |
| BRA | Bite raising appliance |
| BS | Behçet syndrome or Blood sugars or Breathing sounds |
| BSO | Bilateral salpingoophorectomy |
| BSP | Bromsulfalein test |
| BSR | British standard ratio (prothrombin index) |
| BUN | Blood urea nitrogen |
| BW | Bitewing |
| Bx | Biopsy |
| C | Complement |
| c | With |
| c/c | Completed case |

| c/o | Complaining of |
|---|---|
| CA | Competent Authority or Carcinoma |
| Ca | Cancer ($Ca^{2+}$ = calcium) |
| CABG | Coronary artery bypass graft |
| CAC | Chronic atrophic candidosis |
| CAD | Coronary artery disease |
| CAH | Chronic active hepatitis |
| Cal | Calorie |
| cap | capsule |
| CAPD | Continued ambulatory peritoneal dialysis |
| CAT scan | Computerized axial tomography |
| CBC | Complete blood count |
| Cc | Chief complaint or cubic centimeter |
| CCF | Congestive cardiac failure |
| CCU | Coronary care unit |
| CDH | Congenital dislocation of hip |
| CDO | Chief Dental Officer |
| CFT | Complement fixation test |
| CHC | Community Health Council |
| CHD | Congenital heart disease |
| CHF | Congestive heart failure |
| cho | Carbohydrate |
| CJD | Creutzfeldt-Jakob disease |
| CLL | Chronic lymphatic leukaemia |
| CLP | Cleft-lip palate |
| CMC | Chronic mucocutaneous candidosis |
| CMI | Cell-mediated immunity |
| CML | Chronic myeloid leukaemia |
| CMO | Chief Medical Officer |
| CMV | Cytomegalovirus |
| CNS | Central nervous system |
| CO | Complaining of |
| COAD | Chronic obstructive airways disease |
| COCET | Committee on Dental Continuing Education and Training |
| COPD | Chronic obstructive pulmonary disease |
| COREC | Central Office for Research Ethics Committees UK |
| CPC | Clinicopathological conference |
| CPD | Continuing Professional Development |

| | |
|---|---|
| CPK | Creatine phosphokinase |
| CPM | Continued passive motion |
| CPME | Council for Postgraduate Medical Education |
| CPR | Cardiopulmonary resuscitation |
| cr | Creatinine |
| CREST | See CRST |
| CRF | Chronic renal failure |
| CRHIPOV | Cleared from head injury point of view |
| CRST | Calcinosis, Raynaud's, scleroderma, telangiectasia |
| CSAG | Clinical Standards Advisory Group |
| CSF | Cerebrospinal fluid |
| CSSD | Central sterile supplies department |
| CT Scan | Computerized axial tomography |
| CT | Computerized tomography |
| CTA | Clinical Trial Authorisation |
| CV | Curriculum Vitae |
| CVA | Cerebrovascular accident |
| CVP | Central venous pressure |
| CVS | Cardiovascular system |
| CWR | Cardiolipin Washerman reaction |
| Cx | Cervix |
| CXR | Chest X-ray |
| Cysto | CystosCopy |
| D&C | Dilatation and curettage |
| D/c | Discontinue |
| D/O | Diet order |
| D/T | Due to |
| DASU | Day Ambulatory Surgery Unit |
| DB | Decibels |
| DDAVP | Desmopressin |
| DDD | Pacemaker (type of) |
| DEAC | Dental Education Advisory Committee (Dental Deans) |
| DEB | Dental Estimates Board |
| DH | Delayed hypersensitivity or Dermatitis herpetiformis or Department of Health or dental hygienist |
| DHA | District Health Authority |
| DHCW | Dental Health Care Worker |
| DIC | Disseminated intravascular coagulation |

| DIF | Direct immunofluorescence |
| Diff | WBC differential |
| Dig | Digitalis |
| DLA | Dental Laboratories Association |
| DLE | Discoid lupus erythematosus |
| DM | Diabetes mellitus |
| DMFS | Decayed, missing or filled surfaces |
| DMFT | Decayed, missing or filled teeth |
| DMT | District Medical Team |
| DN | Dental nurse |
| DNA | Did not attend |
| DOA | Dead on arrival |
| DOE | Dyspnoea on exterion |
| DPA | Dental practice advisor |
| DPB | Dental practice board |
| DPF | Dental Practitioners Formulary |
| DPT | Diphtheria, pertussis, tetanus (vaccine) or Dental panoramic tomograph |
| DRS | Dental reference service |
| DS | Disseminated sclerosis |
| DSA | Dental surgery assistant |
| DSA | Digital subtraction angiography |
| DSASTAB | DSA standards and training advisory board |
| DT | Delirium tremens |
| DTETAB | Dental technicians education and training advisory board |
| DTR | Deep tendon reflex |
| Dts | Delirium tremens |
| DUB | Dysfunctional uterine bleeding |
| DVT | Deep vein thrombosis |
| Dx | Diagnosis |
| DXR | Deep X-ray radiation |
| EACA | Epsilon aminocaproic acid |
| EB | Epidermolysis bullosa |
| EBD | Evidence based dentistry |
| EBDSA | Examining board for DSA |
| EBM | Evidence-based medicine |
| EBV | Epstein–Barr virus |
| EC | Ethics Committee |

| ECG | Electrocardiogram |
|------|-------------------|
| ECM | External cardiac massage |
| ECT | Electroconvulsive therapy |
| EDH | Enrolled dental hygienist |
| EDT | Enrolled dental therapist |
| EDTA | Ethylene diamine tetraacetate |
| EEC | Electroencephalogram |
| EEG | Electroencephalogram |
| EENT | Eyes, ears, nose and throat |
| EKS | Electrocardiogram |
| ELISA | Enzyme-linked immunosorbent assay |
| EM | Erythema migrans or erythema multiforme |
| EMAS | Employment Medical Advisory Service |
| EMEA | European Agency for the Evaluation of Medicinal Products |
| EMG | Electromyogram |
| EMU | Early morning urine |
| ENT | Ears, nose and throat |
| EOM | Extraoccular movements |
| ER | Emergency room |
| ERCP | Endoscopic retrograde cholangiopancreatography |
| ES | Extra systoles |
| ESR | Erythrocyte sedimentation rate |
| ESRD | End stage renal disease |
| ETOH | Ethyl alcohol |
| ETP | Elective termination of pregnancy |
| ex | Exercise |
| | |
| FB | Foreign body |
| FBC | Full blood count |
| FBS | Fasting blood sugar |
| FDP | Fibrin degradation products |
| Fe | Iron |
| FEV | Forced expiratory volume |
| FH | Family history |
| FPC | Family Practitioner Committee |
| FRC | Forced residual capacity |
| FTA | Fluorescent treponemal antibody (test) |
| FTI | Free thyroxine index |
| FTP | Fitness To Practise |

| | |
|---|---|
| FUO | Fever of unknown origin |
| Fx | Fracture |
| g | Gram |
| G6PD | Glucose-6-phosphate dehydrogenase |
| GA | General anaesthesia |
| Gamma GT | glutamyl transpeptidase |
| GB | Gallbladder |
| Gc | Gonorrhoea |
| GCP | Good Clinical Practice |
| GDC | General Dental Council |
| GDP | General Dental Practitioner |
| GDPA | General Dental Practitioners Association |
| GDSC | General Dental Services Committee |
| GFR | Glomerular filtration rate |
| GGT | Gamma glutamyl transpeptidase |
| GI | Gastrointestinal |
| GIT | Gastrointestinal tract |
| GM | *Grand mal* |
| GMH | General medical history |
| GMP | General Medical Practitioner |
| GMP | Good Manufacturing Practice |
| GP | General practitioner |
| GPI | General paralysis of the insane |
| Gr | Grain |
| Grav | Gravida |
| Gtt | Drop |
| GTT | Glucose tolerance test |
| GU | Genito-urinary |
| GUM | Genito-urinary Medicine |
| GVHD | Graft-versus-host disease |
| Gyn | Gynaecology |
| H&N | Head and neck |
| H&P | History and physical |
| HA | Headache |
| HAA | Hyperalimentation |
| HANE | Hereditary angioneurotic edema (oedema) |
| HAV | Hepatitis A virus |

| Hb | Haemoglobin |
|----|----|
| HbS | Haemoglobin S (sickle-cell) |
| HB$_c$Ag | Hepatitis B core antigen |
| HB$_e$Ag | Hepatitis B 'e' antigen |
| HBsAg | Hepatitis B surface antigen |
| HBD | Hydroxybutyrate dehydrogenase |
| HBP | High blood pressure |
| HBV | Hepatitis B virus |
| HCP | Health Care Professional |
| HCTZ | Hydrochlorothiazide |
| HCV | Hepatitis C virus |
| HCVD | Hypertensive cardiovascular disease |
| HCW | Health Care Worker |
| HAD | Health Development Agency |
| HDL | High density lipoproteins |
| HDV | Hepatitis D virus |
| HEENT | Head, ears, eyes, nose and throat |
| hgt | Height |
| HGV | Hepatitis G virus |
| HHB | Hand held nebulizer |
| Hib | *Haemophilus influenzae* type b |
| HITF | Healthcare Industries Task Force |
| HIV | Human immunodeficiency virus(es) |
| HLA | Human leucocyte antigen |
| HMEC | Hospital Medical Executive Council |
| HO | House officer |
| HOCM | Hypertrophic obstructive cardiomyopathy |
| HOH | Hard of hearing |
| HP | Hot packs |
| HPA | Health Protection Agency |
| HPC | History of present complaint |
| HPI | History of present illness |
| HPV | Human papillomavirus |
| h | Hour |
| hs | At bedtime |
| HS | House surgeon |
| HSC | Health and Safety Committee |
| HSE | Health and Safety Executive |

| HSV | Herpes simplex virus |
| HTLV | Human T cell lymphotrophic virus (HTLV-III=HIV) |
| HTN | Hypertension |
| HU | Herpetiform ulcers |
| Hx | History |
| Hz | Hertz |
| I&D | Incision and drainage |
| I&O | Intake and output |
| IA | Intra-arterial |
| IBW | Ideal body weight |
| IC | Immune complex or Intermittent claudication |
| ICH | International Conference on Harmonisation; European Union, Japan, Canada and USA |
| ICP | Intracranial pressure |
| ICU | Intensive care unit |
| IDD | Insulin-dependent diabetes |
| IF | Immunofluorescence or intrinsic factor or injury factor |
| IFN | Interferon |
| Ig | Immunoglobulin (e.g. IgG, IgA, IgM, IgE) |
| IHD | Ischaemic heart disease |
| IIF | Indirect immunofluorescence |
| IITs | Investigator Initiated Trials |
| IL | Interleukin |
| IM | Intramusculary |
| IMF | Intermaxillary fixation |
| IMP | Investigational Medicinal Product |
| IMPD | Investigational Medicinal Product Dossier |
| INR | International normalized ratio (see BSR) |
| IPD | Intermittent peritoneal dialysis |
| IPPB | Intermittent positive pressure breathing |
| IQE | International Qualifying Examination |
| ITU | Intensive treatment unit |
| IUD | Intrauterine device |
| IUP | Intrauterine pregnancy |
| IV | Intravenously |
| IVC | Inferior vena cava |
| IVD | Intravenous drug misuser |
| IVP | Intravenous pyelography |
| IVU | Intravenous urogram |

| | |
|---|---|
| JC | Jakob–Creutzfeldt disease |
| JCSTD | Joint Committee for Specialist Training in Dentistry |
| JODM | Juvenile onset diabetes mellitus |
| jt | Joint |
| JVP | Jugular venous pressure |
| | |
| K | Potassium |
| KCCT | Kaolin cephalin clotting time |
| Kg | Kilogram |
| KPTT | Kaolin partial thromboplastin time |
| KS | Kaposi's sarcoma |
| KUB | Flat film of kidney ureters, bladder |
| | |
| L or l | Litre |
| LA | Local anaesthesia/analgesia |
| lab | Laboratory |
| LAD | Linear IgA disease |
| LAS | Lymphadenopathy syndrome |
| LATS | Long-acting thyroid stimulator |
| LAV | Lymphadenopathy associated virus (HIV) |
| LBBB | Left bundle branch block |
| LBP | Low back pain |
| LDC | Local Dental Committee |
| LDH | Lactic dehydrogenase |
| LDL | Low density lipoproteins |
| LE | Lower extremity or Lupus erythematosus |
| LFH | Left femoral hernia |
| LFT | Liver function tests (usually serum bilirubin plus several 'liver enzymes' such as AST and GGT) |
| LGV | Lymphogranuloma venereum |
| LH | Luteinizing hormone |
| LHF | Left heart failure |
| LIF | Left iliac fossa |
| LIH | Left inguinal hernia |
| LKKS | Liver, kidneys, spleen (liver, both kidneys and spleen) |
| LL | Lower limb or Lower left |
| LLB | Long leg brace |
| LLC | Long leg cast |
| LLL | Left lower lobe |

| | |
|---|---|
| LLQ | Left lower quadrant |
| LLSD | Lower labial set down |
| LMN | Lower motor neurone |
| LMP | Last menstrual period |
| LOA | Left occiput anterior |
| LOP | Left occiput transverse |
| LP | Lumbar puncture or lichen planus |
| LPN | Licensed Practical Nurse |
| LS | Lumbosacral |
| LSSP | Lumbosacral spine and pelvis |
| Lt | Left |
| LUL | Left upper lobe |
| LUQ | Left upper quadrant |
| LVF | Left ventricular failure |
| LVH | Left ventricular hypertrophy |
| Lytes | Electrolytes |
| | |
| m | Murmur or metre |
| MAE | Moving all extremities |
| MAOI | Monoamine oxidase inhibitors |
| MaRAS | Major aphthae |
| max | Maximal |
| MCA | Medicines Control Agency |
| mcg | Microgram |
| MCH | Mean corpuscular haemoglobin concentration |
| MCV | Mean corpuscular volume |
| MDU | Medical Defence Union |
| MEA | Multiple endocrine adenoma |
| Meq | Milliequivalent |
| MG | Myasthenia gravis |
| mg or mgm | milligram |
| MHRA | Medicines and Healthcare products Regulatory Agency |
| MI | Myocardial infarct or if referring to valvular lesion, Mitral insufficiency |
| MIC | Medical Intensive Care |
| MICU | Medical Intensive Care Unit |
| min | Minimal (or minute) |
| Mini-hep | Subcutaneous heparin |

| MiRAS | Minor aphthae |
| MLSO | Medical laboratory scientific officer |
| MMC | Modernizing Medical Careers |
| MMP | Mucous membrane pemphigoid |
| MMR | Measles, Mumps, Rubella (vaccine) |
| MMT | Manual muscle test |
| MND | Motor neurone disease |
| mod | Moderate |
| MOM | Milk of magnesia |
| MOV | Multiple oral vitamin |
| MPD | Mandibular pain-dysfunction |
| MPS | Medical Protection Society |
| MR | Magnetic resonance |
| MRC | Medical Research Council |
| MRI | Magnetic resonance imaging |
| MRSA | Meticillin resistant *Staphylococcus aureus* |
| MS | Multiple sclerosis or mitral stenosis |
| MSE | Mental state examination |
| MSM | Man who has sex with men |
| MSU | Mid-stream urine |
| | |
| N & V | Nausea and vomiting |
| N/B | Newborn |
| N/S | Normal saline |
| NAD | No abnormality detected |
| NANB(H) | Non-A, non-B hepatitis |
| NB | Note well |
| NBM | Nil by mouth |
| NCCPC | National Collaborating Centre for Primary Care |
| NCVQ | National Council for Vocational Qualifications |
| neg | Negative |
| NG | Nasogastric |
| NHL | Non-Hodgkin's lymphoma |
| NHS | National Health Service |
| NHSTA | National Health Service Training Authority |
| NICE | National Institute for Clinical Excellence |
| NIDDM | Non insulin dependent diabetes mellitus |
| NJC | National Joint Council for the Craft of Dental Technicians |

| nl | Normal |
| NMR | Nuclear magnetic resonance (=MRI) |
| NP | Proper name (of drug) |
| NPO | Nothing by mouth |
| NRPB | National Radiation Protection Board |
| NSAIDs | Non-steroidal anti-inflammatory drugs |
| NSF | National Service Framework |
| NSR | Normal sinus rhythm |
| NSU | Non-specific urethritis |
| Ntg | Nitroglycerin |
| NTN | No treatment needed |
| NTR | No treatment required |
| | |
| O | Orally |
| OA | Osteoarthritis |
| OAF | Oro-antral fistula or osteoclast activating factor |
| OB | Obstetrics |
| OD | Right eye or every day (o.d.) |
| OFG | Orofacial granulomatosis |
| OHS | Open heart surgery |
| OI | Opportunistic infection |
| OM | Occipitomental (radiograph) |
| OMFS | Oral and maxillofacial surgery |
| OOB | Out of bed |
| OPD | Outpatient Department |
| OPT | Orthopantomograph (or OPG or DPT or OPTG) |
| OR | Operating room |
| ORF | Orthograde root filling |
| OS | Left eye |
| OT | Occupational therapy |
| OU | Both eyes |
| | |
| P | Wave on ECG or pulse |
| P&A | Percussion and auscultation |
| PA | Pleomorphic adenoma, Pernicious anaemia, periapical or postero-anterior (radiograph) |
| PACU | Post-anaesthesia care unit |
| PAN | Polyarteritis nodosa |
| PAT | Paroxysmal atrial tachycardia |

| PBC | Primary biliary cirrhosis |
| pc | after meals |
| PCA | Patient cancelled appointment or Patient controlled analgesia |
| PCM | Protein calorie malutrition |
| $PCO_2$ | Partial pressure of carbon dioxide |
| PCP | *Pneumocystis carinii* pneumonia |
| PCR | Polymerase chain reaction |
| PCT | Primary Care Trust |
| PCV | Packed cell volume |
| PDA | Patent ductus arteriosus |
| PDH | Past dental history |
| PE | Physical examination or Pulmonary embolism |
| PEEP | Positive and expiration pressure |
| PEN V | Penicillin V |
| PERLA | Pupils equal reacting to light and accommodation (i.e. normal) |
| PET | Pre-eclamptic toxaemia (in pregnancy) |
| PGL | Persistent generalized lymphadenopathy |
| Pgv | Pregnancy |
| PH | Past history |
| PHT | Pulmonary hypertension |
| phys ther | Physical therapy |
| PID | Pelvic inflammatory disease |
| PLS | Persistent lymphadenopathy syndrome (HIV) |
| pm | In the evening |
| PM | *Petit mal* (epilepsy) |
| PMD | Private physician |
| PMH | Past medical history |
| PMI | Point of maximal impulse |
| PMNR | Periadenitis mucosa necrotica recurrens (major aphthae) |
| PND | Postnasal drip or Paroxysmal nocturnal dyspnoea |
| PO | Postoperative or per-oral |
| $PO_2$ | Partial pressure of oxygen |
| POC | Polythene occlusal cover |
| POMR | Problem orientated medical reports |
| Pos or + | Positive |
| PP | Post partum |
| PPD | Purified protein derivative |

| PR | Per rectum or pulse rate |
| PRBLs | Packed red blood cells |
| PRHO | Pre-Registration House Officer |
| PRIST | Paper radioimmunosorbent test |
| prn | as necessary |
| pro | Protein |
| PROM | Passive range of motion |
| PS | Pulmonary stenosis |
| PSA | Pleomorphic salivary adenoma |
| PSE | Porto-systemic encephalopathy (in liver failure) |
| PSP | Phenosulfonphthalein |
| PSVT | Paroxysmal supraventricular tachycardia |
| PT | Physical therapy or Physiotherapy or Prothrombin time |
| PTA | Prior to admission |
| PTH | Parathyroid hormone |
| PUO | Pyrexia or unknown origin |
| PV | Per vaginam (or pemphigus vulgaris) |
| PVC | Premature ventricular contractions |
| PVD | Peripheral vascular disease |
| PWA | Person with AIDS |
| Q | Wave on ECT |
| Q2d | Every second day |
| qid or qds | Four times a day |
| qod | Every other day |
| R | Wave on ECT or respiration |
| R/O | Rule out |
| RA | Rheumatoid arthritis or relative analgesia or reason for admission |
| RAS | Recurrent aphthous stomatitis |
| RAST | Radioallergosorbent test |
| RBBB | Right bundle branch block |
| RCN | Royal College of Nursing |
| RCS | Royal College of Surgeons |
| RCST | Regional Committee on Specialist Training |
| RCT | Root canal treatment |
| RCU | Respiratory Care Unit |
| Retics | Reticulocytes |

| | |
|---|---|
| RF | Rheumatoid factor or rheumatic fever |
| RFH | Right femoral hernia |
| RFT | Renal function tests |
| Rh | Rhesus |
| RHA | Regional Health Authority |
| RHD | Rheumatic heart disease |
| RhF | Rheumatic fever |
| RHF | Right heart failure |
| RIF | Right iliac fossa |
| RITA | Record of In-Training Assessment |
| RLL | Right lower lobe |
| RLQ | Right lower quadrant |
| RML | Right middle lobe |
| ROA | Right occiput anterior |
| ROM | Range of Motion |
| ROP | Right occiput posterior |
| ROS | Review of systems |
| ROT | Right occiput transverse |
| ROU | Recurrent oral ulcers |
| RPA | Radiation Protection Advisor |
| RPCFT | Reiter protein complement fixation test |
| RPS | Radiation Protection Supervisor |
| RRF | Retrograde root filling |
| RROM | Resisted range of motion |
| RT | Radiation therapy |
| Rt | Right |
| RTA | Road traffic accident |
| RTC | Return to clinic |
| RU | Retrograde urogram |
| RUL | Right upper lobe |
| RUQ | Right upper quadrant |
| RVF | Right ventricular failure |
| Rx | Treat |
| | |
| s | Without |
| S/M | Statement |
| S/T | States that |
| S1 | First heart sound |

| | |
|---|---|
| S2 | Second heart sound |
| S3 | Third heart sound |
| S4 | Fourth heart sound |
| SA | Subarachnoid |
| SAC | Standing Advisory Committee (of JCHTD) |
| SBE | Subacute bacterial endocarditis |
| SBFT | Small bowel follow through |
| SC | Subcutaneous |
| SCOPME | Standing Committee on Postgraduate Medical Education in England |
| Sed rate | Erythrocyte sedimentation rate |
| SERC | Science and Engineering Research Council |
| SG | Specific Gravity |
| SGGT | see GGT |
| SGOT | see AST |
| SGPT | see ALT |
| SHA | Strategic Health Authority |
| SHHD | Scottish Home and Health Dept |
| SHO | Senior house officer |
| SI | International system of units |
| SICU | Surgical Intensive Care Unit |
| Sig | Directions |
| SLB | Short leg brace |
| SLC | Short leg cast |
| SLE | Systemic lupus erythematosus |
| SLR | Straight leg raising |
| SMV | Submentovertex (radiograph) |
| SNF | Skilled Nursing Facility |
| SOA | Swelling of ankles |
| SOB | Shortness of breath |
| SOL | Space-occupying lesion (usually neoplasm) |
| SpR | Specialist Registrar |
| SRN | Staff Registered Nurse |
| SS | Sjögren's syndrome or systemic sclerosis or sagittal split (osteotomy) |
| SSRI | Selective serotonic reuptake inhibitor |
| ST | Segment of ECG record |

| STD | Sexually transmitted diseases (or STI—sexually transmitted infections) |
| SUBQ | Subcutaneous |
| SUSAR | Suspected, Unexpected Serious Adverse Reactions |
| SVC | Superior vena cava |
| SVD | Spontaneous vaginal delivery |
| | |
| T | Temperature or wave on ECG |
| TAH | Total abdominal hysterectomy |
| TASS | Technical and supervisory staff section |
| TB | Tuberculosis |
| TCA | Tricyclic antidepressants |
| TDS or tid | Three times a day |
| TFT | Thyroid function tests |
| THR | Total hip replacement |
| TI | Tricuspid incompetence |
| TIBC | Total iron binding capacity |
| TKR | Total knee replacement |
| TKVO | To keep vein open |
| TLC | Tender loving care or total lung capacity |
| TLE | Temporal lobe epilepsy |
| TM | Tympanic membrane |
| TMJ | Temporomandibular joint |
| TNF | Tumour necrosis factor |
| TPHA | *Treponema pallidum* haemaqqlutination (test) |
| TPI | *Treponema pallidum* immobilization (test) |
| TPN | Total parenteral nutrition |
| TPR | Temperature, pulse and respiration |
| TRH | Thyroid-releasing hormone |
| TS | Tricuspid stenosis |
| TSH | Thyroid-stimulating hormone |
| TSSU | Theatre sterile supplies unit |
| TUR | Transurethral resection |
| | |
| U | Regarding |
| U&E | Urea and electrolytes |
| U&L | Upper and lower |
| U/A | Urinalysis |
| UC | Ulcerative colitis |

| UE | Upper extremity |
| UGI | Upper gastrointestinal |
| UGS | Urogenital system |
| UHA | University Hospitals Association |
| UL | Upper limb |
| UMN | Upper motor neurone |
| URI | Upper respiratory infection |
| Urol | Urology |
| URTI | Upper respiratory tract infection |
| US | Ultrasound |
| USB | Ultrasonic nebulizer |
| USDAW | Union of Shop, Distributive and Allied Workers |
| UTI | Urinary tract infection |
| | |
| VA | Visual acuity |
| VAcC | Visual acuity with correction |
| VC | Vital capacity |
| VCsC | Visual acuity without correction |
| VDRL | Venereal Disease Research Laboratories (test) |
| VF | Ventricular fibrillation |
| vit/min | vitamin/mineral |
| VNA | Visiting Nurses' Association |
| vs | Vital signs |
| VSD | Ventricular septal defect |
| VSS | Vertical subsigmoid |
| VT | Ventricular tachycardia or Vocational training |
| VV | Varicose veins |
| VZV | Varicella zoster virus |
| | |
| w/c | Wheelchair |
| W/D | Well developed |
| W/N | Well nourished |
| W/u | Work-up |
| WBC | White blood count |
| WCC | White cell count |
| WFL | Within functional limits |
| WNL | Within normal limits |
| WR | Wasserman reaction or ward round |
| wt | Weight |

# Eponymous diseases

| Term | Meaning |
| --- | --- |
| Addison's disease | Primary adrenocortical insufficiency |
| Alzheimer's disease | Senile dementia |
| Berger's disease | IgA nephropathy |
| Bornholm disease | Epidermic myalgia |
| Budd–Chiari syndrome | Obstruction of the hepatic vein |
| Buerger's disease | Thromboangiitis obliterans |
| Chagas' disease | American trypanosomiasis |
| Caisson disease | Decompression sickness |
| Charco–Marie–Tooth syndrome | Peroneal muscular atrophy |
| Christmas disease | Factor IX deficiency |
| Churg–Strauss syndrome | Eosinophilic granulomatous vasculitis |
| Conn's syndrome | Primary hyperaldosteronism |
| Crohn's disease | Regional enteritis |
| Cushing's disease | Pituitary dependent adrenocortical hypoplasia |
| Devic's disease | Neuromyelitis optica |
| Dressler's syndrome | Post-myocardial infarction syndrome |
| Eaton–Lambert syndrome | Paraneoplastic myasthenia |
| Erb's paralysis | Injury of the upper root of the brachial plexus |
| Fabry's disease | Galactosidase-A deficiency |
| Friedreich's ataxia | Spinocerebellar ataxia |
| Gardner's syndrome | A type of familial adenomatous polyposis |
| Gelineau's syndrome | Narcolepsy |
| Grave's disease | Autoimmune thyrotoxicosis |
| Guillain–Barré syndrome | Post-viral polyneuropathy |
| Hanot's disease | Primary biliary cirrhosis |
| Hansen's disease | Leprosy |
| Kallman's disease | Hypogonadotrophic hypogonadism |
| Kartagener's syndrome | Situs inversus (organs on wrong side of body) |
| Klumpke's paralysis | Injury of the lower root of the brachial plexus |
| Koch's infection | Tuberculosis |
| Loeffler's syndrome | Simple pulmonary eosinophilia |
| McArdle's syndrome | Type V glycogen storage disease |

| | |
|---|---|
| Marchiafava–Michell syndrome | Paroxysmal nocturnal haemoglobinuria |
| Mayer–Betz syndrome | Paroxysmal myoglobinuria |
| Osler–Weber–Rendu syndrome | Hereditary haemorrhagic telangectasia |
| Pickwickian syndrome | Obstructive sleep apnoea |
| Pott's disease | Spinal tuberculosis |
| Sheehan's disease | Postpartum hypopituitarism |
| Sjögren's syndrome | Keratoconjunctivitis sicca |
| Tietze's syndrome | Idiopathic costochondritis |
| von Reckinghausen's disease | Neurofibromatosis |
| Wilson's disease | Hepatolenticular degeneration |
| Wolff–Parkinson–White syndrome | Abberant atrioventricular pre-excitation |

# Glossary of important terms in pathology

**Abscess**   A closed cavity containing pus.

**Atypical**   In a diagnosis, the use of the term atypical is a vague warning to the physician that the pathologist is worried about something.

**Carcinoma**   A malignant neoplasm whose cells are derived from epithelium.

**Dysplasia**   An atypical proliferation of cells, loosely thought of as intermediate between hyperplasia and neoplasia.

**Epithelium**   A specialized type of tissue that normally lines the surfaces and cavities of the body.

**Granuloma**   Inflammation characterized by accumulations of macrophages, some of which coalesce into 'giant cells.' Granulomatous inflammation is especially characteristic of tuberculosis, sarcoidosis, Crohn's disease, orofacial granulomatosis, reaction to foreign bodies and deep fungal infections (like histoplasmosis).

**Hyperplasia**   A proliferation of cells which is not neoplastic.

**Inflammation**   A reaction manifest clinically by swelling, pain, tenderness, redness, heat, and/or loss of function. The infiltration of inflammatory cells including: (1) neutrophils, in acute inflammation, (2) lymphocytes, in more chronic or long-standing inflammations, and (3) macrophages (histiocytes), which are also seen in chronic inflammation.

**Lesion**   This is a vague term meaning 'the thing that is wrong with the patient.'

**Metastatic**   Of or pertaining to metastasis, or the process by which malignant neoplasms can shed individual cells, which can travel through the lymph vessels or blood vessels, lodge in some distant organ, and grow into tumours in their own right.

**Necrosis**   Death of tissue.

**Neoplasm, or Neoplasia**   A 'new growth' of cells no longer under normal control. These may be 'benign' or 'malignant.' Benign neoplasms are typically tumours (lumps or masses) that, if removed, never recur or metastasise. Malignant neoplasms, or 'cancers', are those whose natural history is to cause death by (1) local invasion, in which the neoplasm extends into vital organs and interferes with their function; (2) metastasis; and/or (3) paraneoplastic syndromes, in which the neoplasm secretes inappropriately large amounts of hormones.

**-Oma**  This suffix means 'tumour' or 'lump.' It typically, but not invariably, refers to a neoplasm ('GRANULOMA' is an exception).

**Polyp**  A structure consisting of a rounded head attached to a surface by a stalk (also called a 'pedicle' or 'peduncle'). Polyps may be hyperplastic, metaplastic, neoplastic, inflammatory, or none of the above.

**Sarcoma**  A malignant neoplasm whose cells are derived from those other than epithelium.

**Suppuration**  A type of acute inflammation characterized by infiltration of neutrophils at the microscopic level and formation of pus at the gross level. An abscess is a special type of suppurative inflammation.

**Tumour**  A mass or lump that can be seen or felt.

## Other terminology

100 $\underline{120}$ 60: blood pressure: standing 120/80
    80

(systolic/diastolic); lying 100/60

| | |
|---|---|
| *Nocte* | in the night |
| *mane* | in the morning |
| 2° | Metastasis |
| # | Fracture |
| 5LICSMCL | Usually refer to apex beat situation: in the 5th left intercostal space in the mid-clavicular line |
| *Stat* | immediately |
| *bd* | twice daily (bis die) |
| *od* | every day |
| *qds, qid* | four times daily (quater die sumendum, quater in die) |
| *tds* | three times daily (ter die sumendum) |
| *prn* | as required (pro re nata) |
| BTS | Reflexes: biceps, triceps, supinator |
| KAP | Reflexes: knee, ankle, plantar |
| Babinski reflex | plantar reflex |
| Specific infection | syphilis |
| Mitotic lesion | malignant neoplasm |
| Lymphoproliferative state | sometimes used instead of 'leukaemia' |
| Special clinic | clinic for sexually transmitted diseases |
| Vital signs | Temperature, blood pressure, pulse, respiration |
| Inoculation risk | patient infected with HBV, HCV or HIV |
| Retrovirus | often used instead of 'HIV' |

| | |
|---|---|
| ♀ | Female |
| ♂ | Male |
| 1° | Primary |
| 2° | Secondary |
| > | Greater than |
| < | Lesser than |
| >= | Greater than or equal to |
| <= | Less than or equal to |
| + | Positive |
| – | Negative |
| ↑ | Increased |
| ↓ | Decreased |
| ° | Nil |

# Some qualifications in dentistry and medicine

| | | |
|---|---|---|
| BA | Bachelor of | Arts |
| Bch | Bachelor of | Surgery |
| BChD | Bachelor of | Dental Surgery |
| BDS | Bachelor of | Dental Surgery |
| BS | Bachelor of | Surgery |
| Bsc | Bachelor of | Science |
| ChM | Master of | Surgery |
| Dip Bact | Diploma in | Bacteriology |
| DA | Diploma in | Anaesthetics |
| DCH | Diploma in | Child Health |
| DDPH | Diploma in | Dental Public Health |
| DDR | Diploma in | Dental Radiology |
| DDS | Diploma in | Dental Science |
| DDS | Doctor of | Dental Science |
| DLO | Diploma in | Laryngology and Otology |
| Dorth | Diploma in | Orthodontics |
| DMRD | Diploma in | Medical Radiodiagnosis |
| Dphil | Doctor of | Philosophy |
| DPM | Diploma in Psychological | Medicine |
| DRCOG | Diploma of Royal College of | Obstetricians and Gynaecologists |
| DRD | Diploma in Restorative | Dentistry |
| DSc | Doctor of | Science |
| DTM+H | Diploma in | Tropical Medicine and Hygiene |
| FDS | Fellow in | Dental Surgery (FDS, RCS, FDS, RCPS, FDS, RCSE) |
| FFARCS | Fellow in | Faculty of Anaesthesia, Royal College of Surgeons |
| FFCM | Fellow in | Faculty of Community Medicine |
| FFD | Fellow in | Faculty of Dental Surgery |
| FFR | Fellow in | Faculty of Radiology |
| FMEDsci | Fellow of the | Academy of Medical Sciences |
| FRACDS | Fellow of the | Royal Australasian College of Dental Surgeons |
| FRCGP | Fellow of Royal College of | General Practitioners |
| FRCOG | Fellow of Royal College of | Obstetricians & Gynaecologists |
| FRCP | Fellow of Royal College of | Physicians |
| FRCPath | Fellow of Royal College of | Pathologists |
| FRCPsych | Fellow of Royal College of | Psychiatrists |
| FRCS | Fellow of Royal College of | Surgeons |

| LDS | Licentiate in | Dental Surgery |
| LRCP | Licentiate of Royal College of | Physicians |
| LRCS | Licentiate of Royal College of | Surgeons |
| MA | Master of | Arts |
| MB | Bachelor of | Medicine |
| MCCD | Membership in Clinical | Community Dentistry |
| MClinDent | Master of | Clinical Dentistry |
| MD | Doctor of | Medicine |
| MDS | Master in | Dental Surgery |
| MFDS | Membership in | Faculty of Dental Surgery |
| MGDS | Membership in | General Dental Surgery |
| Morth | Master in | Orthodontics |
| Mphil | Master of | Philosophy |
| MRCGP | Member of Royal College of | General Practitioners |
| MRCOG | Member of Royal College of | Obstetricians & Gynaecologists |
| MRCP | Member of Royal College of | Physicians |
| MRCPath | Member of the Royal College | of Pathologists |
| MRCPsych | Member of the Royal College | of Psychiatrists |
| MRCS | Member of the Royal College | of Surgeons |
| MS | Master of Surgery (In USA, | Master of Science) |
| MSc | Master of | Science |
| PhD | Doctor of | Philosophy |

# Appendix 2  Reflexes

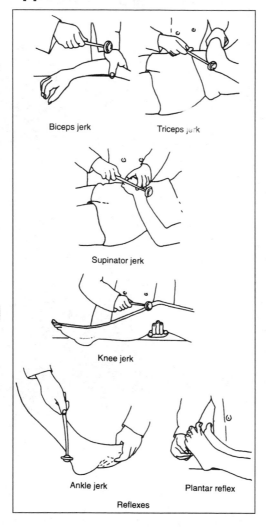

Biceps jerk

Triceps jerk

Supinator jerk

Knee jerk

Ankle jerk

Plantar reflex

Reflexes

# Appendix 3   Cephalometric points and planes

Anterior nasal spine (ANS): The tip of the anterior nasal spine

Articulare (Ar): The projection on a lateral skull radiography of the posterior outline of the condylar process on to the interior outline of the cranial base

Glabella: The most prominent point over the frontal bone

Gnathion (Gn): The most anterior inferior point of the bony chin

Gonion (Go): The most posterior inferior point at the angle of the mandible

Menton (Me): The most inferior point on the bony chin

Nasion (N): The most anterior point on the frontonasal suture

Orbitale (Or): The lowest point on the bony margin of the orbit

Pogonion (Pog): The most anterior point on the bony chin

Point A: The deepest point on the maxillary profile between the anterior nasal spine and the alveolar crest

Point B: The deepest point on the mandibular profile between the pogonion and the alveolar crest

Porion (Po): The uppermost, outermost point on the bony external acoustic meatus

Posterior nasal spine (PNS): The tip of the posterior nasal spine

Sella (S): The mid-point of the sella turcica

Frankfort plane: The plane through the orbitale and porion. This is meant to approximate the horizontal plane when the head is in the free postural position but this varies appreciably (substitutes for maxillary plane on clinical examination)

Mandibular plane: The plane through the gonion and menton

Maxillary plane: The plane through ANS and PNS (substitutes for Frankfort plane on clinical examination)

# Appendix 4  Abdominal examination

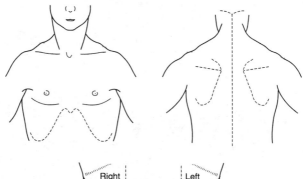

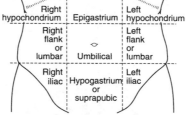

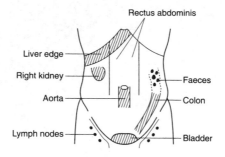

Palpation of the abdomen: some normal findings

# Appendix 5 Sterilization in the dental surgery

| Method | Temperature | Time | Comments |
| --- | --- | --- | --- |
| Autoclave | 121°C at 15 lb/in$^2$ or 134°C at 32 lb/in$^4$ | 15 min 3 min | Most efficient form of sterilization for metal instruments and fabrics |
| Hot-air oven | 160°C or 180°C | 60 min 20 min | Effective but time-consuming and chars fabrics |
| Glutaraldehyde | 20°C | 60 min | Does **not** sterilize but kills most bacteria, spores, and viruses |
| | | | Useful for heat-sensitive equipment |
| | | | Deteriorates rapidly with time |

# Appendix 6   Changes in vital signs of serious significance

| Sign | Change | Possible interpretation |
|------|--------|------------------------|
| Fever | Alone or with increased pulse rate | Infection |
| | With rapid, thready pulse, rapid breathing, and lethargy | Serious infection—a 'toxic' patient |
| | With rapid, thready pulse and falling BP | Serious infection and possibly septicaemia |
| | With thirst, lethargy, rising pulse rateand falling BP, and falling urine output | Dehydration |
| Pulse rate and BP | Rising pulse rate and falling BP | Bleeding, possibly hidden, e.g. into abdominal cavity; shock or anaphylaxis |
| | Falling pulse rate and rising BP | Rising intracranial pressure, e.g. intracranial bleeding |
| | Absent pulse | Cardiac arrest |
| Consciousness | Irritability, vomiting, and/or decreasing consciousness with or without other signs | Rising intracranial pressure or other causes of coma, e.g. hypoglycaemia |
| | Fits appearing after a head injury | Brain damage or rising intracranial pressure |
| | Severe headache, particularly if associated with neck stiffness, vomiting, and drowsiness | Meningeal irritation, e.g. from meningitis |
| | Cranial neuropathy appearing in a patient with head injury | Direct damage to nerve, or rising intracranial pressure |
| Respiration | Stridor | Laryngeal obstruction, e.g. foreign body or laryngospasm |
| | Wheezing alone | Bronchial or bronchiolar obstruction,e.g. foreign body, bronchospasm |
| | Wheezing with collapse, falling BP and weak, thready pulse with or without oedema | Anaphylaxis |
| | Hyperventilation | Hysteria; pain; cardiovascular disease; neurological disease or metabolic disease |

# **Appendix 6** Contd.

| Sign | Change | Possible interpretation |
|------|--------|------------------------|
| | Dyspnoea | Respiratory disease or obstruction, cardiac disease |
| | Irregular respiration | Respiratory obstruction, brain damage, drugs or metabolic disorders |
| Urine output | Persistent polyuria | Overhydration; diabetes mellitus; diabetes insipidus or hyperpara-thyroidism |
| | Oliguria | Dehydration or renal failure |
| Collapse | Collapse | See Emergencies (Chapter 6) |

# Appendix 7 Changes in vital signs in patients with infection

| Vital sign | Normal range | Changes associated with infection indicative of | |
|---|---|---|---|
| | | Mild to moderate infection | Serious infection[a] |
| Temperature[d] | 35.5–37.5°C | 37.5–39.5°C[b] | Above 40°C |
| Pulse | 60–80/min | 90–100/min[c] | Above about 100/min |
| BP | Systolic: 120–140 mmHg; | No change | If falling may indicate shock |
| | Diastolic: 60–90 mmHg | | |
| Respiration | | | |
| Airways | Clear | Clear | If not clear |
| Rate | 12–18/min | 18–20/min | Above about 22/min |
| Rhythm | Regular | No change | Any change in rhythm or depth |

[a] Admit to hospital. CNS changes are also indications for admission. These include decreasing consciousness, intensive headache with stiff neck and/or vomiting, eyelid oedema, visual disturbances.
[b] If the temperature is above 38.5°C and a bacterial infection is suspected, consider taking blood cultures (pages 92–93).
[c] Often higher in children.
[d] Oral temperature.

# Appendix 8   Common symptoms and signs of cardiac disease

| Symptoms | Cardiac disease | Other causes |
|---|---|---|
| Breathlessness (dyspnoea) | Cardiac failure | Respiratory disease: anaemia; renal failure |
| Ankle swelling | Cardiac failure | Venous obstruction; renal failure; liver disease |
| Angina | Myocardial ischaemia in coronary artery disease | Other cardiac diseases; severe anaemia |
| Palpitations | Often insignificant but may indicate cardiac disease | Tachycardias |
| Cyanosis | Cardiac disease including right to left shunts | Respiratory disease |
| Finger clubbing | Cyanotic heart disease | Various (see page 25) |
| Bradycardia | Heart block | The elderly, athletes, drugs |
| Tachycardia | Cardiac disease | Pyrexia, hyperthyroidism, drugs |
| Extra beats (extra-systoles) | Rare | Idiopathic |
| Irregularly irregular pulse | Atrial fibrillation | Drugs |
| Small volume pulse | Aortic or mitral stenosis Cardiac failure | Hypotension |

# Appendix 9 Common symptoms and signs of respiratory disease

| Symptoms and signs | Respiratory causes | Other causes |
|---|---|---|
| Breathlessness (dyspnoea) | Obstructive airways disease<br>Pneumothorax<br>Pulmonary embolism | Cardiac disease<br>Anaemia<br>Renal failure |
| Stridor | Laryngeal obstruction | — |
| Wheezing | Bronchial or bronchiolar spasm (e.g. asthma) | — |
| Cough | Bronchitis<br>Asthma<br>Carcinoma<br>Bronchiectasis | Cardiac failure |
| Cyanosis | Severe respiratory disease | Cardiac disease |
| Rapid breathing (tachypnoea) | Pulmonary fibrosis<br>Emphysema | Intra-abdominal lesions<br>Hysteria<br>Metabolic acidosis |
| Finger clubbing | Bronchiectasis<br>Carcinoma | Cirrhosis<br>Cardiac disease<br>GI disorders<br>Idiopathic |

| Signs | Collapse due to obstruction of | | Pleural effusion | Pneumothorax | Emphysema | Consolidation (as in lobar pneumonia) |
|---|---|---|---|---|---|---|
| | Major bronchus | Peripheral bronchus | | | | |
| Chest movement | Reduced on affected side | Reduced on affected side | Reduced or absent on affected side | Reduced or absent on affected side | Symmetrically diminished | Reduced on affected side |
| Mediastinal displacement | Towards side of lesion | ± towards side of lesion | Towards opposite side | Towards opposite side | — | — |
| Percussion | Dull | Dull | Stony dull | Normal or hyperresonant | Normal or hyperresonant over both lungs | Dull |
| Breath sounds | Reduced or absent | Bronchial | Usually reduced or absent | Usually reduced or absent | Reduced vesicular with prolonged expiration | Bronchial |
| Voice sounds | Reduced or absent | Increased | Reduced or absent | Reduced or absent | Normal or reduced | Increased |
| Added sounds | None | None early | ± pleural rub | None | Rhonchi and coarse crepitations (from associated bronchitis) | Crepitations |

# Appendix 10  Infectious diseases

| Disease | Major manifestations | Oral manifestations | Laboratory diagnosis | Specific treatment used |
|---|---|---|---|---|
| AIDS (see page 192) | Pneumonia, Kaposi's sarcoma, lymphomas | Candidosis, herpes simplex, hairy leucoplakia, periodontal disease, ulcers, Kaposi's sarcoma, cervical lymphadenopathy | Lymphopenia, HIV antibodies | None; nucleoside analogues or protease inhibitors may prolong life |
| Cat scratch | Tender papule, regional lymph nodes enlarge, mild fever | Cervical lymphadenopathy | Leucocytosis, ESR raised. Skin test | None |
| Chickenpox (varicella)[a] | Rash evolves through macule, papule, vesicle and pustule; rash crops and is most dense on trunk | Oral ulcers | Complement fixation antibody titres (not usually needed) | Zoster immune globulin in high risk patients ± aciclovir |
| Cytomegalo virus[a] | Glandular fever type of syndrome (Paul-Bunnell negative) | — | Serology | Ganciclovir; foscarnet |
| Diphtheria | Tonsillar or pharyngeal exudate; cervical lymph nodes enlarged; myocarditis | Tonsillar exudate, palatal palsy | Culture. *Corynebacterium diphtheriae* toxigenic strain | Antitoxin Penicillin |
| Erysipelas | Rash (confluent erythema and oedema) | — | Culture *Streptococcus pyogenes* | Penicillin |
| Hand, foot and mouth disease | Rash, minor malaise | Oral ulceration (usually mild) | Serology | None |
| Hepatitis[a] (see page 156) | Jaundice, malaise, pale stools, dark urine | — | Serology | Interferon; immune globulin in some patients |
| Herpangina | Fever, sore throat, enlarged cervical lymph nodes | Vesicles and ulcers on soft palate | Serology | None |
| Herpes simplex[a] | Fever, oral ulceration, gingivitis, cervical lymph node enlargement | Gingivostomatitis, herpes labialis (secondary infection) | Serology; viral isolation | Aciclovir or valaciclovir |

# Appendix 10 Contd.

| Disease | Major manifestations | Oral manifestations | Laboratory diagnosis | Specific treatment used |
|---|---|---|---|---|
| Herpes zoster[a] (shingles) | Rash like chicken pox but limited to dermatome, severe pain | Oral ulceration in zoster of maxillary or mandibular division of trigeminal nerve. Ulcers on palate and in pinna of ear in Ramsay–Hunt syndrome | Not needed | Aciclovir or valaciclovir. Zoster immune globulin in high risk patients |
| Impetigo | Rash (bullous) spreading to other areas rapidly | Lesions on lips may resemble recurrent herpes labialis | Culture streptococci and/or staphylococci | Flucloxacillin |
| Infectious mononucleosis | Fever, lymph node enlargement, pharyngitis | Tonsillar exudate, palatal petechiae, oral ulceration | Blood film (atypical mononuclear cells), Monospot test, Paul-Bunnell test | None |
| Measles | Rash (maculo papular), fever, acute respiratory symptoms | Koplik's spots, pharyngitis | Not usually needed | Immune globulin in high risk patients |
| Mucocutaneous lymph node syndrome (Kawasaki disease) | Rash, hands and feet desquamation, lymph node enlargement, myocarditis | Strawberry tongue, labial oedema, pharyngitis | — | None |
| Mumps | Fever, malaise, parotitis | Sialadenitis, trismus, papillitis at salivary duct orifices | Complement fixing antibody titres to S and V antigens rise; not usually needed | None |
| Mycoplasmal pneumonia (atypical pneumonia) | Sore throat, fever, pneumonia | Erythema multiforme (occasionally) | Culture mycoplasma, complement fixing antibodies, cold agglutinins | Erythromycin or tetracycline |
| Pertussis[b] (whooping cough) | Cough, fever | Occasionally ulceration of lingual fraenum | Culture *Bordetella pertussis* | Ampicillin for secondary infection |

# **Appendix 10** Contd.

| Disease | Major manifestations | Oral manifestations | Laboratory diagnosis | Specific treatment used |
|---|---|---|---|---|
| Poliomyelitis | Paralyses | — | Serology | None |
| Rubella | Rash (mainly macular), fever, enlarged posterior cervical lymph nodes | Pharyngitis | Serology | None |
| Scarlet fever | Sore throat, fever, rash (macular), enlarged cervical lymph nodes, desquamation | Tonsillar punctate exudate, ± palatal petechiae, strawberry tongue | Culture *Streptococcus pyogenes* antistreptolysin O titre | Penicillin |
| Toxoplasmosis[a] | Glandular fever type of syndrome (Paul–Bunnell negative) | Sore throat | Sabin–Feldman dye test | Sulphonamide plus pyrimethamine |

[a] Prevalent and often widespread infections in the immunocompromised high risk patients such as renal transplant or leukaemic patients.
[b] Some cases are caused by *Bordetella parapertussis*, or by viruses.

# Appendix 10: Notifiable diseases

# Appendix 11    Notifiable diseases

Doctors must notify the Proper Officer of the local authority (usually the consultant in communicable disease control) when attending a patient suspected of suffering from any of the diseases listed below; a form is available from the Proper Officer

Anthrax
Cholera
Diphtheria
Dysentery (amoebic or bacillary)
Encephalitis, acute
Food poisoning
Haemorrhagic fever (viral)
Hepatitis, viral
Leprosy
Leptospirosis
Malaria
Measles
Meningitis
Meningococcal septicaemia (without meningitis)
Mumps
Ophthalmia neonatorum
Paratyphoid fever
Plague
Poliomyelitis, acute
Rabies
Relapsing fever
Rubella
Scarlet fever
Smallpox
Tetanus
Tuberculosis
Typhoid fever
Typhus
Whooping cough
Yellow fever

# Appendix 12  Antibiotic prophylaxis for infective endocarditis

| Recommended for antibiotic prophylaxis | Not recommended for antibiotic prophylaxis |
| --- | --- |
| Periodontal probing | Preventive procedures |
| Sialography | Fissure sealants |
| Polishing teeth with a rubber cup | Fluoride treatments |
| Oral irrigation with water jet | Dental examination with mirror and probe |
| Light scaling | Intra-oral radiographs |
| Deep scaling | Extra-oral radiographs |
| Scaling teeth with hand instrument | Air polishing |
| Scaling with ultrasonic instrument | Infiltration local anaesthesia |
| Intraligamentary local anaesthesia | Nerve block local anaesthesia |
| Extractions | Oral airways for GA |
| Rubber dam placement | Nasal airways for GA |
| Matrix band and wedge placement | Laryngeal mask airway for GA |
| Gingival retraction cord placement | Slow and fast drilling of teeth (without rubber dam) |
| Root planning | Root canal instrumentation within canal |
| Antibiotic fibres or strips placed subgingivally | Pulpotomy of primary molar |
| Gingivectomy | Pulpotomy of permanent tooth |
| Periodontal Surgery | Alginate impressions |
| Root canal instrumentation beyond the root apex | Orthodontic band placement and cementation |
| Avulsed tooth reimplantation | Orthodontic band removal |
| Tooth separation | Adjustment of fixed appliances |
| Expose OR expose and bond of tooth or teeth | Incision and drainage of an abscess |
| Mucoperiosteal flap to gain access to tooth or lesion | Biopsy |
| Dental Implant placement | Dental Implants Transmucosal fixture Suture removal Removal of Surgical Packs |

Adapted from British Cardiac Society 2004.

# Appendix 13   Patient referral proforma

**Eastman Dental Institute**
256 Gray's Inn Road
London WC1X 8LD

**PATIENT REFERRAL FORM** (to be completed by referring **PRACTITIONER**)

**PERSONAL DETAILS OF PATIENT**

Surname _____ First names _____ Sex: M/F
Date of Birth:        /        /
Address:_____
_____
Postcode: _____
Telephone: (Home) _____ (Work) _____
Mobile phone _____ (Fax) _____
E-mail: _____
Hospital No. (if known) _____

**REFERRING PRACTITIONER**

Name: _____
Telephone No.:_____ Mobile phone _____
Address: _____
_____
Postcode: _____
Fax: _____
E-mail: _____

**REFERRAL**
**Urgency with which you wish patient to be seen** (please circle)

Immediately [    ] if possible within:  1 week [    ]   1 month [    ]   3 months [    ]

Purpose of referral: _____
Patient main complaint _____
Comments _____

**HISTORY**
Medical: does the patient have   [        ]        [        ]

|  | No | Yes |  |  | No | Yes |  |  | No | Yes |
|---|---|---|---|---|---|---|---|---|---|---|
| Allergies |  |  | Bleeding tendency |  |  | Medication |  |  |  |  |
| Heart problems |  |  | Diabetes |  |  | Any other problem |  |  |  |  |

Salient points from medical history _____
Other (Specify) _____

**Please enclose other relevant information such as radiographs, study casts (if available)**

Date : _____              Signature of Practitioner: _____

# Index

# For Reference

**Not to be taken from this room**

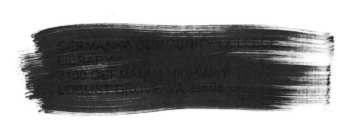